Commissioning Editor: Timothy Horne
Project Development Manager: Janice Urquhart
Project Manager: Nancy Arnott
Designer: Erik Bigland
Page layout: Jim Farley

PATHOLOGY ILLUSTRATED

Robin Reid BSc MB ChB FRCPath
Consultant Pathologist, Western Infirmary; Senior Lecturer, Glasgow University,
Glasgow, UK

Fiona Roberts BSc MD MRCPath
Consultant Pathologist, Western Infirmary; Senior Lecturer, Glasgow University,
Glasgow, UK

Original illustrations by

Robin Callander FFPh FMAA AIMI
Formerly Director, Medical Illustrations Unit, University of Glasgow, Glasgow, UK

New illustrations by

Ian Ramsden
Formerly Head of Medical Illustration, University of Glasgow, Glasgow, UK

SIXTH EDITION

ELSEVIER
CHURCHILL
LIVINGSTONE

EDINBURGH LONDON NEW YORK OXFORD PHILADELPHIA ST LOUIS SYDNEY TORONTO 2005

ELSEVIER
CHURCHILL
LIVINGSTONE

© Longman Group Limited 1981, 1986, 1991, 1995
© Harcourt Publishers Limited 2000
© 2005, Elsevier Limited. All rights reserved.

First edition 1981   Fourth edition 1995
Second edition 1986   Fifth edition 2000
Third edition 1991   Sixth edition 2005

ISBN 0 443 07336 8

International edition ISBN 0 443 07337 6

British Library Cataloguing in Publication Data
A catalogue record for this book is available from the British Library

Library of Congress Cataloging in Publication Data
A catalog record for this book is available from the Library of Congress

Note
Medical knowledge is constantly changing. Standard safety precautions must be followed, but as new research and clinical experience broaden our knowledge, changes in treatment and drug therapy may become necessary or appropriate. Readers are advised to check the most current product information provided by the manufacturer of each drug to be administered to verify the recommended dose, the method and duration of administration, and contraindications. It is the responsibility of the practitioner, relying on experience and knowledge of the patient, to determine dosages and the best treatment for each individual patient. Neither the Publisher nor the authors assume any liability for any injury and/or damage to persons or property arising from this publication.
The Publisher

Working together to grow
libraries in developing countries

www.elsevier.com | www.bookaid.org | www.sabre.org

ELSEVIER   **BOOK AID** International   Sabre Foundation

your source for books, journals and multimedia in the health sciences

www.elsevierhealth.com

The publisher's policy is to use **paper manufactured from sustainable forests**

Printed in China by RDC Group Limited

PREFACE

'We believe that communication by verbal and written methods is the fundamental basis for study and learning. Nevertheless, in the modern setting where knowledge is increasing so rapidly and in a subject where morphological changes are a major component, we consider that the visual image has an important facilitating role.'

Since these comments were written in the preface to the first edition of 1981, undergraduate medical education has evolved greatly, notably in the widespread adoption of topic- or problem-based curricula and the generally diminished allocation of time, at least in a formal sense, to pathology.

We do not believe, however, that there has been any reduction in the importance of pathology as one of the foundations of clinical medicine.

In this sixth edition, the general layout and style of the book and its division into general and systemic chapters have been retained. The volume aims to be simple yet comprehensive and provide relevant information that can be assimilated in a reasonable time scale. We have concentrated on 'core' topics and on what we regard as clinically important pathology, not solely in 'Western' countries. Whilst including significant developments in each area we have tried to avoid 'information overload' not least in the vast field of molecular and cell biology. We recognize that our attempts at simplification do not tell the whole story.

We are indebted to our predecessors, Alasdair Govan, Peter Macfarlane and Robin Callander whose vision inspired the original concept of *Pathology Illustrated*. Much of their work from earlier editions remains with, we hope, appropriate modification. The credit for the book remains due to them; the shortcomings of this revision are our responsibility.

The most recent illustrations are the work of Ian Ramsden, to whom we are grateful. Many thanks are also owed to Janice Urquhart, Development Editor at Elsevier for her considerable efforts in bringing this project to completion.

R. Reid
F. Roberts

CONTENTS

Pathology is the study of disease. It describes the effects, progress and consequences of the disease and attempts to determine the cause (aetiology) and underlying mechanisms (pathogenesis). It forms a bridge between basic science and clinical practice and has traditionally had the same role in linking pre-clinical and clinical study for medical students.

Disease occurs when there are variations of function or structure outside the normal range.

The manifestations of the disease are the sum of the damage done by the precipitating cause and the body's response (which may be helpful or unhelpful or both). The variations in these components account for the great diversity of disease, which can then be classified into four main groups:

DEVELOPMENTAL   INFLAMMATORY   NEOPLASTIC   DEGENERATIVE

The relative importance of these groups varies with the age of the individual:

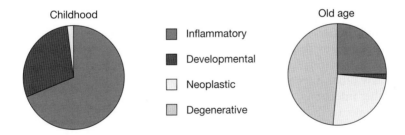

Different diseases affect different age groups. Developmental disorders and degenerative diseases affect the opposite extremes of life while tumours, in general, affect an ageing population.

Physiological ageing itself implies a gradual loss of cellular and body vitality usually associated with atrophy of tissues and organs. This process is aggravated and mimicked by the degenerative diseases of old age so that the physiological and pathological states tend to merge. Nonetheless, the student should attempt to identify the distinctions between ageing and disease. Additionally, in old age multiple diseases often coexist and interact with one another, and drug induced disorders are also common in this age group.

CAUSES OF DISEASE

The various factors involved are considered in two broad groups:
1) Environmental and 2) Genetic.

1. **ENVIRONMENTAL FACTORS** are numerous and can be classified under the following general headings:

Physical agents. Among these are trauma, radiation, both ionising and non-ionising, extremes of temperature, electrical power, i.e. the application to the body of excess (or insufficiency) of physical energy in any form.

Chemical poisons. Historically, these increased in importance with advances in industrial processing, but their effects have diminished by legislation to provoke safe working environments. Some, for example cyanide, are toxic to all tissues, while others target certain organs – paraquat affects the lungs and organic solvents damage especially the kidneys and liver. Others, for example strong acids and alkalis, act locally.

Iatrogenic diseases are an increasingly important subgroup as powerful drugs often have undesirable side effects, either predictably in a dose-dependent fashion or in an unpredictable idiosyncratic manner.

Nutritional deficiencies and excesses. These may arise from an inadequate supply, due to interference with absorption, inefficient transport within the body or defective utilisation. The effects may be general in distribution as in starvation or in severe hypoxia or they may damage specific tissues, e.g. vitamin deficiencies. Dietary excess plays an increasingly important role in Western countries, the rapidly increasing prevalence of diabetes mellitus being noteworthy.

Infections and infestations. Viruses, bacteria, fungi, protozoa and metazoa all cause disease. They may do so by destroying cells directly, for example in malaria. Infection with HIV destroys T cells resulting in severe immunodeficiency which renders the individual susceptible to many other infections, often due to organisms of low virulence (opportunistic infections). In other infections, the damage is done by toxins produced by the infecting agent such as tetanus, cholera and diphtheria; these may have a general or local effect.

Abnormal immune reactions. The normally protective immune system can in certain circumstances become deranged and damage the individual. Hypersensitivity to foreign substances can lead to anaphylactic shock or to more localised but nonetheless potentially lethal disorders such as asthma. If the process of 'tolerance' by which the immune system recognises the body's own tissues as self breaks down, then autoimmune diseases such as thyroiditis and pernicious anaemia result.

Psychological factors. These cause and influence disease processes in several ways. Psychological stress may lead to mental illness, and may alter the individual's symptoms and response to somatic diseases. They are important components of diseases caused by addiction such as alcohol, tobacco and drugs. Finally, it is thought that psychological factors may be causally related to diseases such as hypertension, coronary thrombosis and, perhaps because of its effects on the immune system, to ulcerative colitis. It is worth noting, however, that the importance ascribed to stress in the pathogenesis of duodenal ulcers became much less when the pathogenic effects of *helicobacter pylori* were discovered in the 1980's.

2. **GENETIC FACTORS** are the results of actions of single genes or groups of genes.

Research, including the human genome product, has lead to a rapid expansion in our knowledge. Both variations in 'normal' genes and mutations which radically affect the function of 'abnormal genes' influence the development of disease.

Normal genes. There is considerable genetic variation among individuals, both within and between races and even within families. These genetic polymorphisms strongly influence SUSCEPTIBILTY and RESISTANCE to disease. For example:

a) The susceptibility of fair skin to damage by ultra-violet light and the development of skin cancer is well known and the mechanism – lack of the protective pigment melanin – is obvious and presumably determined on evolutionary grounds.

b) The human leucocyte antigen (HLA) system is a complex of genes on chromosome 6 in which there is great allelic variation. An individual's HLA type strongly influences the development of many disorders, especially autoimmune diseases, and of course determines whether a transplanted organ from a potential donor will be rejected or not.

Abnormal genes. The mutations which give rise to disease vary from point mutations which affect a single base pair (e.g. sickle cell anaemia) through chromosomal translocations found in many tumour types such as Burkitt's lymphoma to the presence of an entire extra chromosome (e.g. trisomy 21 – Down's syndrome). Many mutations appear to arise spontaneously while others follow exposure to irradiation (in the survivors of Chernobyl and those who have received radiotherapy) or chemicals. Some mutations arise in the somatic tissues, whilst others are transmitted in the germline. These give rise to INHERITED diseases such as cystic fibrosis where the mutation directly determines the disease. In many other diseases, there is a genetic component, often contributed to by multiple genes, and an environmental contribution.

There is also variation in the rate at which mutations occur within individuals, often determined by variations in the genes responsible for DNA repair.

METHODS IN PATHOLOGY

The traditional methods of careful naked eye and light microscopic examination of organs at autopsy have been supplemented by the much wider use in clinical practice of biopsy and cytology where tissue or cells are removed during life for diagnosis. Endoscopic and fine needle techniques allow biopsies to be obtained from most parts of the body. In addition, technological advances have allowed examination at more detailed levels:

Naked eye examination — Colonic cancer

Light microscopy – morphology — Adeno-carcinoma

Immunocytochemistry – demonstration of specific proteins — Epithelial membrane antigen

Electron microscopy – organelles — Junctional complexes

Molecular biology – chromosomal analysis and chip technology — TTAGCTA — Sequencing

These increasingly sophisticated methods tend to influence the student to focus on detailed mechanisms at the molecular levels. It should not be forgotten that simple methods of gross examination and histological assessment are fundamental to the study of diseases. The following descriptions begin therefore with gross and microscopic pathology and proceed to the more detailed cellular changes when they are known. The student will find that such an approach is the basis of their learning in clinical practice.

CHAPTER 1

CELL AND TISSUE DAMAGE

CELLULAR PHYSIOLOGY AND PATHOLOGY

To understand diseases of the body systems or individual organs, requires knowledge of the function and dysfunction of individual cells. This is a topic of great complexity and only the basic principles can be outlined.

Cellular physiology is characterised by:
(a) Close interdependence of the various cellular components and activities (though it is convenient to describe them separately).
(b) Balancing control mechanisms aimed at maintaining constant conditions (i.e. homeostasis).
(c) Very efficient compensatory and repair mechanisms to minimise damage.

PLASMA MEMBRANES

Main functions.
1. Maintain integrity of cell.
2. Contact with extracellular environment
   e.g. cell surface receptors.

3. (a) Passage of ions through permeable channels e.g. Na$^+$, K$^+$
   or (b) Passage of complex molecules by pinocytosis or phagocytosis.

Any disorder may lead to dysfunction or cell death.

MITOCHONDRIA These are the main sites of ENERGY production.

Disorder of energy production affects all cellular functions.

Source	Production	Utilisation
	ADP → ATP	

O$_2$ + glucose → (oxidative phosphorylation) → release of energy → for all cellular activities

NUCLEUS

The nucleus controls all cellular activities through the action of at least 10 000 genes, each of which encodes a protein with structural, enzymatic or control functions.

Damage to DNA (e.g. by ionising radiation) is particularly likely in dividing cells. There are effective repair mechanisms but severe damage usually leads to cell death by apoptosis (see p.4).

Germ cell DNA damage (i.e. to spermatogonia or oocytes)
1. Severe damage to chromosomal structure — Prevention of conception / Early abortion
2. Less severe damage to groups of genes or single genes — Developmental abnormalities / Hereditary disease / Susceptibility to diseases

Somatic cell DNA damage
This is acquired during life. Damage to stem cells is especially important.
The development of cancer (p.151) through activation of oncogenes or loss of tumour suppressor genes is the most important example.

LYSOSOMES

These membrane bound organelles contain hydrolytic enzymes and are responsible for digestion and disposal of complex substances. — Disorder may lead to escape of enzymes or to cellular overloading (e.g. storage disorders).

2

CONTROL OF CELL NUMBER

In adult life the CELL NUMBER is fairly constant: this is achieved by complex control mechanisms which evenly balance the continuing formation of new cells with cell loss.

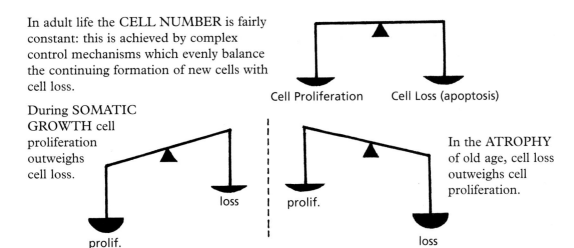

Cell Proliferation   Cell Loss (apoptosis)

During SOMATIC GROWTH cell proliferation outweighs cell loss.

loss   prolif.

In the ATROPHY of old age, cell loss outweighs cell proliferation.

prolif.   loss

Also in many diseases the balance is lost.

Cell proliferation – the Cell Cycle

In adult life, cells fall into 3 main groups in respect of their proliferation potential.

	Proliferation potential	Examples
1. LABILE CELLS	rapid proliferation and cell turnover	gut lining epithelial cells
2. STABLE CELLS	slow proliferation and cell turnover	hepatocytes
3. PERMANENT CELLS	NOT able to proliferate	neurones

In preparation for division, a cell passes through 4 consecutive phases (G_1, S, G_2, M) ending in **Mitosis (M)**.

G_2 (Gap 2) cell prepares for division

2 daughter cells produced

These cells may continue in the cycle – this applies to LABILE cells,

(a)

or (b) temporarily leave to cycle into a resting phase (G_0). Stimulation by e.g. growth factors is required for re-entry – this applies to STABLE cells.

S (synthesis) phase DNA content doubles

G_1 (Gap 1) cell prepares for DNA synthesis

Various growth promotors, inhibitors and drugs influence the cycle at various stages.

Knowledge of the cycle underlies the understanding of mechanisms involved in HEALING and REPAIR and in CARCINOGENESIS.

APOPTOSIS

Apoptosis (programmed cell death) (Greek: apoptosis = falling off, like leaves from a tree) is an important process in health and disease by which effete, abnormal or unwanted cells are eliminated. It differs from necrosis (p.5) and is an active process. A few examples are:

Apoptosis in health

In embryogenesis and development

(i) Metamorphosis of tadpole to frog.
(ii) Loss of autoreactive response of 'T' cells in the **thymus** preventing auto-immune attack.

Apoptosis of cells

Shedding of tail

(iii) In atrophy and involution, often on withdrawal of hormones, e.g. menstrual breakdown of endometrium.

Apoptosis in disease

(i) Irradiation, (ii) Virus infection, (iii) Action of cytotoxic 'T' cells, e.g. in rejection of transplanted organs.
(iv) In tumours, apoptosis and proliferation rates together control the rate of tumour growth.

Apoptosis is a rapid process usually affecting single cells scattered in a population of healthy cells. It is considered in 2 stages:

Stage 1: **The dying process**

(a) Active metabolic changes in the cell cause – cytoplasmic and nuclear condensation

Plasma membrane intact

(b) Cell disintegrates into apoptotic bodies – each surrounded by a plasma membrane

Some contain nuclear material

Stage 2: **The elimination process**

Phagocytosis by surrounding cells (e.g. liver cells, tumour cells) followed by rapid digestion

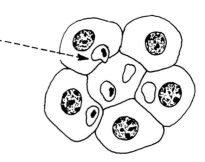

1. The surrounding cells move together to fill the vacant space, leaving virtually no evidence of the process.
2. The presence of intact plasma membranes around the apoptotic bodies explains the absence of inflammation.
3. The process of apoptosis is regulated by many genes including *bcl-2* which prevents apoptosis in damaged cells.

CELL DAMAGE

A wide variety of noxious agents can damage cells. These can be grouped as follows (the individual diseases mentioned are illustrative examples):

1. **Reduced oxygen supply** – respiratory disease, cardiovascular disease, anaemia
2. **Physical agents** – mechanical trauma, excessive heat or cold, radiations
3. **Chemical agents** – these continue to increase enormously with the complexity of industrial processes
4. **Toxins** – bacteria, plants, animals e.g. snakes
5. **Viruses**
6. **Abnormal immunological reaction** – hypersensitivity states, glomerulonephritis
7. **Nutritional deficiencies** – vitamin deficiency and malabsorption syndromes
8. **Genetic abnormalities** – Down's syndrome

The severity of the injury determines the outcome:

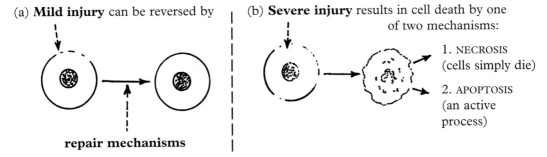

(a) **Mild injury** can be reversed by **repair mechanisms**

(b) **Severe injury** results in cell death by one of two mechanisms:

1. NECROSIS (cells simply die)
2. APOPTOSIS (an active process)

NECROSIS

This term describes death of a cell or group of cells, typically following severe hypoxia, physical or chemical injury. Death of the cell is associated with rapid depletion of intracellular energy systems. Initially there are no morphological changes, but within a few hours the cell membrane and intracellular organelles are disrupted. Electron microscopy demonstrates these changes earlier than light microscopy.

Group of necrotic cells

Passage into cell of Ca^{2+} and Na^+

Loss of PLASMA MEMBRANE BARRIER FUNCTION

Passage out of cell of K^+ and ENZYMES

Blood vessel

Concentration of enzymes increases in blood – used in diagnostic tests

What we recognise as necrosis is due to denaturation and coagulation of protein and/or digestion of the cell by released enzymes. There are several naked eye appearances depending on which of these predominates.

NECROSIS

COAGULATIVE NECROSIS

This type of necrosis is frequently caused by lack of blood supply and is exemplified well in infarcts of solid organs, e.g. heart, spleen and kidney.

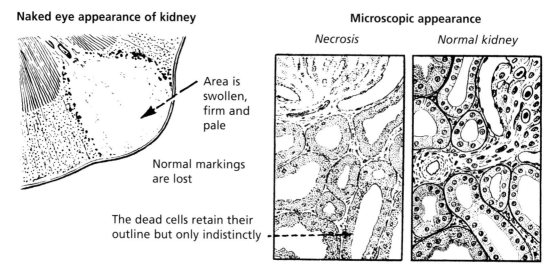

Naked eye appearance of kidney

Area is swollen, firm and pale

Normal markings are lost

The dead cells retain their outline but only indistinctly

Microscopic appearance

Necrosis   *Normal kidney*

At *light microscopic level* the following changes in the cell are seen:

1. The nucleus shows one of two changes (a) Karyolysis (b) Karyorrhexis.
2. The cytoplasm becomes opaque and strongly eosinophilic (affinity for the red dye, eosin).

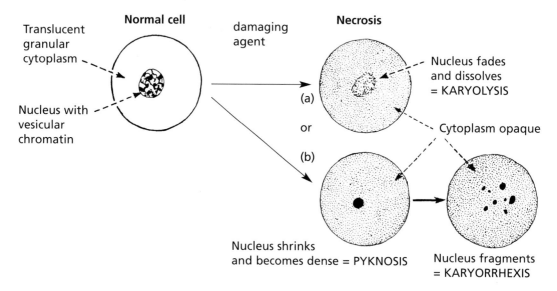

Translucent granular cytoplasm

Normal cell

Nucleus with vesicular chromatin

damaging agent

Necrosis

(a)

Nucleus fades and dissolves = KARYOLYSIS

Cytoplasm opaque

or

(b)

Nucleus shrinks and becomes dense = PYKNOSIS

Nucleus fragments = KARYORRHEXIS

At *electron microscope (E.M.)* level, in addition to the above nuclear changes, disorganisation and disintegration of the cytoplasmic organelles and severe damage to the plasma membrane are seen.

NECROSIS

COLLIQUATIVE NECROSIS

In the brain consistently, and in other tissues when they contain a large amount of fluid and enzyme activity is marked, necrotic areas undergo softening and are filled with pigmented or turbid fluid, with complete loss of structure.

An **abscess** (see p.39, 40) is an example of colliquative necrosis caused by the enzymatic action of polymorphonuclear leucocytes.

GANGRENE

This is a complication of necrosis. In certain circumstances necrotic tissue is liable to be invaded by putrefactive organisms which are both saccharolytic and proteolytic. Foul-smelling gases are produced and the tissue becomes green or black due to breakdown of haemoglobin. Obstruction of the blood supply to the bowel is almost inevitably followed by gangrene, e.g.:

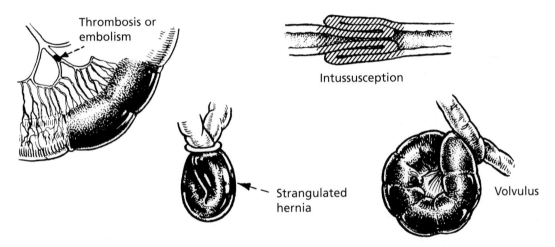

Thrombosis or embolism

Intussusception

Strangulated hernia

Volvulus

Gangrene also occurs on the skin surface following arterial obstruction. It is particularly liable to affect the limbs, especially the toes in diseases such as diabetes.

A special type of gangrene follows infection with clostridial organisms (gas gangrene; see p.70).

NECROSIS

CASEOUS NECROSIS (CASEATION)

The necrotic tissue assumes a cream-cheesy appearance, slightly greasy to the touch. It is commonly seen in tuberculosis (see p.72).

FAT NECROSIS

Adipose tissue is damaged in pancreatitis and occasionally due to trauma. The special appearances are due to the action of lipases on triglycerides as follows:

TRIGLYCERIDES (released from necrotic fat) $\longrightarrow$ FATTY ACIDS + Ca^{2+} $\longrightarrow$ Insoluble SOAPS

LIPASE usually pancreatic

E.g. Appearances in omentum and mesenteries.

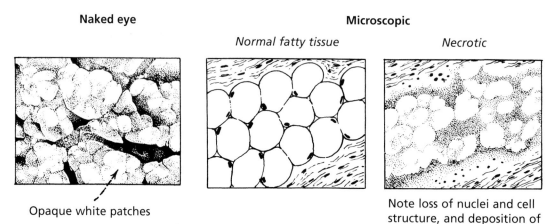

Naked eye

Opaque white patches

Microscopic

Normal fatty tissue

Necrotic

Note loss of nuclei and cell structure, and deposition of insoluble soaps.

FIBRINOID NECROSIS

This is a descriptive term in which connective tissues and especially arterial walls are infiltrated by a strongly eosinophilic hyaline material which shows some of the characteristics of fibrin. Any actual necrosis is usually inconspicuous.

NECROSIS – AUTOLYSIS

SEQUELS OF NECROSIS

1. When small numbers of cells are involved, the cellular debris is removed by PHAGOCYTOSIS (see p.36).
2. With larger numbers of dead cells, there is an inflammatory response with organisation and fibrous repair (see p.40).
3. When the necrotic tissue cannot be completely removed or organised, deposition of calcium may be an additional feature, for example in TUBERCULOUS CASEOUS NECROSIS. This feature is important in radiological diagnosis. It is sometimes described as 'dystrophic' (p.25).

AUTOLYSIS

The process of 'self-digestion' begins after the death of the cell (as described above) and proceeds at a rate dependent on the local enzyme content; it is an inevitable sequel of necrosis. However, the term is more commonly applied to the changes which take place in tissues removed from the body and in the whole body after death:

In practice, autolysis can be modified or inhibited as follows:

(1) by REFRIGERATION
↓
ENZYME activity
slowed down
↓
Whole body
'preserved'
↓
AUTOPSY performed
without undue
haste

(2) by FIXATION
↓
CHEMICALS added
(e.g. formalin)
or HEAT
↓
ENZYMES and PROTEINS
DENATURED
↓
AVAILABLE for PATHOLOGICAL
PROCESSING

CELL DAMAGE – HYDROPIC SWELLING

The various agents which can cause cell necrosis may also cause lesser cell damage which is reversible when the injurious agent is removed.

The appearances and effects are considered under these headings: (1) **hydropic swelling,** (2) **fatty change,** (3) **radiation** and (4) **atrophy.**

HYDROPIC SWELLING

Hydropic swelling – formerly called Cloudy swelling – proceeds to hydropic vacuolation.

The damaged organs become swollen and on section have a pale and swollen appearance.

Electron microscopic (E.M.) appearances indicate the mechanisms:

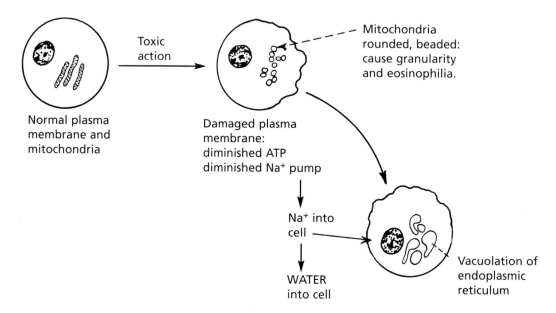

CELL DAMAGE – FATTY CHANGE

This is accumulation of fat in non-fatty tissues, especially the parenchymatous organs, skeletal muscles and the heart, which have a high metabolic rate.

The essential problem is the inability of the non-fatty tissues to metabolise the amount of lipid presented to them, resulting in its accumulation within the cells. The most important causes range from direct cell poisons through clinical conditions associated with reduced cellular energy.

CELL POISONS
Bacterial,
Chemical e.g. Chloroform, Alcohol.

REDUCED cellular **ENZYME** activity → Inability to metabolise fat → Accumulation of fat in cells

CLINICAL DISORDERS
Anoxia due to anaemia,
    cardiac failure, respiratory disease.
Diabetes mellitus, Chronic malnutrition.

In normal non-fatty tissues the intracellular fat is not visible by light microscopy using conventional fat stains.

In fatty change, the accumulated fat is visualised using frozen sections and fat-soluble dyes: in routine paraffin sections the fat has been dissolved and is indicated by clear vacuoles.

For example, in the **LIVER**, the increase of deposited fat causes enlargement of the organ. Its distribution varies with the cause, e.g.:

(1) Lack of Oxygen – in anaemia and cardiac failure

Hepatic a.
Portal v.
Bile duct

Fats tend to be deposited furthest from the arterial blood supply (hepatic arteriole) around the efferent vein (hepatic venule)

(2) Poison, Toxins etc – alcohol, infections, organic solvents

Fat is found nearest the afferent blood supply (portal venule and hepatic arteriole)

EFFECTS OF FATTY CHANGE
Impairment of cellular function is usually due to the pathological process causing the fatty change (e.g. anoxia in severe anaemia) and not to the physical presence of fat within the cell. In the liver, for example, very large accumulations of fat do not impair basic liver functions.

A possible exception is the myocardium in certain circumstances.

(a) **Rapid or large transfusion** → Increased ventricular pressure → Dilatation of heart → Cardiac failure
    +
Fatty myocardium → Weak muscle fibres

(b) **Sudden excessive exertion** → Rise in blood pressure → Temporary left sided cardiac embarrassment
    +
Fatty myocardium → Weak muscle fibres

11

CELL DAMAGE – FREE RADICALS

The formation of free radicals is now thought to be an important contributory factor in many disease processes.

Free radicals are molecules with a single unpaired electron in an outer orbital position: they react vigorously with and modify a wide range of molecules affecting particularly lipids (of cell membranes), DNA and proteins.

A dot above the chemical symbol indicates the presence of a free radical:
e.g. $OH^\bullet$ = hydroxyl radical: $O_2^\bullet$ = superoxide radical.

Formation

(i) Radiation

$$H_2O \xrightarrow{\text{hydrolysis}} H^\bullet + OH^\bullet$$
Water

(ii) Killing of bacteria by neutrophils and macrophages (see p.36).

$$O_2 \longrightarrow O_2^\bullet$$
Oxygen   Superoxide

(iii) Poisons
e.g. carbon tetrachloride

$$CCl_4 \longrightarrow CCl_3^\bullet + Cl$$

Chain reaction can AUGMENT effects

Effects

Damage to
LIPIDS : DNA : PROTEINS
contributes to

INFLAMMATION – acute and chronic

AGEING

RADIATION DAMAGE

Re-perfusion injury (following thrombolytic therapy for coronary thrombosis)

Defence mechanisms to free radicals
Some free radicals decay spontaneously (e.g. $O_2^\bullet$) but they can also be removed by ANTIOXIDANTS e.g. Vitamin E and also by the action of enzymes such as superoxide mutase and catalase.

Mutase   Catalase

$O_2^\bullet$
Superoxide $\xrightarrow[\text{hydrogen}]{\text{contributes}}$ H_2O_2 Hydrogen peroxide $\xrightarrow[\text{oxygen}]{\text{releases}}$ H_2O Water

CELL DAMAGE – RADIATION

High energy (ionising) radiation, particularly in the form of gamma (γ) or X-rays can cause serious cellular and tissue damage. At cellular level there are 2 mechanisms involving:

1. The cell **CYTOPLASM**

   A large dose of radiation hydrolyses water producing damaging **free hydroxyl** radicals: acute cell death follows

2. The cell **NUCLEUS**

   Lower doses damage DNA with 2 results:
   (a) failure to replicate
   (b) mutation with variable genetic abnormalities

These effects will be considered under 3 headings:

1. The **localised effects** complicating radiotherapy in the tissues adjacent to the therapeutic field.
   Following any reparable acute damage a latent period precedes persistent injury. This is caused by:
   (a)   damage to blood vessels ⎱
   (b)   damage to fibroblasts   ⎰ leading to   (a) *ischaemia*
                                                   (b) *dense fibrosis*

   Injury to organs which are difficult to shield is seen, for example, in skin, eyes, alimentary tract, bladder, lungs, gonads and spinal cord.
   In surgical practice, wound healing is seriously impaired.
2. Some of the mutations may lead to cancer, particularly leukaemias and lymphomas. (About 2% of all malignancies are associated with radiation.)
   The mechanisms are described on page 148.
3. **Whole body radiation** is usually the result of atomic explosion. The acute effects which are related to large doses are summarised below.

Note: Total body irradiation is used in treatment of some leukaemias.

Dose (Grays)	Result		Mechanism
above 50	Death in a few hours		All cells damaged but particularly **CNS**: CEREBRAL OEDEMA ↓ COMA
5–10	Death 3–7 days		Mucous lining of **intestine** destroyed: DIARRHOEA: SEPTICAEMIC SHOCK
2–5	Death 2–3 weeks		**Bone marrow** destroyed: LEUCOPENIA THROMBOCYTOPENIA ↓ INFECTION: HAEMORRHAGE
0.2–1	Damage to fetus in early pregnancy		Embryonal cell mutation

13

ATROPHY

This is a simple decrease in cell size or number, resulting in a shrinkage of affected tissues and organs. The most common example is atrophy of old age (see p.15).

Causes

(1) **Gradual diminution** ⟶ Reduction in oxygen ⟶ General fall in cell activity and
    in blood supply   supply and nutrients   shrinkage, e.g. narrowing of
     coronary arteries → myocardial
     atrophy

Normal   Accumulation of lipofuscin around nucleus

Lipofuscin ('wear and tear' pigment) is a golden yellow pigment representing undigested lipid material derived from cellular metabolism.

(2) **Reduced functional activity** ⟶ Diminished demand ⟶ Atrophy of cells
    (disuse atrophy)   for nutrition

    E.g. Lack of exercise ⟶ Atrophy of skeletal muscle
    E.g. Obstruction of gland duct ⟶ Atrophy of gland (Apoptosis is important here)

(3) **Interrupted nerve supply** ⟶ Reduced reflex and metabolic activities, e.g. atrophy of skeletal muscles after destruction of motor nerves as in poliomyelitis.

Normal   Loss of structure and shrinkage

(4) **Endocrine deficiency** ⟶ Loss of trophic mechanism ⟶ Reduced metabolic activity
     in dependent tissues

    E.g. Pituitary deficiency ⟶ Atrophy of ⟶ Thyroid
     ⟶ Adrenals
     ⟶ Gonads and genital organs

(5) **Pressure** ⟶ Interruption of blood supply and interference with function, e.g. neoplasm pressing on surrounding tissues.

Atrophy is reversible provided the cause is eliminated or deficiencies restored.

AGEING

The distinction between 'true' ageing and ageing complicated by disease processes may be difficult; since therapy can be directed at the latter the distinction is important in clinical practice.

The changes associated with *true* ageing would be seen in a theoretical 'ideal' environment (minimal stress).

The following diagram is illustrative. The main controlling factors are *intrinsic*, i.e. genetic:
　　? associated with expression of ageing genes in mitochondria:
　　? loss of cells' ability to divide due to telomeric shortening (ends of chromosomes).

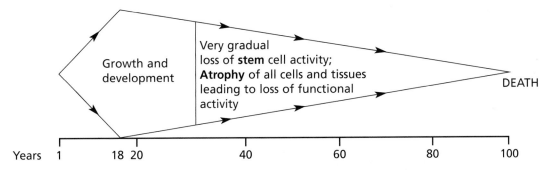

In the real environment this theoretical concept of ageing is accelerated and aggravated by two groups of *extrinsic* factors:

Ageing accelerated and aggravated

Note: Death is only very rarely, if ever, due to 'pure' ageing. It is the result of disease – either a single process or, with increasing age, more often several causes.

HEREDITY, GENES AND DISEASE

CELL NUCLEUS AND CHROMOSOMES

Knowledge of the GENETIC influence on disease is expanding very rapidly. The following can only be a brief outline of basic facts:

The cell **NUCLEUS** contains structures, CHROMOSOMES, which transmit hereditary traits from one generation to the next and also control the synthesis of all the proteins in the body.

The 46 chromosomes which most human nuclei contain are not identifiable in differentiated cells or cells in the non-proliferating phase of the cell cycle (G_0).

The different morphological appearances of nuclei in histological sections indicate to some extent the amount of nuclear activity.

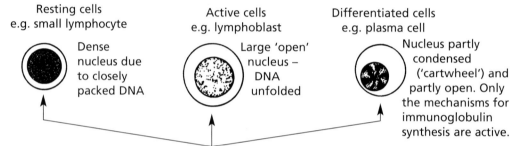

Resting cells
e.g. small lymphocyte
Dense nucleus due to closely packed DNA

Active cells
e.g. lymphoblast
Large 'open' nucleus – DNA unfolded

Differentiated cells
e.g. plasma cell
Nucleus partly condensed ('cartwheel') and partly open. Only the mechanisms for immunoglobulin synthesis are active.

Individual chromosomes NOT identifiable. (Can be demonstrated by molecular methods e.g. Fluorescent-in-situ hybridisation (FISH).)

CHROMOSOMES

During MITOSIS the chromosomes condense into specific morphological forms which are identifiable by light microscopy: when colchicine is added to a cell culture, mitosis is arrested at the metaphase: chromosomes are then separable and can be studied.

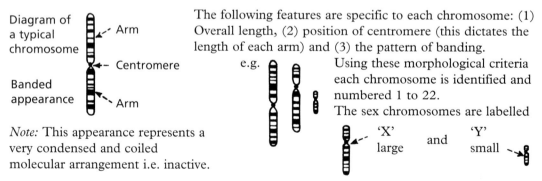

Diagram of a typical chromosome — Arm

— Centromere

Banded appearance — Arm

Note: This appearance represents a very condensed and coiled molecular arrangement i.e. inactive.

The following features are specific to each chromosome: (1) Overall length, (2) position of centromere (this dictates the length of each arm) and (3) the pattern of banding.

e.g. Using these morphological criteria each chromosome is identified and numbered 1 to 22.

The sex chromosomes are labelled 'X' large and 'Y' small

A typical normal chromosome map (karyotype) shows 22 pairs of different but identifiable chromosomes .... plus 2 sex chromosomes,

Each pair is called an AUTOSOME and consists of a PATERNAL and MATERNAL chromosome.

×22

either 2 large X = FEMALE *or*

1 large X and 1 small Y = MALE

HEREDITY, GENES AND DISEASE

DEOXYRIBONUCLEIC ACID (DNA)

Since Watson and Crick defined the molecular structure of DNA in 1953, there has been a great increase in knowledge of the 'genetic code'. Each chromosome is a very long single molecule of deoxyribonucleic acid (DNA), condensed during mitosis.
It is extended to its characteristic structure when active:

The **DOUBLE HELIX**

2 long spirals of nucleotides [consisting of a deoxyribose (sugar) + phosphate] around a central axis, complementary but running in opposite directions.

Diagram of a very small part of a very long molecule.

Extending to millions of base pairs

Joined by purine and pyrimidine base pairs

The essential function is to initiate and control the synthesis of proteins from amino-acids. All types of protein (structural proteins, hormones, receptors, intra-cellular messengers etc.) are ENCODED along the molecule.

A **GENE** is the unit of the chromosome responsible for the synthesis of a single SPECIFIC PROTEIN. Genes vary in length but on average occupy about 20 000 base pairs of the molecule.

There are over 10 000 genes in all the human chromosomes, not all are active: some are repetitive: some form clusters subserving related activities [e.g. MHC (HLA) locus, see p.91].

There is a complex REGULATION of gene activity involving stop and start signals, promotor and enhancer functions all within the DNA structure. The entire human genome has now been sequenced.

Gene expression and protein synthesis

A gene consists of coding regions (EXONS) interspersed with non-coding regions (INTRONS). In transcription the introns are eliminated and all the exons are transcribed to a ribonucleic acid form (mRNA) which is a copy of the DNA-code sequencing the amino-acids required for the production of a specific protein.
The simplified diagram illustrates:

In the cell nucleus
Start signal 'switches on' gene

(1) **TRANSCRIPTION**

In the cell cytoplasm

(2) **TRANSLATION**

Coding regions (EXONS)

RNA copy

mRNA

(a) Coded message to RIBOSOME
(b) Sequencing amino-acids to protein

Non-coding regions (INTRONS)

SPLICING

(Introns removed)

Note smaller molecule

17

MITOSIS AND MEIOSIS

MITOSIS is the process by which SOMATIC cells proliferate ensuring *exact replication of the daughter cells*. Following the stimulus to proliferate, the chromosomes condense and replicate exactly.

PROPHASE
All chromosomes
condense and replicate

METAPHASE
All chromosomes
are aligned along
equatorial plate:
nuclear membrane
'dissolves'.

ANAPHASE
Chromatids are
'pulled apart'
and become
chromosomes.

TELOPHASE
2 daughter cells
are about to form,
each containing
identical
chromosomes.

2 pairs only
are shown

Exact replicates
joined at
centromeres (called
CHROMATIDS).

MEIOSIS is a complex process occurring during GAMETOGENESIS: it involves the reduction and division of chromosomes in such a way that (1) a random mixture of both parental genes is present in the gamete and that (2) the chances are equal for fertilisation to result in either sex.

This simple diagram shows the important results of meiosis.

Primitive germ cell
contains 46 chromosomes
(i.e. 22 autosomes
+ XX or XY)

One illustrative AUTOSOME
consisting of a pair of chromosomes,
one from each parent.

(1) During MEOSIS the
chromosomes come
close together and
random segments
are exchanged

Cell division without replication

(2) During MEOSIS
the sex
chromosomes
are similarly
distributed

Gametes contain 22 single
chromosomes. On fertilisation
22 autosomes are restored.

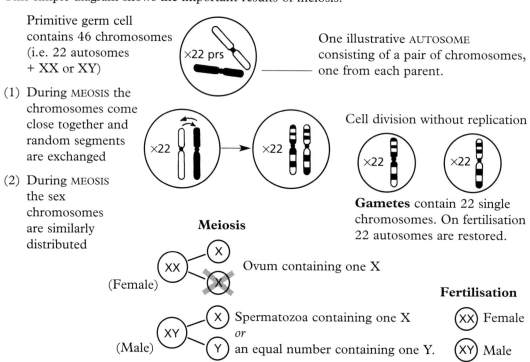

Meiosis

(Female) — XX — X / Ovum containing one X

Fertilisation

(Male) — XY — X Spermatozoa containing one X
or
Y an equal number containing one Y.

XX Female

XY Male

Note: In this simplified diagram a preliminary replication before meiosis and mitotic divisions after meiosis are omitted. The chances of error can be seen to be greatly increased.

GENETIC ABNORMALITIES AND ASSOCIATED DISORDERS

It is not surprising that errors arise during these complex genetic activities. GERM CELLS and proliferating SOMATIC CELLS (including STEM CELLS) are susceptible to such errors.
They may occur spontaneously or be potentiated by external influences.
It is important to distinguish between germ cell and somatic cell abnormalities.

GERM CELL ABNORMALITIES

Errors which have arisen during germ cell development are transferred to the fertilised ovum and thence to all cells including the germ cells of the new individual.

ABNORMALITIES arising in SOMATIC CELLS

These tend to cause restricted effects: they are not transmitted to the next generation.

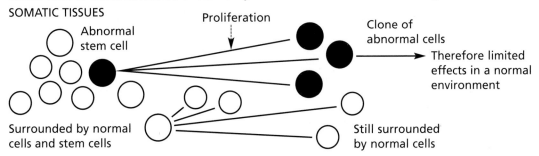

TYPES OF GENETIC ABNORMALITIES

They range from large, involving whole chromosomes, through parts of chromosomes, to gene clusters and single genes.

CHROMOSOMAL ABNORMALITIES

(1) *Polyploidy* – when the chromosomal numbers are increased by an exact multiple of the normal (23) e.g. $23 \times 3 = 69$ chromosomes. Such nuclei are seen in hypertrophied muscle cells and ageing liver cells (i.e. somatic cell polyploidy).
Such gross chromosomal abnormalities occurring during gametogenesis or at fertilisation are usually incompatible with life and are a common cause of spontaneous abortion.

(2) *Aneuploidy* – where the number of chromosomes is increased usually by one (TRISOMY) or decreased by one (MONOSOMY). Early spontaneous abortion is again common: survivors show mental retardation and varied physical abnormalities.
Down's syndrome is a good example of AUTOSOMAL TRISOMY and is due to an extra chromosome (i.e. Trisomy 21 – karyotype 47XX + 21 or 47XY + 21).
The abnormality occurs in utero after fertilisation of the ovum and is therefore autosomal. Increasing maternal age is a potentiating factor in Down's syndrome and many other genetic defects.

19

GENETIC ABNORMALITIES AND ASSOCIATED DISORDERS

CHROMOSOMAL ABNORMALITIES *(continued)*

(3) *Structural abnormalities*

Despite the existence of efficient repair mechanisms structural errors do arise when the long DNA molecules are accidentally broken during the dramatic physical changes occurring at replication. They include, for example, duplication and deletion of gene clusters and single genes: and translocation of fragments of DNA between chromosomes.

SINGLE GENE DISORDERS

Factors regulating the production of the final specific protein are extremely complex and interacting:

1. *In the nucleus*   *In the cytoplasm*

Activity of other genes

promotion / enhancement / start/stop signals → single gene activity (including RNA transcription and movement) → *or* ← detailed control of each step in protein synthesis

Therefore GENETIC EXPRESSION very VARIABLE

2. The corresponding genes on each parental chromosome exert important influences on each other. The inheritance of the Rhesus blood group D is illustrative: there are two possibilities at the D locus on the chromosome – 'D' or 'd'. The 3 possible combinations give rise to the actual blood group (phenotype) as follows:

	Homozygous		Heterozygous	
Genotype	DD	dd	Dd	The presence of one D confers the
Blood group (phenotype)	D	d	D	blood group D i.e. D is DOMINANT.

The presence of two d's is required to confer the blood group d, i.e. d is RECESSIVE.

This concept is important in *inherited single gene disorders*.

(1) In DOMINANT inheritance any HETEROZYGOUS offspring bearing the abnormal trait will be affected: mating with a normal partner statistically produces 50% of normal offspring and 50% affected.

(2) In RECESSIVE inheritance only HOMOZYGOTES for the trait are affected. Such cases usually arise from the mating of 2 heterozygous CARRIERS who, by definition, are themselves unaffected.

The results of mating are as follows: (A = affected gene, N = normal gene)
NN = normal individual: NA = carrier: AA = affected individual.

Heterozygote – Heterozygote
NA ———— NA
NN   NA   NA   AA
Statistically 1 normal, 2 carriers, 1 affected

Monozygote – Normal
AA ———— NN
NA   NA   NA   NA
All offspring are carriers.

Heterozygote – Normal
NA ———— NN
NN   NA   NA   NN
2 are normal, 2 are carriers.

20

GENETIC ABNORMALITIES AND ASSOCIATED DISORDERS

The concept of dominant and recessive traits is useful in genetic counselling. Long lists of dominant and recessive disorders are available: only a few important examples are given.

Autosomal dominant – neurofibromatosis, Huntington's disease: polyposis coli: congenital spherocytosis.

Autosomal recessive – cystic fibrosis, congenital deafness, mucopolysaccharidoses.

Sex-linked disorders are usually recessive and are carried on the X-chromosome: males are affected and females are carriers. Important disorders are haemophilia and muscular dystrophy.

METABOLIC DISORDERS (inborn errors of metabolism)

These are inherited disorders of single genes which code for the enzymes concerned in many metabolic pathways. The clinical effects show considerable variation in severity.

Examples are: disorders of carbohydrate (including glycogen storage), lipid and amino-acid metabolism: lysosomal storage: and membrane transport (including cystic fibrosis).

Note: Not all single gene abnormalities cause, by themselves, significant pathological effects. As indicated above, the controlling factors are complex and include the important effects of 'modifying genes'. It seems likely that abnormal recessive genes exist in the normal population but only present as clinical disorders in rare special circumstances.

MULTIFACTORIAL DISORDERS

Most human diseases have a genetic component but environmental factors usually play a very important part in the pathogenesis.

COMBINED ACTIVITY
of SEVERAL GENES   **+**   ENVIRONMENTAL ⟶ DISEASE
(both normal and abnormal)   FACTORS

Examples are: atopic (allergic) disorders: diabetes mellitus, hypertension, rheumatoid arthritis and various infections.

SOMATIC CELL GENETIC DISORDERS

When mutation occurs after fertilisation of the ovum and at any stage throughout life the effects are limited to the disordered cell(s) and progeny. The clinical effects tend to be localised.

NEOPLASMS and hamartomas are examples of somatic cell genetic disorders (see Carcinogenesis).

Note: In the systematic section of this book significant genetic contribution to the pathogenesis of diseases will be recorded.

AMYLOID DEPOSITION

Amyloid is a waxy substance deposited in the extracellular tissues, particularly around blood vessels and in basement membranes. Various forms of amyloid are seen and they have varying effects. Amyloid is resistant to degradation and its deposition tends to progress relentlessly.

Nature of Amyloid
Chemical: amyloid fibrils are made up of
(i) A major variable component >90%.
(ii) A minor constant component, AMYLOID P PROTEIN – a glycoprotein normally found in serum.
Physical: whatever its composition, amyloid fibrils are arranged in a β-pleated configuration: this accounts for its resistance to degradation and its staining properties.

Detection
At *post-mortem*, the affected organs are pale, enlarged and have a firm, waxy texture.

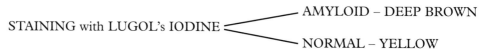

STAINING with LUGOL's IODINE — AMYLOID – DEEP BROWN / NORMAL – YELLOW

On *biopsy* material, specific stains and electronmicroscopy are needed.

(i) **Light microscopy**

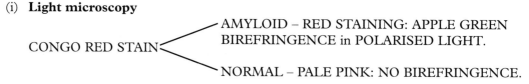

CONGO RED STAIN — AMYLOID – RED STAINING: APPLE GREEN BIREFRINGENCE in POLARISED LIGHT. / NORMAL – PALE PINK: NO BIREFRINGENCE.

IMMUNOSTAINING – for specific constituents e.g. P protein.

(ii) **Electronmicroscopy** – specific appearance: closely packed interlacing fibrils 70–100 nm in diameter.

Pathological effects

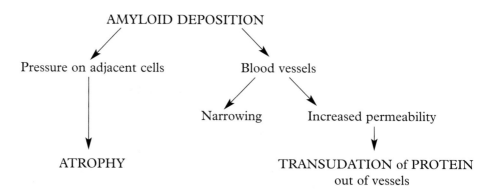

AMYLOID DEPOSITION

Pressure on adjacent cells → ATROPHY

Blood vessels → Narrowing / Increased permeability → TRANSUDATION of PROTEIN out of vessels

AMYLOID DEPOSITION

Almost any tissue in the body may be affected by amyloid deposition, but the most important changes occur in the kidney, gastrointestinal tract and the heart. Other organs, such as the liver and spleen, may also be grossly affected without serious functional impairment.

KIDNEY

In severe cases the kidneys are pale, firm and waxy, and with the iodine test the glomeruli stand out as brown dots to the naked eye.

Renal biopsy is useful in the diagnosis of amyloidosis.

Deposits around:
(a) Glomerular capillaries

(b) Basement membranes of atrophic tubules

(c) Blood vessel

Effects: Glomerular capillary permeability altered

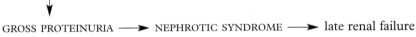

GROSS PROTEINURIA ⟶ NEPHROTIC SYNDROME ⟶ late renal failure

GASTROINTESTINAL TRACT

Due to altered permeability of the capillaries, the patient suffers from diarrhoea and protein loss. There may also be malabsorption, nutritional deficiencies and electrolyte imbalance.

Rectal biopsy is useful in the diagnosis of amyloidosis.

HEART

Amyloid deposition occurs around the cardiac muscle fibres and the capillary basement membranes. The heart is enlarged with apparently thick muscular walls but much of the thickness is due to amyloid deposition.

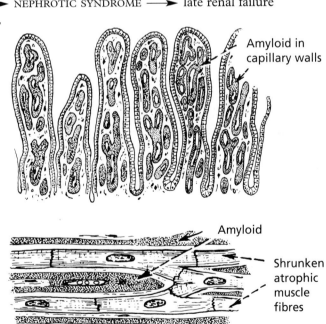

Amyloid in capillary walls

Amyloid

Shrunken atrophic muscle fibres

Effects: Cardiac failure develops mainly due to the mechanical effect of amyloid, making the heart muscle stiff and preventing cardiac filling (restrictive defect). The blood supply to the muscle fibres is also impaired.

AMYLOID CLASSIFICATION

Amyloid was previously classified into 2 main groups.

(i) Primary i.e. without known cause.
(ii) Secondary i.e. associated with chronic inflammatory disease.

Knowledge of the mechanisms of amyloid deposition has made this classification obsolete. Instead:

1. SYSTEMIC AMYLOIDOSIS

(a) *Associated with monoclonal plasma cell proliferation*
    (e.g. myeloma, monoclonal gammopathy, Waldenstrom's macroglobulinaemia).

Increased production of:
    Variable protein – AL (Amyloid Light chain derived) – from fragments of immunoglobulin, especially lambda light chains.

(b) *Associated with chronic inflammation*
    (e.g. tuberculosis, osteomyelitis, rheumatoid arthritis, bronchiectasis and the genetically inherited familial Mediterranean fever.).

Increased production of:
    Variable protein – AA (Amyloid A protein) – derived from serum AA protein, an acute phase reactant in many inflammatory conditions.

Summary of formation of amyloid

Abnormal (monoclonal) proliferation of plasma cells

↓

Abnormal immunoglobulins esp. lambda light chains

Proteolysis ⟶ ↓

AMYLOIDOGENIC PROTEIN > 90%
(AL)
+ Amyloid P glycoprotein < 10%

↓

SYSTEMIC AMYLOID (AL)

Long continued active inflammation

↓

Acute phase reactant protein

↓ ⟵ Proteolysis

AMYLOIDOGENIC PROTEIN > 90%
(AA)
+ Amyloid P glycoprotein <10%

↓

SYSTEMIC AMYLOID (AA)

2. LOCALISED AMYLOIDOSIS

In ENDOCRINE TUMOURS – amyloid derived from polypeptide hormones e.g. medullary carcinoma of thyroid – calcitonin derived amyloid.

In OLD AGE – the amyloidogenic protein is related to pre-albumin. Deposits of amyloid occur in the heart, brain and joints. In Alzheimer's disease (p.549) local amyloid deposition in the brain is important.

CALCIFICATION

Abnormal deposits of calcium salts occur in 2 circumstances: dystrophic calcification and metastatic calcification.

1. DYSTROPHIC CALCIFICATION

Local deposits of calcium may occur in:

(a) **Necrotic tissue which is not absorbed** e.g. old caseous lesions of tuberculosis; old infarcts; old collections of pus; dead parasites; in fat necrosis associated with pancreatitis.

(b) **Tissues undergoing slow degeneration** e.g. hyaline areas in benign tumours e.g. fibroids (p.498); in arteries due to atheromatous degeneration or in old age; in old thrombi; diseased or abnormal heart valves.

The mechanism may be as follows:

Note: The presence of radio-opaque Ca^{2+} is of diagnostic use particularly in old healed disease (e.g. tuberculosis) and also in some tumours, e.g. breast cancer where very small deposits of calcium may be present.

2. METASTATIC CALCIFICATION

In this case the essential feature is an increase in the calcium phosphate product in the blood (usually hypercalcaemia).

The mechanisms are complex: the 2 usual mechanisms are simplified as follows:

(1)
Parathyroid overactivity
due to:
(a) Tumour (adenoma)
(b) Hyperplasia (tertiary) – associated with phosphate retention in severe prolonged chronic renal failure.

(2)
Vitamin D overdosage

MOBILISATION of Ca^{2+} from bone

Increased absorption of Ca^{2+}

↑ Increased blood Ca^{2+} ↑

Deposition may be widespread occurring at sites where the local environment tends to be alkaline, favouring precipitation. ⟶ KIDNEYS ARTERIES LUNGS
(renal stones)

About 5% of MALIGNANCY cases – particularly with carcinoma of the breast and lung – have HYPERCALCAEMIA, although most do not live long enough to have significant systemic deposition.

The mechanisms are (1) secretion by the tumour of a protein [parathyroid hormone related peptide (PTHrP)] which mimics the action of parathormone and (2) of less importance, the local release of bone resorbing cytokines by tumour metastases in bones.

ENDOGENOUS PIGMENTATION

IRON-CONTAINING PIGMENT

Two main pigments are derived from the breakdown of red blood cells.
(1) HAEMOSIDERIN and (2) BILIRUBIN.

The detailed mechanism is described on page 341 in relation to JAUNDICE.

HAEMOSIDERIN

The iron derived from red cell breakdown is held in the spleen, liver and bone marrow, combined with apoferritin. In the plasma it is transported by transferrin. The two mechanisms maintain an equilibrium between the iron contents in these three sites. When the amount of iron within the cells becomes excessive and overloads the ferritin system, it is deposited in a brown granular form – haemosiderin. This occurs in 2 situations:

1. Local breakdown of red cells in tissues e.g. in

The colour changes in a 'black' eye exemplify this mechanism

Local haemorrhage into loose tissues
↓
Extravasated red cells
↓
Phagocytosis of red cells by macrophages
↓   ↓
Haemosiderin   Iron free pigments

RED
↓
GREENISH BLUE
↓
YELLOW

2. Visceral siderosis

(a) *Haemosiderosis*

This is seen in the liver, spleen and sometimes the kidneys in cases of haemolytic anaemia, and in patients requiring repeated blood transfusion. The change is most strikingly seen in the liver, which becomes deep brown. Iron is found in the Kupffer cells first and, later, in liver cells. Easily demonstrated by the Prussian blue reaction, these iron deposits very rarely cause organ damage, in contrast to haemochromatosis.

Granules of haemosiderin in liver cells in later stages

Kupffer cell

ENDOGENOUS PIGMENTATION

Haemosiderin *(continued)*

(b) *Haemochromatosis (Bronzed diabetes)*

The absorption of iron from the intestine is controlled by the ferritin-transferrin mechanism already mentioned.

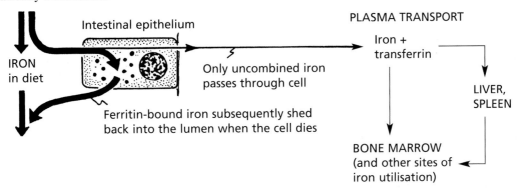

The ferritin content of the intestinal epithelium, iron saturation of the plasma, stores of iron in the liver and spleen and the demand for iron by the bone marrow form a balancing mechanism preventing overloading of any part of the system.

In haemochromatosis the absorption of iron is virtually uncontrolled, due to an inherited defect on chromosome 6. The system becomes overloaded and iron is deposited as haemosiderin in many sites, the main ones being:

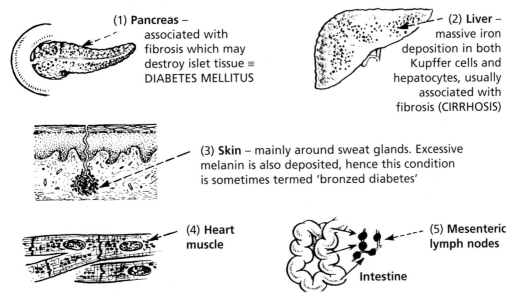

(1) **Pancreas** – associated with fibrosis which may destroy islet tissue ≡ DIABETES MELLITUS

(2) **Liver** – massive iron deposition in both Kupffer cells and hepatocytes, usually associated with fibrosis (CIRRHOSIS)

(3) **Skin** – mainly around sweat glands. Excessive melanin is also deposited, hence this condition is sometimes termed 'bronzed diabetes'

(4) **Heart muscle**

(5) **Mesenteric lymph nodes**

Intestine

Haemosiderin may be found in almost any site in the body.

ENDOGENOUS PIGMENTATION

Haemoglobin

Occasionally, intravascular haemolysis occurs. Haemoglobin appears in the urine, giving it a dull red colour – in the severe acute situation (e.g. incompatible blood transfusion) acute renal tubular necrosis occurs. If the condition is chronic, as in paroxysmal haemoglobinuria, some of the haemoglobin is reabsorbed and subsequently broken down so that iron, as haemosiderin, appears in the renal tubular epithelium.

(Demonstrated by the Prussian blue reaction)

Haematin (or haemazoin)

This is a brown pigment produced by malarial parasites from haemoglobin. It is taken up by the monocytes in the blood and subsequently deposited in the liver and spleen.

Red-cell – containing malarial parasite

Monocyte – containing haematin

Lipofuscin

This is a yellowish brown pigment having a high lipid content, often found in the atrophied cells of old age – 'wear and tear' pigment. It is particularly common in the heart muscle, and the term 'brown atrophy' is often applied.

Thin myocardial fibre
Pigment granules around nucleus

It is also found in liver cells, testes and nerve cells.

EXOGENOUS PIGMENTATION – DEGENERATIONS

EXOGENOUS PIGMENTATION

Pigments may be introduced by inhalation, ingestion or injection. The most important are those introduced by inhalation of dusts in industrial processes.

Inhalation

The commonest substances inhaled are COAL DUST (carbon) – black, and STONE DUST (silica) – grey.

The particles reach the alveoli especially if the bronchial ciliary action is disturbed by chronic bronchitis.

Particles taken up by macrophages in alveoli

Transported into lymph channels and deposited in small focal aggregates throughout lungs and hilar lymph nodes

The effects are described in detail under PNEUMOCONIOSIS.

Ingestion

Pigmentation can be caused by chronic ingestion of metals such as silver or lead. In both, the skin has a metallic hue, and in the case of lead a blue line appears on the gums due to interaction between lead and hydrogen sulphide. Excessive intake of carrots can lead to yellowish red skin pigmentation caused by carotene.

Injection

Tattooing is the most striking example of pigmentation following injection.

DEGENERATIONS

(1) Hyaline

This is a descriptive term meaning a glossy, refractile appearance, seen in sections stained with haematoxylin and eosin. It is most commonly encountered in the form of dense collagen, particularly in benign tumours such as leiomyomas where the collagen has replaced muscle fibres, and in blood vessels in arteriosclerosis.

The term 'Mallory's hyaline' refers to an *intra*cellular accumulation of cytoskeletal proteins e.g. in alcoholic liver disease.

(2) Mucoid

This is a common change in epithelial tumours which secrete mucin. In these cases the epithelial cells undergo degeneration and appear to dissolve in the mucin.

Connective tissue may also accumulate mucin. Spaces filled with mucopolysaccharides (e.g. hyaluronic acid) appear between the fibres. The change is common in some tumours and the term 'myxomatous' may be used.

29

INFLAMMATION

INFLAMMATION

Inflammation is the dynamic process by which living tissues react to injury. They concern vascular and connective tissues particularly.

Causes:
Various agents may kill or damage cells:

PHYSICAL

Trauma   Heat   Radiation
          or cold

CHEMICAL

Simple chemical   Organic poisons,
poisons, e.g. acids   e.g. paraquat

INFECTIVE

Bacteria   Viruses   Parasites

IMMUNOLOGICAL

Antigen-antibody   Cell-mediated

... and any other circumstance leading to tissue damage, e.g. VASCULAR or HORMONAL DISTURBANCE.

The inflammatory reaction takes place in the surviving adjacent vascular and connective tissues; the specialised parenchymal cells do not directly participate.

The initial stages are known as the **acute** inflammatory reaction. Where the process is prolonged the inflammation may be **subacute** or **chronic**.

ACUTE INFLAMMATION
The classical signs are:

REDNESS (rubor)
HEAT (calor)
SWELLING (tumor)
PAIN (dolor)
LOSS OF FUNCTION (functio laesa).

e.g. Boil

These gross signs are explained by changes occurring at microscopic level. Three essential features are:

1. **HYPERAEMIA**
2. **EXUDATION OF FLUID**
3. **EMIGRATION OF LEUCOCYTES**

ACUTE INFLAMMATION

HYPERAEMIA

The hyperaemia in inflammation is associated with the well known microvascular changes which occur in Lewis' triple response – a FLUSH, a FLARE and a WEAL. It occurs when a blunt instrument is drawn firmly across the skin and illustrates the vascular changes occurring in acute inflammation.

The stroke is marked momentarily by a white line due to VASOCONSTRICTION.
The flush, a dull red line, immediately follows and is due to CAPILLARY DILATATION.
The flare, a bright red irregular surrounding zone, is due to ARTERIOLAR DILATATION.

Mechanisms
involved are:

HYPERAEMIA explains the classical signs of REDNESS and HEAT.

ACUTE INFLAMMATION

EXUDATION

Exudation is the increased passage of protein-rich fluid through the vessel wall into the interstitial tissue. It explains the **weal** in Lewis' triple response.

Advantageous results

Fluid increase

↓

Dilution of toxins

Contents of fluid

(a) Globulins ➤ protective antibodies

(b) Fibrin deposition ➤ Helps to limit spread of bacteria

(c) Various factors promoting subsequent healing

Mechanism

(1) *Protein passage*

Chemical mediators ⟨ Endothelial contraction – formation of gaps

↓

Increased permeability

Direct endothelial injury (all vessels), e.g. burns ⟶ Increased permeability

Post-capillary venule

Leak of **proteins**, roughly in proportion to their molecular size: *albumin* (smallest) greatest in amount, but all plasma proteins present. If capillary damage is severe, FIBRINOGEN (largest molecule) escapes.

(2) *Fluid movement*

Hyperaemia	Loss of protein from capillaries	Interstitial tissue protein increase
↓	↓	↓
Capillary blood pressure rises	Reduced plasma osmotic pressure	Increased tissue osmotic pressure

INCREASED FILTRATION PRESSURE

↓

Local swelling (OEDEMA) – 3rd classical sign

↓

Increased lymph flow from area

ACUTE INFLAMMATION

EMIGRATION OF LEUCOCYTES

Neutrophils and mononuclears pass between the endothelial cell junctions by amoeboid movement through the venule wall into the tissue spaces. In this process both neutrophils and endothelial cells are activated and both express cell adhesion molecules, initially SELECTINS and then INTEGRINS.

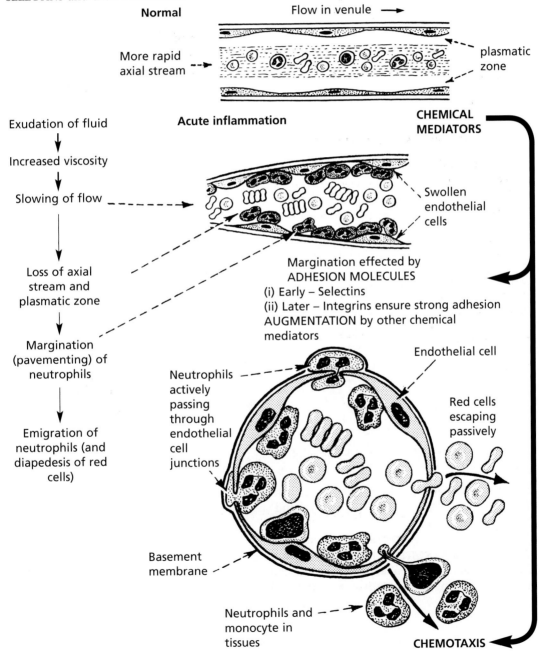

Normal

Flow in venule →

More rapid axial stream

plasmatic zone

Exudation of fluid
↓
Increased viscosity
↓
Slowing of flow

Acute inflammation

CHEMICAL MEDIATORS

Swollen endothelial cells

↓

Loss of axial stream and plasmatic zone

↓

Margination (pavementing) of neutrophils

↓

Emigration of neutrophils (and diapedesis of red cells)

Margination effected by
ADHESION MOLECULES
(i) Early – Selectins
(ii) Later – Integrins ensure strong adhesion
AUGMENTATION by other chemical mediators

Neutrophils actively passing through endothelial cell junctions

Endothelial cell

Red cells escaping passively

Basement membrane

Neutrophils and monocyte in tissues

CHEMOTAXIS ←

35

ACUTE INFLAMMATION

CHEMOTAXIS

The initial margination of neutrophils and mononuclears is potentiated by slowing of blood flow and by increased 'stickiness' of the endothelial surface.

After penetration of the vessel wall, the subsequent movement of the leucocytes is controlled by CHEMOTAXIS. The cell moves in response to an increasing concentration gradient of the particular chemotactic agent, usually a protein or polypeptide.

Increasing concentration of ⎯⎯⎯ Chemotactic agent

Cell movement

Bacteria

Important examples of chemotactic agents are:

Fractions of the COMPLEMENT SYSTEM (esp. C5a)
Factors derived from arachidonic acid by the neutrophils – LEUKOTRIENES (e.g. LTB4)
Factors derived from pathogenic BACTERIA
Factors derived from sensitised lymphocytes – CYTOKINES (e.g. IL-8).

The process helps to explain the apparently purposeful movement of leucocytes and their aggregation in large numbers in inflammation.

PHAGOCYTOSIS

This is the process by which neutrophils and macrophages clear the injurious agent. It is an important defence mechanism in bacterial infections particularly.

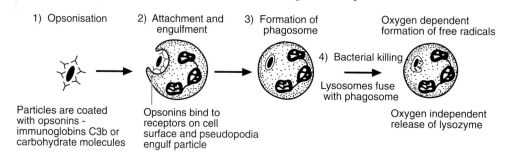

1) Opsonisation 2) Attachment and engulfment 3) Formation of phagosome Oxygen dependent formation of free radicals

4) Bacterial killing

Lysosomes fuse with phagosome

Particles are coated with opsonins - immunoglobins C3b or carbohydrate molecules

Opsonins bind to receptors on cell surface and pseudopodia engulf particle

Oxygen independent release of lysozyme

Factors influencing the efficiency of phagocytosis:
(1) OPSONINS – antibodies of both natural and specific immune type, especially antibodies of IgG class (p.96).
(2) Fractions of the COMPLEMENT system.
(3) The PHYSICAL STATE of the cellular environment.
The opsonic activity is enhanced when it is confined within a solid organ or rigid medium such as a fibrin network; where conditions are looser and more fluid, activity is diminished.

ACUTE INFLAMMATION

CHEMICAL MEDIATORS

Various chemical mediators have roles in the inflammatory process. They may be circulating in plasma and require activation or they may be secreted by inflammatory cells. Many of these mediators have overlapping actions.

Mediators dervived from:

1. Inflammatory cells

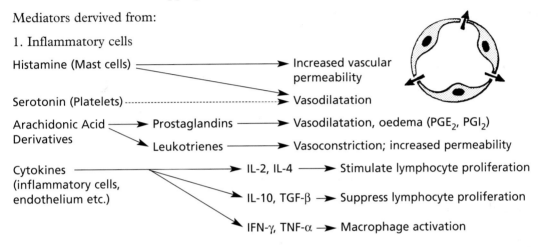

Histamine (Mast cells) ⟶ Increased vascular permeability

Serotonin (Platelets) ⟶ Vasodilatation

Arachidonic Acid Derivatives ⟶ Prostaglandins ⟶ Vasodilatation, oedema (PGE_2, PGI_2)

⟶ Leukotrienes ⟶ Vasoconstriction; increased permeability

Cytokines (inflammatory cells, endothelium etc.) ⟶ IL-2, IL-4 ⟶ Stimulate lymphocyte proliferation

⟶ IL-10, TGF-β ⟶ Suppress lymphocyte proliferation

⟶ IFN-γ, TNF-α ⟶ Macrophage activation

2. Plasma. These pathways are all interrelated.

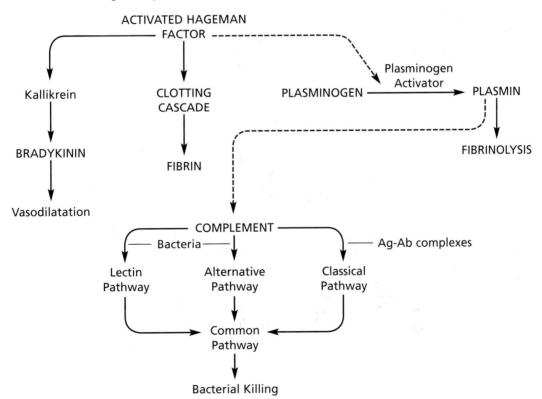

SEQUELS OF ACUTE INFLAMMATION

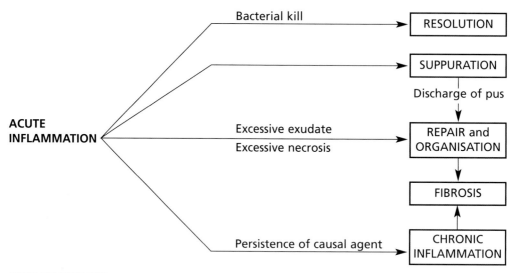

RESOLUTION

This means the complete restoration of normal conditions after the acute inflammation. The three main features which potentiate this sequel are:

1. minimal cell death and tissue damage
2. rapid elimination of the causal agent, e.g. bacteria
3. local conditions favouring removal of fluid and debris.

Resolution of lobar pneumonia (bacterial inflammation of lung alveoli) is a good example:

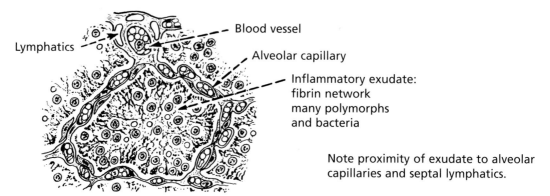

Following bacterial kill the mechanism is as follows:

1. Solution of fibrin by enzyme action (polymorphs and fibrinolysin)
2. Removal of fluid by blood vessels and lymphatics
3. Removal of all debris by phagocytes to hilar lymph nodes
4. The capillary hyperaemia diminishes and restoration to normal is complete

SEQUELS OF ACUTE INFLAMMATION

SUPPURATION

This means the formation of PUS; where pus accumulates an ABSCESS forms.

Infection by pyogenic (pus-forming) bacteria is the usual cause, e.g. staphylococcal abscess (or boil). The pus in this case is a thick, creamy yellow fluid which, on centrifugation, separates thus:

Supernatant fluid → { Inflammatory exudate containing proteins and the products of protein breakdown.

Deposit (solids) → { Polymorphs (pus cells) } Living and Bacteria } and dead

Fragments of cell
Globules of fat
and other
particulate matter

Evolution of an abscess

The usual evolution of an abscess is as follows:

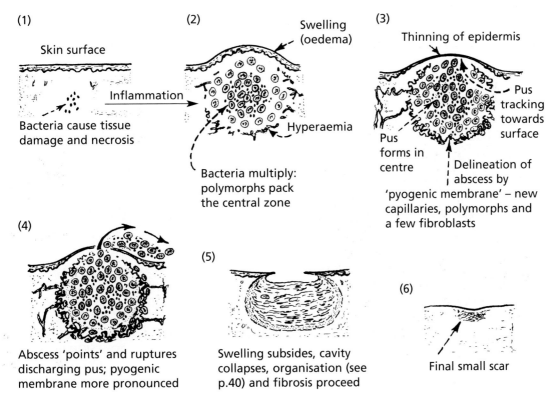

(1)

Skin surface

Bacteria cause tissue damage and necrosis

→ Inflammation →

(2)

Swelling (oedema)

Hyperaemia

Bacteria multiply: polymorphs pack the central zone

(3)

Thinning of epidermis

Pus tracking towards surface

Pus forms in centre

Delineation of abscess by 'pyogenic membrane' – new capillaries, polymorphs and a few fibroblasts

(4)

Abscess 'points' and ruptures discharging pus; pyogenic membrane more pronounced

(5)

Swelling subsides, cavity collapses, organisation (see p.40) and fibrosis proceed

(6)

Final small scar

39

SEQUELS OF ACUTE INFLAMMATION

Evolution of an abscess *(continued)*

When the abscess is deep-seated, the process may be modified as follows:

Chronic discharging SINUS ← Deep-seated abscess → Localised collection of pus

Discharge via long tortuous track

Pyogenic membrane

Failure to discharge all the abscess contents, especially if foreign matter is retained

Small → Absorption of pus → Scar

Large → Inspissation of pus and walling off by fibrous tissue → Calcium salts

ORGANISATION AND FIBROSIS

Organisation occurs when, during the acute inflammatory process, (a) there is excessive exudation or necrosis or (b) when local conditions are unfavourable for the removal of exudate and debris. The term also applies to the local reaction to the presence of thrombus and also the necrosis associated with infarction.

The changes are similar to those described in wound healing viz – the growth of new capillaries into the inert material (exudate or thrombus), the migration of macrophages and the proliferation of fibroblasts resulting in FIBROSIS.

A good example of organisation following acute inflammation is seen in the pleura overlying pneumonia. The inflammation of the lung tissue proper usually resolves completely (p.264); in contrast the pleural exudate is not easily removed and organisation takes place.

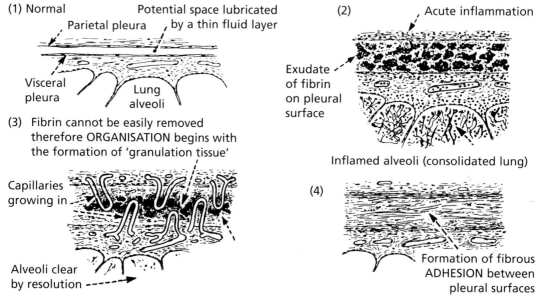

(1) Normal — Parietal pleura, Potential space lubricated by a thin fluid layer, Visceral pleura, Lung alveoli

(2) Acute inflammation — Exudate of fibrin on pleural surface, Inflamed alveoli (consolidated lung)

(3) Fibrin cannot be easily removed therefore ORGANISATION begins with the formation of 'granulation tissue' — Capillaries growing in, Alveoli clear by resolution

(4) Formation of fibrous ADHESION between pleural surfaces

Other good examples of organisation are seen after infarction (see p.164).

CHRONIC INFLAMMATION

Chronic Inflammation may (a) follow acute inflammation if the causal agent is not removed: or (b) be 'primary' i.e. there is no pre-existing acute stage.

The essential changes are

1. Absence of polymorphs (natural life span of 1–3 days); the appearance of lymphocytes and plasma cells. Macrophages play an increasingly important role including removing dead polymorphs, presentation of antigenic material and granuloma formation.
2. Proliferation of vascular endothelium by 'budding' – formation of new capillaries (angiogenesis).
3. Proliferation of fibroblasts with collagen production leading to
4. Fibrosis.

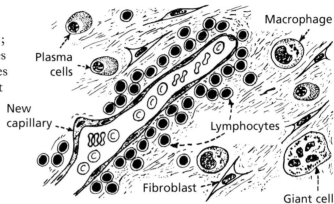

Common causes of 'primary' chronic inflammation include:

(a) Persistent infections e.g. tuberculosis, leprosy – where the organisms are resistant to neutrophil attack and bacteria survive within macrophages.
(b) Foreign material e.g. silicates, including asbestos.
(c) Auto-immune diseases e.g. auto-immune thyroiditis.
(d) Conditions of unknown aetiology e.g. sarcoidosis: Crohn's disease.

Cellular interactions

The various cells in chronic inflammation release messengers e.g. cytokines, which influence each other's behaviour.

In the illustrative diagram below, ↓ denotes one cell type changing to another: ⌇ denotes activity of a messenger.

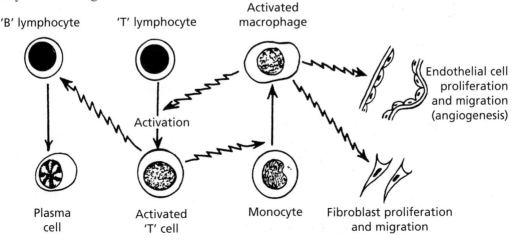

CHRONIC INFLAMMATION

GRANULOMATOUS INFLAMMATION

This is the term given to forms of chronic inflammation in which modified macrophages (epithelioid cells) accumulate in small clusters surrounded by lymphocytes. The small clusters are called GRANULOMAS. The basic lesion in TUBERCULOSIS is a good example.

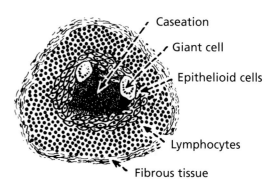

Caseation

Giant cell

Epithelioid cells

Lymphocytes

Fibrous tissue

Similar granulomas are seen in:

Sarcoidosis – a rare inflammatory disease of unknown aetiology affecting especially the lymph nodes and lungs, but also many other organs

'Talc' granuloma – where particular silicates introduced into the tissues evoke an inflammatory reaction after a latent period (usually years)

Crohn's disease – a chronic inflammatory disease affecting the terminal ileum and colon (see p.309).

Lymph nodes draining ulcerated areas in which breakdown of lipid is occurring.

N.B. In all of these granulomatous diseases the basic lesion may be identical, but CASEATION only occurs in tuberculosis.

The epithelioid cells of the granulomas are modified macrophages, and giant cells are derived from macrophages usually by cell fusion but occasionally by nuclear division without cytoplasmic separation.

The Langhans' giant cell – seen in chronic granulomata, e.g. tuberculosis and sarcoidosis.

Nuclei in horse-shoe arrangement

The foreign body giant cell – seen in association with particulate insoluble material.

Nuclei scattered throughout cytoplasm

Mechanism of granuloma formation

Indigestible material in MACROPHAGE

+

IMMUNE RESPONSE via ACTIVATED 'T' LYMPHOCYTE

Proinflammatory cytokines including IFNγ, TNF-α and IL-1

PROLIFERATION and ACTIVATION of MACROPHAGES

GRANULOMA FORMATION

ULCERATION – BENIGN

ULCERATION is a complication of many disease processes.

An **ulcer** is formed when the surface covering of an organ or tissue is lost due to necrosis and replaced by inflammatory tissue.

The most common sites are the alimentary tract and the skin.

Ulcers are divided into two main groups: (1) BENIGN (inflammatory) and (2) MALIGNANT (cancerous).

The word 'benign' is used here in the limited sense of contrasting with 'malignant': 'benign' ulcers may have serious consequences.

Evolution of a benign ulcer

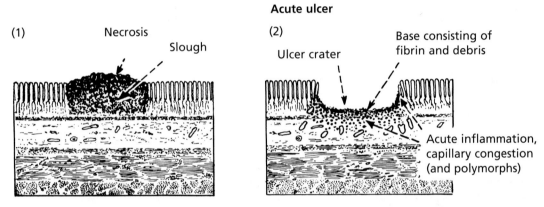

Healing can occur at this stage with restoration to normal, but if irritation (e.g. bacterial action, slight trauma, digestive juices and acid) continues, a CHRONIC ULCER forms.

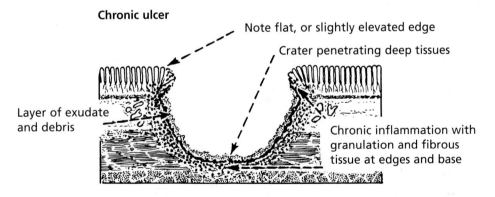

Healing of a chronic ulcer may be impeded by the secondary obliterative changes in the blood vessels due to the chronic inflammation, and it is inevitably associated with a variable amount of scarring.

ULCERATION – MALIGNANT

Evolution of a malignant ulcer (ulcerated tumour)

Such an ulcer is the result of the growth of a malignant tumour.

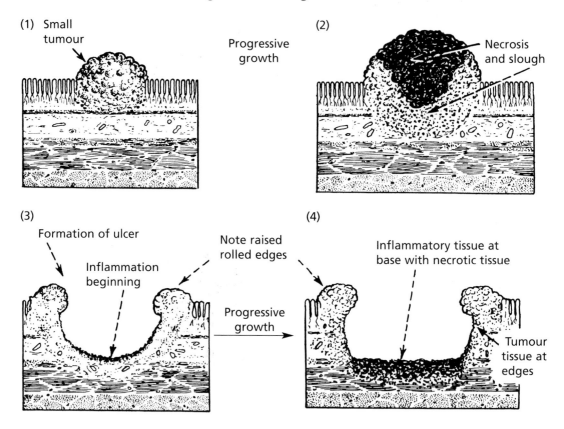

(1) Small tumour

Progressive growth

(2) Necrosis and slough

(3) Formation of ulcer

Inflammation beginning

Note raised rolled edges

Progressive growth

(4) Inflammatory tissue at base with necrotic tissue

Tumour tissue at edges

The differences between benign and malignant ulcers are most prominent at the edges – from which a diagnostic biopsy should be taken.

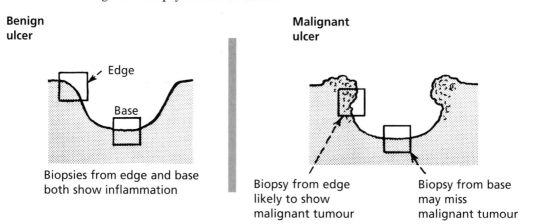

Benign ulcer

Edge

Base

Biopsies from edge and base both show inflammation

Malignant ulcer

Biopsy from edge likely to show malignant tumour

Biopsy from base may miss malignant tumour

INFLAMMATION – ANATOMICAL VARIETIES

SINUS

A sinus is a tract lined usually by granulation tissue leading from a chronically inflamed cavity to a surface. In many cases the cause is the continuing presence of 'foreign' or necrotic material.

Examples include:

- **Sinuses associated with osteomyelitis** (inflammation of bone).
  Where necrosis of bone occurs, chronic sinuses form over it.
- **Pilonidal sinus** (pilonidal = nest of hairs).
  Seen in the mid-line over the sacrum (natal cleft) where hairs which have penetrated deeply under the skin are associated with chronic relapsing inflammation.

FISTULA

A fistula is a track open at both ends, through which abnormal communication between two surfaces is established.

There are two main types:
1. **Congenital** – due to developmental abnormality: any inflammation is superimposed.
2. **Acquired** – due to:

An **EMPYEMA** is a collection of pus in a body cavity or hollow organ. The term refers usually to the pleural cavity or the gall bladder.

CELLULITIS occurs when inflammation spreads in the connective tissue planes.

HEALING

HEALING

Healing is the final stage of the response of tissue to injury.

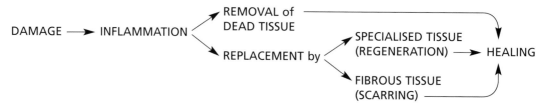

The capacity of a tissue for REGENERATION depends on its PROLIFERATIVE ABILITY and on the type and severity of the damage.

Three broad GROUPS of cells are considered in the context of the cell cycle (p.3).

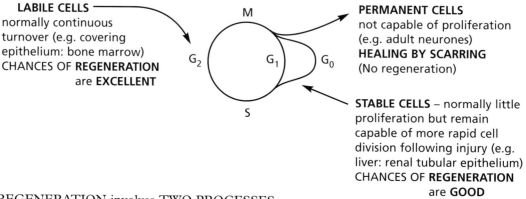

LABILE CELLS —
normally continuous turnover (e.g. covering epithelium: bone marrow)
CHANCES OF **REGENERATION** are **EXCELLENT**

PERMANENT CELLS
not capable of proliferation (e.g. adult neurones)
HEALING BY SCARRING
(No regeneration)

STABLE CELLS – normally little proliferation but remain capable of more rapid cell division following injury (e.g. liver: renal tubular epithelium)
CHANCES OF **REGENERATION** are **GOOD**

REGENERATION involves TWO PROCESSES

1. PROLIFERATION of SURVIVING CELLS to replace lost tissue.
2. MIGRATION of SURVIVING CELLS into the vacant space.

The FACTORS which CONTROL healing and repair are complex: they include the production of a variety of **growth factors.**

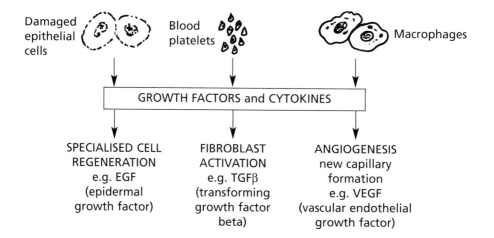

WOUND HEALING

Healing of a wound demonstrates both epithelial regeneration (healing of the epidermis) and repair by scarring (healing of the dermis).

Two patterns are described depending on the amount of tissue damage. These are essentially the same process varying only in amount.

1. Healing by first intention (primary union)

This occurs in clean, incised wounds with good apposition of the edges – particularly planned surgical incisions.

Immediately: Blood clot and debris fill the small cleft.

Movement of epithelial cells across wound

2–3 hours: Early inflammation close to edges. Mild hyperaemia and a few polymorphs.

Epithelium growing across

Mitotic activity

2–3 days: Macrophage activity removing clot. Proliferation of blood vessels. Fibroblastic activity.

10–14 days: Scab loose and epithelial covering complete. Fibrous union of edges, but wound is still weak.

Weeks: Scar tissue still slightly hyperaemic. Good fibrous union, but not full strength.

Months – years: Devascularisation. Remodelling of collagen by enzyme action. Scar is now minimal and merges with surrounding tissues.

WOUND HEALING

2. Healing by second intention (secondary union)

This occurs in open wounds, particularly when there has been significant loss of tissue, necrosis or infection.

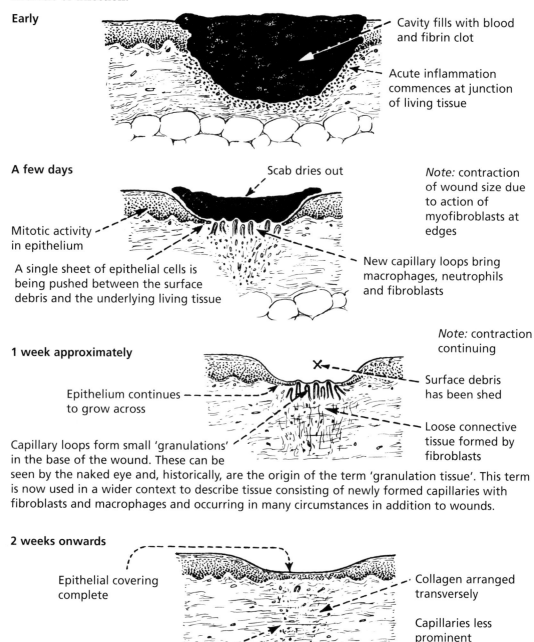

Early

Cavity fills with blood and fibrin clot

Acute inflammation commences at junction of living tissue

A few days

Scab dries out

Note: contraction of wound size due to action of myofibroblasts at edges

Mitotic activity in epithelium

A single sheet of epithelial cells is being pushed between the surface debris and the underlying living tissue

New capillary loops bring macrophages, neutrophils and fibroblasts

Note: contraction continuing

1 week approximately

Surface debris has been shed

Epithelium continues to grow across

Loose connective tissue formed by fibroblasts

Capillary loops form small 'granulations' in the base of the wound. These can be seen by the naked eye and, historically, are the origin of the term 'granulation tissue'. This term is now used in a wider context to describe tissue consisting of newly formed capillaries with fibroblasts and macrophages and occurring in many circumstances in addition to wounds.

2 weeks onwards

Epithelial covering complete

Collagen arranged transversely

Capillaries less prominent

Fewer cells

WOUND HEALING

Healing by second intention *(continued)*

Months

Full thickness of epithelium restored

Varying depth of surface depression

Thick collagenous scar tissue becoming less vascular

Note that the differences in the two types of wound healing are quantitative: the essential pathological processes are the same.

Wound contraction

Wound contraction, which is beneficial and begins early, is due mainly to the young, specialised 'myofibroblasts' in the granulation tissue exerting a traction effect at the wound edges. The exposed surface is reduced by gradual regeneration of the surface epithelium. The remodelling of the collagen continues for many months.

COMPLICATIONS

Contracture

Later, CONTRACTURE with distortion due to thickening and shortening of collagen bundles may cause serious cosmetic and functional disability, particularly in deep and extensive skin burns and around joints if muscles are seriously damaged.

Occasional complications

1. At the edges and base of a wound granulation tissue may form in excess and prevent proper healing ('exuberant granulations': 'proud flesh').

Contracture following burn of neck and jaw

2. The formation of excess collagen in the form of thick interlacing bundles which causes marked swelling at the site of the wound is known as a KELOID. The essential cause is unknown. It is particularly common in black people.

51

HEALING – FIBROSIS

FIBROSIS is the end result of WOUND HEALING, CHRONIC INFLAMMATION and ORGANISATION.

Formation of fibrous tissue

FIBROCYTES
- - - - - - - - - - →
    (and primitive stem cells) situated around capillaries and loose connective tissues

STIMULUS –
growth factor e.g. TGFβ (see p.48) derived from damaged cells and macrophages.

Enlarge to become active
FIBROBLASTS
and active PROTEIN SYNTHESIS begins

(1) INTRACELLULAR PRODUCTION of COLLAGEN precursors.
(a) Hydroxylation of proline and lysine (vit C required)
(b) Triple helix formation.

(2) adhesive glyco-proteins – FIBRONECTINS which provide a scaffolding and contribute to the progress of the repair process

Secretion to EXTRACELLULAR SITE

(c)   cleavage of terminal peptides

(d) Cross-linking
+
polymerisation

COLLAGEN FIBRE

REMODELLING follows: Action of COLLAGENASE ⟶ SCAR TISSUE
+ secretion of COLLAGEN

Factors delaying healing

1. Local
INFECTION, a POOR BLOOD SUPPLY, excessive movement and presence of foreign material DELAY HEALING.
2. General
DEFICIENCY of VITAMIN C
DEFICIENCY of AMINO ACIDS (in malnutrition)
DEFICIENCY of ZINC
EXCESS of ADRENAL GLUCOCORTICOIDS
DEBILITATING CHRONIC DISEASE
} Failure of proper collagen synthesis with delayed healing and weak scars.

HEALING – SPECIAL SITUATIONS

INTERNAL SURFACES

The regeneration of the covering epithelium is very similar to that of the skin, as seen for example in the alimentary tract.

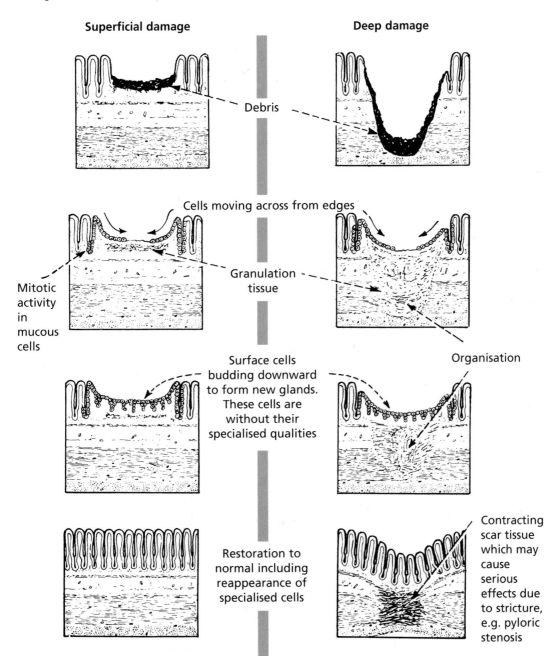

Superficial damage

Deep damage

Debris

Cells moving across from edges

Mitotic activity in mucous cells

Granulation tissue

Organisation

Surface cells budding downward to form new glands. These cells are without their specialised qualities

Restoration to normal including reappearance of specialised cells

Contracting scar tissue which may cause serious effects due to stricture, e.g. pyloric stenosis

HEALING – SPECIAL SITUATIONS

SOLID EPITHELIAL ORGANS

1. Following gross tissue damage – including supporting tissue (post-necrotic scarring).

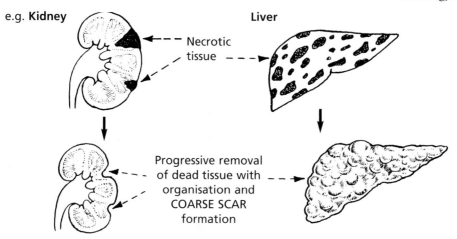

e.g. **Kidney**　　　　　　　　　　　**Liver**

Necrotic tissue

Progressive removal of dead tissue with organisation and COARSE SCAR formation

2. Following cell damage with survival of the supporting (reticular) tissues

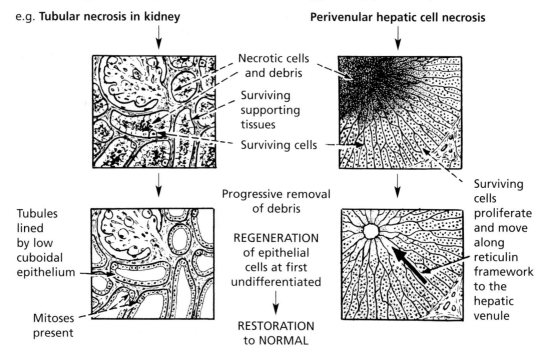

e.g. **Tubular necrosis in kidney**　　　　**Perivenular hepatic cell necrosis**

Necrotic cells and debris

Surviving supporting tissues

Surviving cells

Tubules lined by low cuboidal epithelium

Mitoses present

Progressive removal of debris

REGENERATION of epithelial cells at first undifferentiated

↓

RESTORATION to NORMAL

Surviving cells proliferate and move along reticulin framework to the hepatic venule

HEALING – SPECIAL SITUATIONS

MUSCLE

Muscle fibres of all 3 types – skeletal, cardiac and visceral – have only limited capacity to regenerate.

When a MASS of muscle tissue is damaged, repair by SCARRING occurs. This is particularly important in the HEART after infarction.

If the damage affects individual muscle fibres diffusely and with varying severity, then regeneration of the specialised fibres is possible (e.g. the myocardium may recover completely from the effects of diphtheria toxin and virus infection).

NERVOUS TISSUE

Central nervous system

Regeneration does not occur when a neurone is lost.

In cases of acute damage, the initial functional loss often exceeds the loss of actual nerve tissue because of the reactive changes in the surrounding tissue. As these changes diminish, functional restoration commences.

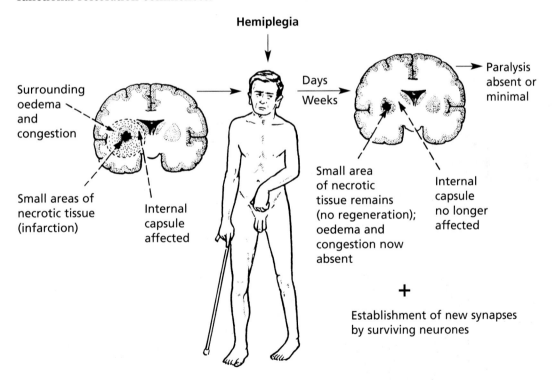

Scarring within the CNS is by proliferation of ASTROCYTES and the production of fibrillary glial acidic protein – a process known as GLIOSIS.

HEALING – SPECIAL SITUATIONS

NERVOUS TISSUE *(continued)*

Peripheral Nerves

When a peripheral nerve is damaged, the axon and its myelin sheath rapidly degenerate distally. The supporting tissues of the nerve (neurilemma) degenerate slowly.

Regeneration can occur because the central neurone of which the axon is a peripheral extension is remote from the site of damage.

A spinal motor nerve is taken as an example.

Normal spinal cord

Results of damage

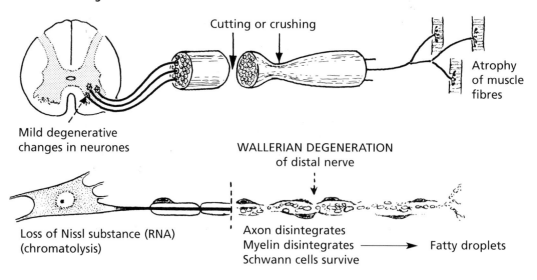

HEALING – SPECIAL SITUATIONS

Peripheral Nerves *(continued)*

Regeneration takes the form of a sprouting of the cut ends of the axons.

Sprouting
of axons

Growth along the track
of the degenerate nerve
(about 1 mm per day)

**The results depend on the apposition of the
distal remnant with the sprouting axons.**

Good apposition

Good restoration

**The best results are seen in crushing injuries
where the sheaths remain in continuity.**

Poor apposition

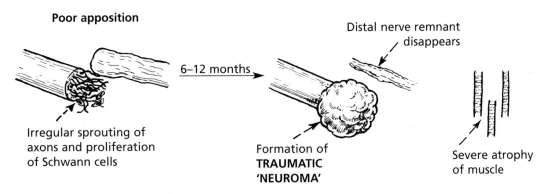

Distal nerve remnant
disappears

6–12 months

Irregular sprouting of
axons and proliferation
of Schwann cells

Formation of
**TRAUMATIC
'NEUROMA'**

Severe atrophy
of muscle

HEALING – SPECIAL SITUATIONS

BONE

A fracture is usually accompanied by damage to or haemorrhage into adjacent soft tissues which are repaired by the process of organisation (p.40), while the bone is repaired by regeneration.

Events following a fracture

(1) *Immediate effects*

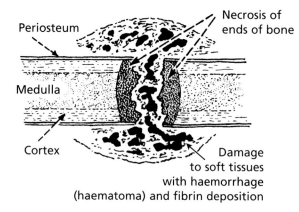

Periosteum

Necrosis of ends of bone

Medulla

Cortex

Damage to soft tissues with haemorrhage (haematoma) and fibrin deposition

(2) *Early reaction-inflammatory*
First 4–5 days

Phagocytosis of debris and necrotic tissues

Early organisation: capillaries and fibroblasts

(3) *Formation of callus*
(early bone regeneration) –
after 1 week.

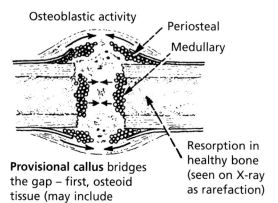

Osteoblastic activity

Periosteal

Medullary

Resorption in healthy bone (seen on X-ray as rarefaction)

Provisional callus bridges the gap – first, osteoid tissue (may include cartilage) then woven bone

(4) *Mature callus*
– from 3 weeks onwards

Cortical gap healed by ossification

Osteoblastic and osteoclastic activity proceeding

(5) *Remodelling of callus*
Definitive – weeks into months

Osteoblasts and osteoclasts active

Lamellar bone

(6) *Final reconstruction*
Months later

Fracture site may be almost invisible

HEALING – SPECIAL SITUATIONS

Events following a fracture *(continued)*

Complications

1. *Fat embolism* may occur in fracture of long bones due to entry of fat from the marrow cavity into the torn ends of veins.

2. *Infection*
   If the overlying skin is breached in any way, i.e. the fracture is 'compound', the risk of infection is greatly increased; this is an important adverse factor in the healing process. E.g.

By sharp bone ends

Penetrating injury from outside

PATHOLOGICAL FRACTURE

When the break occurs at the site of pre-existing disease of the bone, the term 'pathological fracture' is applied.

A common condition is a secondary tumour growing in and destroying the bone

Mixture of tumour and haematoma – healing inhibited

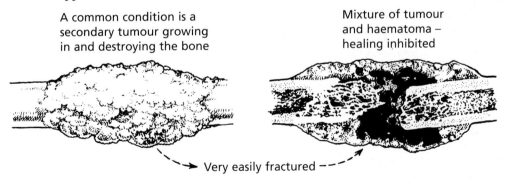

Very easily fractured

HEALING – SPECIAL SITUATIONS

FACTORS INFLUENCING HEALING OF FRACTURES

| | ADVERSE | FAVOURABLE |

1. Local factors

(a) *Infection* ⎱ See previous
(b) *Pathological fracture* ⎰ page

(c) *Poor apposition and alignment* . . . . *Good apposition*

— There may be interposition
of soft tissue, e.g. muscle

— Large irregular callus:
slow repair, permanent deformity of bone

Small callus,
quick repair

(d) *Continuing movement of bone ends* . . . . *Good immobilisation*

Callus formation
inhibited

Fibrous union

Small callus, good
bone formation

In extreme cases, a rudimentary joint
(pseudoarthrosis)
may form

(e) *Poor blood supply* . . . . *Good blood supply*

This is largely influenced by the anatomical site
of the fracture, for example:
(a) Nutrient artery entering remote from the
 fracture or damaged by fracture
 (e.g. scaphoid, femoral head)
(b) Fracture through area devoid of periosteum
 (e.g. neck of femur)
(c) Minimal adjacent soft tissue (e.g. tibia).

In favourable conditions
blood supply is derived
from:
(a) periosteal arteries
(b) nutrient artery
(c) adjacent soft tissues.

2. General factors

(a) *Old age* . . . . *Youth*
(b) *Poor nutrition* – e.g. famine conditions, ... *Good nutrition* – especially
 malabsorption lead to lack of
 protein, calcium, vit D and vit C.
 protein, calcium, vit D and vit C.

INFECTION

INFECTION

There are very many infections: the chapter will deal only with principles and a few examples.

Type of Infecting Agent	Example	Example of Disease
BACTERIA (a very wide range)	STAPHYLOCOCCUS	ABSCESS
VIRUSES (a wide range)	HERPES ZOSTER	CHICKENPOX and SHINGLES
FUNGI (a limited range)	CANDIDA	BUCCAL and VAGINAL THRUSH
PROTOZOA	PLASMODIUM	MALARIA
Infestation with PARASITES WORMS and FLUKES	ECHINOCOCCUS GRANULOSIS	HYDATID DISEASE

COLONISATION AND COMMENSAL GROWTH

Vast number of bacteria normally colonise the external body surfaces (skin, alimentary and upper respiratory tracts). These **commensal** inhabitants usually do not harm the host. Organisms that injure the host are said to be **pathogenic**. If the host defences are damaged a commensal organism may cause an **opportunistic infection**.

INFECTION AND INFECTIOUS DISEASE

INFECTION occurs when microorganisms invade the sterile internal body tissues. (Multiplication usually follows invasion.)

An INFECTIOUS DISEASE occurs when infection is associated with clinically manifest tissue damage.

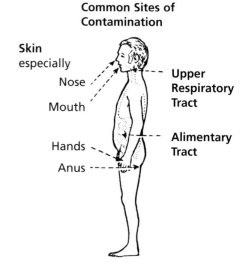

Common Sites of Contamination

Skin especially

Nose

Mouth

Hands

Anus

Upper Respiratory Tract

Alimentary Tract

Routes of entry of infecting organisms

1. Through the *skin* or *mucous membranes*
   (a) By direct close contact, e.g. venereal disease, HIV.
   (b) By contamination of abrasions and wounds, e.g. wound infections, rabies.
   (c) By inoculation, e.g. insect bite – yellow fever, syringe – hepatitis B and C, AIDS.

2. By *ingestion*
   Contaminated food and water, e.g. enteric fever, hepatitis A, poliomyelitis, cholera.

3. By *inhalation*
   Dust and droplets, e.g. influenza: tuberculosis.

INFECTION

Factors influencing the establishment of infection

1. In the HOST

In addition to a good state of general health and nutrition, the following mechanisms operate in preventing and limiting infection.

Physical barriers
e.g. (a) **SKIN**

Cornified squamous epithelium

(b) **FILTRATION** by nostril hairs

Secretions
Washing action by

(a) **TEARS**

(b) **URINE**

(c) **MUCIN** (aided by ciliary action in respiratory tract)

Fluid layer
Cilia

Chemical action
(1) Acid secretion in stomach and urinary tract.
(2) Lysozymes – enzymes capable of dissolving bacterial capsules, e.g. in tears and saliva.
(3) Immunoglobulin A (IgA) – a specialised immunoglobulin (see p.97), – tears, intestinal secretions.
(4) Non-specific inhibitory substances – urine, sweat, sebum.

2. In the MICRO-ORGANISM

Factors potentiating invasive capacity include:

(1) **Quantity of dose** – the larger the dose the more likely that the defences are penetrated.
(2) **Virulence** – describes the degree of pathogenicity, includes:
    (a) Capacity to resist phagocytosis and enzyme attack,
    (b) Adhesive properties,
    (c) Production of exoenzymes which act on host tissues, e.g. hyaluronidase (streptococci), coagulase (staphylococci) and of toxins, e.g. leucocidins, enterotoxins.

INFECTION

Factors influencing the course of infection

Once infection has occurred, important defence mechanisms operate:

1. **Inflammation** in the **acute** local reaction (see p.33) tends to limit the spread of organisms. In some important diseases, there is no acute local inflammatory response at the site of entry, e.g. Brucellosis (undulant fever) and many virus infections. In the **chronic** inflammatory reaction (see p.41), the formation of fibrous tissue also helps to localise infection.
2. **Phagocytosis** (see p.36) *Note:* some organisms may survive or multiply within phagocytes – usually associated with chronic infection. Good examples are tuberculosis, brucellosis, leprosy.
3. **The Immune Response**
    (a) *Humoral antibody* reactions e.g. agglutination, opsonisation, lysis via complement – especially important in *bacterial* infections.
    (b) *Cell-mediated* reactions, e.g. cytotoxic T cells, especially important in viral infections.
4. **Cytokines** – glycoproteins that regulate the immune response to pathogens.

Examples of failure of protective and defence mechanisms

1. **In skin** – direct breach by wounding and burns; softening of the surface by exposure to water and sweat or due to skin disorders.
2. **In the respiratory tract** – inhibition of ciliary movement by nicotine in smokers potentiates infection.
3. **In the stomach** – in achlorhydria (no hydrochloric acid) organisms flourish in the stomach.
4. **When secretions are prevented from flowing freely** by narrowing of natural passages, bacterial growth in the 'stagnant' fluid is potentiated (e.g. enlarged prostate urethral obstruction, urinary infection).
5. **When commensal growth is impaired** by antibiotic treatment, pathogenic bacteria may colonise the 'vacant site'.
6. **Deficiency of the immunological system:**
    (a) natural deficiency due to hereditary defect, e.g. X-linked agammaglobulinaemia
    (b) acquired due to administration of drugs in treatment of disease, e.g. steroids, cytotoxic drugs; specific virus infection, e.g. Human Immunodeficiency Virus (HIV) causing Acquired Immune Deficiency Syndrome (AIDS).
7. **Deficiency of phagocytosis** – especially polymorphs (either low numbers or deficient function – see page 36).
8. **In debilitating diseases** such as diabetes, chronic failure and nutritional deficiency.
9. **Genetic susceptibility** – may be a factor in some infections.

INFECTION

Mechanisms by which disease is produced

The local reaction to infections is usually INFLAMMATORY and is evoked by cellular damage and death. The detailed mechanisms are different in bacteria and viruses.

BACTERIA

1. Production of toxins (poisons)

Exotoxins	Endotoxins
Secreted by living bacteria	Integral part of bactrial cell wall Release on death of organism (usually Gram-negative)
Simple proteins	Lipid-polysaccharide complexes
Neutralised by specific antibody (antitoxin)	Do not stimulate antitoxin production
Often have specific enzyme activity and may act on specific organs or tissues	Cause fever and ENDOTOXIC SHOCK. Act by damaging capillaries and disturbing the coagulation system as well as causing necrosis. Activate fibrinolytic and complement cascades: facilitate release of chemical mediators of acute inflammation.

2. Hypersensitivity reaction causing tissue injury

This is a form of the immune response in which reaction between the bacterial protein and sensitised lymphocytes initiates the inflammatory reaction (see p.101).

3. Tissue invasion: lymphatic spread and invasion of blood stream

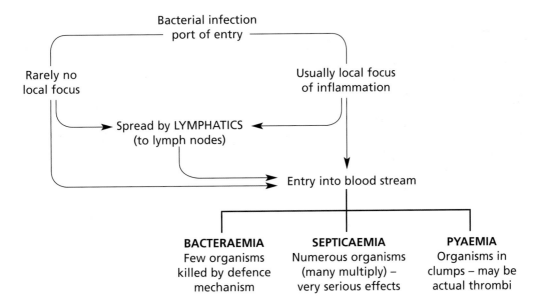

65

INFECTION

BACTERAEMIA
(a) Occurs commonly: usually of no serious significance

(b) An integral part of some infections, e.g. typhoid fever.

Important special cases

(1) *Dental extraction*

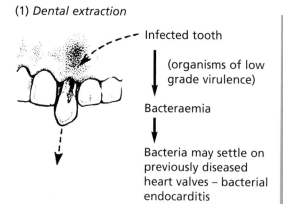

Infected tooth

(organisms of low grade virulence)

Bacteraemia

Bacteria may settle on previously diseased heart valves – bacterial endocarditis

(2) *Established bacterial endocarditis*

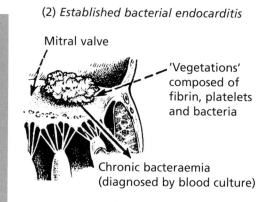

Mitral valve

'Vegetations' composed of fibrin, platelets and bacteria

Chronic bacteraemia (diagnosed by blood culture)

SEPTICAEMIA
Septicaemia is a very serious condition with severe toxaemia and shock. It may:

(a) be primary – usually caused by virulent organisms e.g. *Neisseria meningitides, Streptococcus pyogenes*

(b) complicate the shock syndrome initiated by other causes – especially when the alimentary tract is involved (coliform organisms)

(c) occur during medical treatment when immune mechanisms are disturbed (see opportunistic infections, p.84).

In septicaemia, unless antibiotic treatment is available, the infection is rapidly overwhelming and, at post-mortem, specific damage is difficult to detect. There may be massive adrenal haemorrhage and evidence of disseminated intravascular coagulation (see p.419).

PYAEMIA
Pyaemia is a serious condition with severe toxaemia – the organisms escape into the blood stream in the form of small aggregates – micro-emboli. This results in either (a) PYAEMIC ABSCESSES or (b) SEPTIC INFARCTION.

INFECTION

PYAEMIC ABSCESS

Septic focus – usually staphylococcal

↓

Thrombosis of venules incorporating bacteria

↓

Showers of very small (micro-) emboli

↓

Multiple, very small abscesses in various organs

Especially:

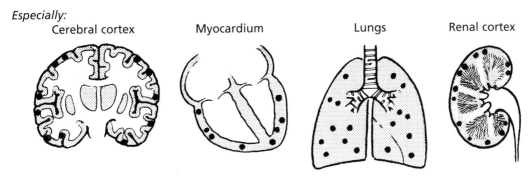

| Cerebral cortex | Myocardium | Lungs | Renal cortex |

SEPTIC INFARCTION

The lesions are larger and less numerous than pyaemic abscesses.

They are associated with:

(a) Septic thrombosis of larger veins (suppurative thrombophlebitis)

(b) Acute infective endocarditis

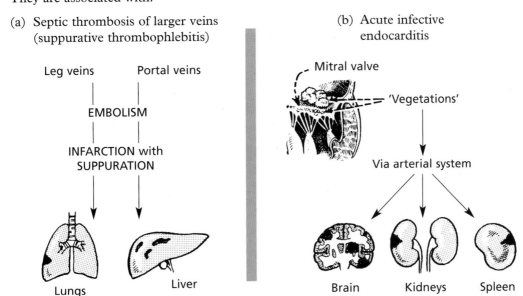

Leg veins   Portal veins

|

EMBOLISM

|

INFARCTION with SUPPURATION

Lungs   Liver

Mitral valve

'Vegetations'

Via arterial system

Brain   Kidneys   Spleen

ACUTE BACTERIAL INFECTION

PYOGENIC BACTERIA

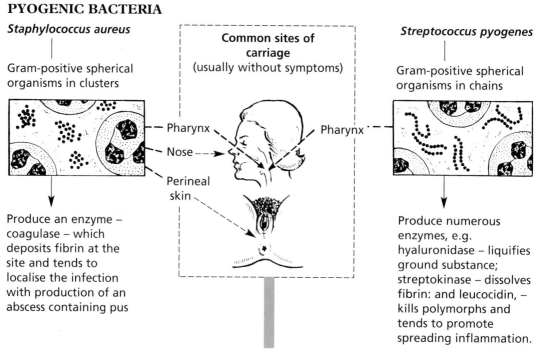

Staphylococcus aureus

Gram-positive spherical organisms in clusters

Common sites of carriage
(usually without symptoms)

Pharynx

Nose

Perineal skin

Streptococcus pyogenes

Gram-positive spherical organisms in chains

Produce an enzyme – coagulase – which deposits fibrin at the site and tends to localise the infection with production of an abscess containing pus

Pharynx

Produce numerous enzymes, e.g. hyaluronidase – liquifies ground substance; streptokinase – dissolves fibrin: and leucocidin, – kills polymorphs and tends to promote spreading inflammation.

Note: In hospitals staphylococci are becoming increasingly resistant to multiple antibiotics (MRSA = methicillin resistant staphylococcus aureus).

Lesions produced

Skin infections – pustules, oils, carbuncles
Wound infection
Staphylococcal broncho-pneumonia may be a serious complication in epidemic influenza
Exotoxin production → food poisoning: toxic shock syndrome.

Skin infections – impetigo, erysipelas, cellulitis
Wound infection
TONSILLITIS and pharyngitis
Exotoxin production
↓
The skin rash of scarlet fever

GENERAL BLOOD SPREAD

PYAEMIA (and septicaemia)
OSTEOMYELITIS – acute inflammation of long bones – particularly in children

SEPTICAEMIA

Note: Rheumatic fever and acute glomerulonephritis are complications of streptococcal infection in which the heart and kidneys are damaged. This is caused by disturbance in the immune mechanisms and is not due to the actual presence of streptococci in the heart and kidneys.

ACUTE BACTERIAL INFECTION

PYOGENIC BACTERIA *(continued)*

NEISSERIA

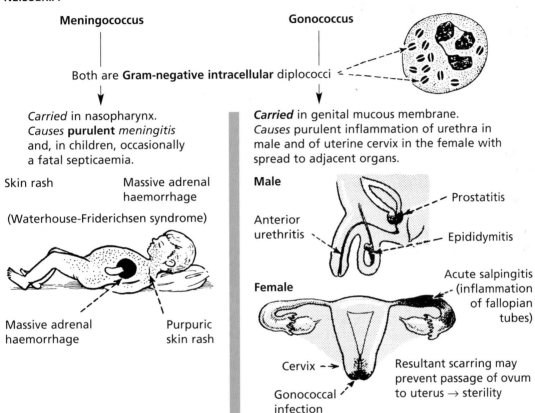

Meningococcus   **Gonococcus**

Both are **Gram-negative intracellular** diplococci

Carried in nasopharynx.
Causes **purulent** *meningitis*
and, in children, occasionally
a fatal septicaemia.

Skin rash   Massive adrenal
                 haemorrhage

(Waterhouse-Friderichsen syndrome)

Massive adrenal
haemorrhage   Purpuric
           skin rash

Carried in genital mucous membrane.
Causes purulent inflammation of urethra in
male and of uterine cervix in the female with
spread to adjacent organs.

Male

Prostatitis

Anterior
urethritis

Epididymitis

Female

Acute salpingitis
(inflammation
of fallopian
tubes)

Cervix

Gonococcal
infection

Resultant scarring may
prevent passage of ovum
to uterus → sterility

Gram-negative bacilli

These are usually commensals in the alimentary tract
and include facultative and obligatory anaerobes.

'Coliform' organisms can cause local
inflammation in the alimentary tract,
the urinary tract and wound infections.

In addition, ENDOTOXINS liberated in the blood
stream cause severe SHOCK (p.172).

FOOD POISONING

E. Coli 0157 – a commensal in cattle is a
human pathogen – production of a powerful
virocytotoxin is associated with the **haemolytic
uraemic syndrome** (see p.480) and may cause
death in the very young and elderly.

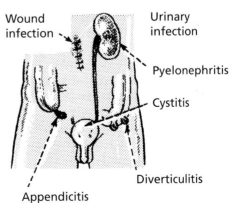

Wound
infection

Urinary
infection

Pyelonephritis

Cystitis

Diverticulitis

Appendicitis

ACUTE BACTERIAL INFECTION

GANGRENE
Gangrene is a form of NECROSIS in which a special type of bacterial activity is superimposed.

The bacteria proliferate in and digest the dead tissues often with the production of gases.

There are two main types: PRIMARY and SECONDARY.

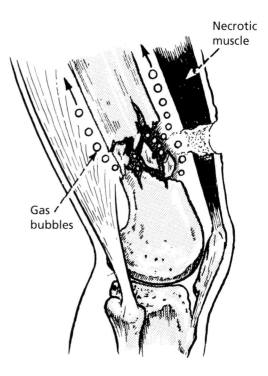

Necrotic muscle

Gas bubbles

Primary (gas gangrene)
This occurs occasionally in civilian practice but is a serious complication of war wounds. It is due to infection of deep contaminated wounds by bacteria of the CLOSTRIDIA group – ANAEROBIC sporulating Gram-positive bacilli (the commonest organism is *Cl. perfringens*). The anaerobic conditions and the presence of necrotic tissue favour the multiplication of these anaerobes with the formation of GAS BUBBLES and further spreading necrosis. Spread is rapid and there is associated TOXAEMIA.

Secondary
This is due to invasion of necrotic tissue usually by a mixed bacterial flora including putrefactive organisms. It occurs in two forms: WET and DRY.

Wet gangrene. The tissues are moist at the start of the process either due to oedema or venous congestion. Examples are in strangulation of viscera and occlusion of leg arteries in obese diabetic patients.

Dry gangrene. Occurs especially in the toes and feet of elderly people suffering from gradual arterial occlusion. The putrefactive process is very slow and only small numbers of putrefactive organisms are present.

ACUTE BACTERIAL INFECTION

TETANUS

This is a toxigenic disease – the organism itself does not cause local tissue damage. The effects are due to a powerful ENDOTOXIN secreted by the organism. This is in contrast to the usual bacterial diseases where tissue damage is important and is due to the local bacterial action.

The infecting organism, *Clostridium tetani*, a STRICT ANAEROBE, is a Gram-positive rod. Often the presence of a terminal spore gives a characteristic drum-stick appearance. The highly resistant spores are widespread in the environment due to contamination by animal faeces.

Method of Infection

Contamination of wounds in which there are anaerobic conditions, e.g. deep-penetrating wounds and wounds with severe soft tissue damage (road traffic accidents and battle casualties); only very occasionally trivial thorn punctures.

In developing communities the umbilical stump of the newborn may be infected by faecal material.

Effects:

The exotoxin is highly potent and causes paroxysmal muscular spasm which becomes progressively more severe and was fatal in many cases: modern therapy including muscle relaxation and ventilation has improved the prognosis dramatically.

Course

Immunity

- Active immunisation by **TOXOID** — prophylactic.
- Passive immunisation by **ANTITOXIN** — therapeutic (only effective before toxin is fixed to nerve tissues).

Other important bacteria producing toxins are: *Clostridium botulinum* (botulism), *Vibrio cholerae* (cholera), *Corynebacterium diphtheriae* (diphtheria).

CHRONIC BACTERIAL INFECTION (GRANULOMAS)

In these infections chronic inflammation is the basic mechanism (see p.42). The detailed evolution of the inflammatory reaction is modified by several factors of which the immune response of the host is important (see p.89).

TUBERCULOSIS

Tuberculosis is caused by the *Mycobacterium tuberculosis* (tubercle bacillus: TB), an organism which has a resistant waxy component in its structure and is acid and alcohol-fast (i.e. resists bleaching with strong acid and alcohol after being stained red with fuchsin). The disease rapidly declined in Western Europe and North America after World War II due to (a) improved nutrition and hygiene, (b) BCG immunisation and (c) chemotherapy (*note:* drug resistance is becoming an increasing problem). Patients with AIDS are at particular risk: other 'at risk' groups are the elderly, the immunosuppressed and alcoholics. The disease remains prevalent in developing countries.

The tuberculous follicle (tubercle)

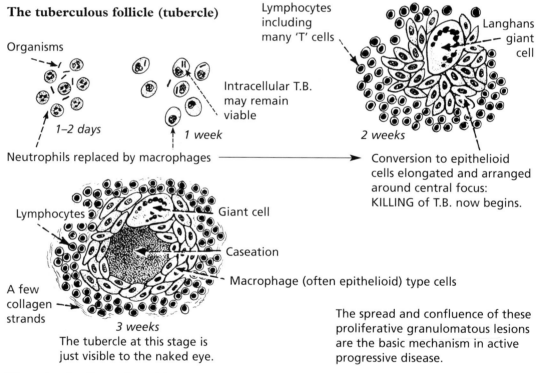

The role of **cell-mediated immunity** (see p.92) in combating infection is well seen in the evolution of the tuberculous follicle.

The caseation is the result of the combined effects of (a) the Type IV hypersensitivity reaction, (b) bacterial activity and (c) ischaemia.

CHRONIC BACTERIAL INFECTION (GRANULOMAS)

TUBERCULOSIS *(continued)*

Primary infection

Usually seen in non-immune children in first contact with tuberculosis. A few bacilli infect the PRIMARY SITE – usually at the periphery of the lung but also occasionally in the pharynx (tonsil) or small intestine.

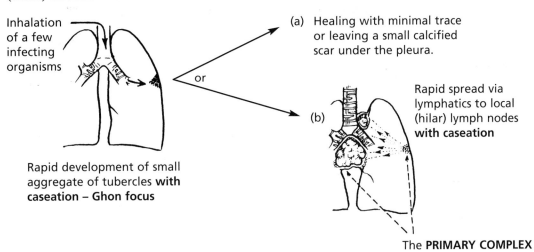

Inhalation of a few infecting organisms

Rapid development of small aggregate of tubercles **with caseation – Ghon focus**

or

(a) Healing with minimal trace or leaving a small calcified scar under the pleura.

(b) Rapid spread via lymphatics to local (hilar) lymph nodes **with caseation**

The **PRIMARY COMPLEX**

Healing can occur at this stage, leaving calcified lymph nodes, or occasionally the disease spreads via blood stream (a) generally or (b) to individual organs.

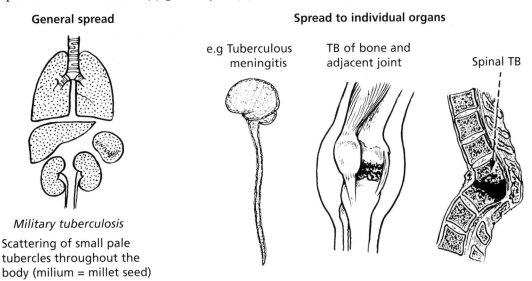

General spread

Spread to individual organs

e.g Tuberculous meningitis

TB of bone and adjacent joint

Spinal TB

Military tuberculosis

Scattering of small pale tubercles throughout the body (milium = millet seed)

CHRONIC BACTERIAL INFECTION (GRANULOMAS)

TUBERCULOSIS *(continued)*

Re-infection tuberculosis
This occurs in older children and adults who have had a primary infection or have received BCG vaccination by which a variable degree of immunity to the tubercle bacillus has been established.

The usual site of reinfection is the lung apex

Gradually progressive disease destroying lung tissue: CAVITATION is common.

The evolution of the disease is much slower than in the primary infection and fibrosis tends to limit the spread, but in untreated cases gradual extension with destruction and scarring of tissues is usual.

If the individual's immunity is impaired for any reason, the disease may spread locally more rapidly with increased caseation or in the miliary form.

Note: In apparently well-healed tuberculosis, the tubercle bacilli can survive for many years in scarred and calcified tissues and are able to re-establish active disease – REACTIVATION of tuberculosis. This is the commonest form in Western countries, occurring in late middle and old age among people who were originally infected when tuberculosis was common.

Variations in the basic mechanism
1. *Exudative* inflammation occurs particularly in serous cavities.

e.g. Pleurisy with effusion

Ascites in abdominal tuberculosis – with adherence of viscera

2. *Cold abscess* – where caseation is marked, the tuberculous pus may track to a surface as a 'cold' abscess and sinus.

3. *Fibrotic tuberculosis* – in this condition the body's reparative mechanism is dominant but not sufficient to ensure complete healing; a slow progressive fibrosis with scarring results. This is seen particularly in lung infections.

4. *Acute caseating 'non-reactive' tuberculosis* is seen when the individual's immunity is seriously impaired; massive caseation with little cellular reaction occurs: macrophages are packed with viable tubercle bacilli.

OTHER MYCOBACTERIAL INFECTIONS
These are of lower pathogenicity than *M.tuberculosis*. *M.avium* and *M.intracellulare* are closely related and are often grouped together *M.avium-intracellulare* (MAI). They may cause pneumonia, lymphadenitis or disseminated disease in immunosuppressed patients.

Other mycobacteria cause skin infections. For example *M.marinum* may cause skin sores in aquarium enthusiasts.

CHRONIC BACTERIAL INFECTION (GRANULOMAS)

ACTINOMYCOSIS

Actinomycosis is a localised but gradually spreading chronic suppuration affecting the lower jaw particularly, the ileocaecal region of the bowel and occasionally the lung.

The organism – *Actinomyces israelii* – widespread in nature, is a Gram-positive, branching, filamentous anaerobe found around the teeth and in the pharyngeal crypts. In the tissues, it forms yellow, densely felted together spherical colonies just visible to the naked eye: the pus is seen to contain 'sulphur granules'.

Sites of infection

Ileocaecal region

Jaw

Tubo-ovarian abscess is strongly associated with the presence of an intra-uterine contraceptive device.

Abscess formation

Sulphur granules

The essential lesion, progressively destructive, is a loculated abscess containing

Neutrophils

Macrophages

Fibrous tissue

Sinuses to the exterior or to internal adjacent surfaces develop

Occasional spread by the blood stream starts abscesses in remote sites

LEPROSY

This slowly progressive disease which causes serious effects by damage to peripheral nerves is still widespread in the tropics and subtropics. The infection is acquired by close, prolonged contact and is due to *Mycobacterium leprae*, a slender acid and alcohol-fast bacillus. The disease presents in two contrasting extreme forms and with cases of intermediate type.

1. Lepromatous leprosy	2. Tuberculoid leprosy
Disfiguring nodularity of the skin – 'leonine facies'. Peripheral nerves affected late. The lesions contain lymphocytes, plasma cells and macrophages – filled with organisms Organisms + + + in tissues.	Focal areas of skin pallor and anaesthesia due to early involvement of nerves. Basic lesion is a follicular granuloma (tubercle) not unlike the true tubercle follicle. Organisms are scanty.

These differences are due in the main to differences in the immune reaction of the host.

Cell-mediated immunity is markedly diminished.	Cell-mediated immunity is well developed.

CHRONIC BACTERIAL INFECTION (GRANULOMAS)

SYPHILIS

Syphilis is a venereal infection; the usual sites of entry of the infection are the penis and the vulva or vagina. Extra-genital infection also occurs.

The organism is a spirochaete (*Treponema pallidum*) with a close set, regular spiral, demonstrated by dark ground illumination, silver staining or immuno-fluorescence. Although it very rapidly dies outside the body it has a highly invasive capacity on contact with mucous membranes.

10μ

PRIMARY SYPHILIS

During the first three weeks after infection, the spirochaetes spread in the blood throughout the body without any noticeable effects. Then the primary lesion – hard chancre – appears at the original site of entry.

Hard chancre –
a painless raised
button-like
nodule

Tightly packed
lymphocytes and
plasma cells

Peri- and
endarteritis

Diagnosis is by examination under dark ground illumination of serum taken from ulcer.

Note: No neutrophils: this is not an abscess. There is minimal tissue destruction and healing occurs without scarring.

The INGUINAL LYMPH NODES present clinically as painless, firm swellings due to proliferation of lymphocytes and plasma cells.

SECONDARY SYPHILIS

During the next 2 or 3 months, the spread of the organisms throughout the body causes secondary stage effects. These are a widespread rash (pox) of varying appearance, ulceration of mucous membranes, generalised lymphadenopathy, damage to various individual organs and tissues. There are constitutional effects – particularly fever and anaemia.

The essential pathology is the presence of very numerous spirochaetes accompanied by focal infiltration of lymphocytes, plasma cells and macrophages with mild arteritis. Infectivity is very high. Tissue destruction is minimal and healing occurs without scarring. A latent stage of long duration is followed in 35% of cases by tertiary syphilis.

TERTIARY (Late) SYPHILIS

The lesions, which may occur at any time for many years after the healing of the secondary phase, offer striking contrasts. This stage is characterised mainly by local destructive lesions, the result of cell-mediated immune reactions (T cells) causing necrosis of tissue. The main forms are:

1. **Gumma**, 2. **Syphilitic Aortitis** and 3. **Neurological Syphilis** (see p.77).

CHRONIC BACTERIAL INFECTION (GRANULOMAS)

TERTIARY SYPHILIS *(continued)*

1. **Gumma**
   This is a localised area of necrosis which may affect large parts of any organ or tissue but particularly bones, testis and liver.

2. **Syphilitic Aortitis**
   The arch and thoracic aorta is damaged with weakening of the media: this leads to ANEURYSM formation (see p.231) which causes serious local pressure effects and may also rupture with severe haemorrhage.

3. **Neurological Syphilis**
   (a) **Meningovascular** – mainly affects the meningeal blood vessels and causes neurological impairment secondarily.

   (b) **Parenchymatous** –

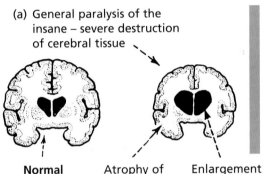

(a) General paralysis of the insane – severe destruction of cerebral tissue

Normal   Atrophy of convolutions   Enlargement of ventricles

(b) Tabes dorsalis – the damage specifically affecting the posterior roots and columns of spinal cord – is associated with characteristic clinical symptoms due to loss of proprioceptive sensation in the legs

CONGENITAL SYPHILIS

Transplacental infection of the fetus occurs with the following possible consequences:

(a) abortion or stillbirth – many organs damaged
(b) birth of marasmic infant – organ and tissue damage at birth and in later childhood.

DIAGNOSIS OF SYPHILIS

1. Demonstration of organisms
   In primary syphilis and early secondary syphilis organisms may be detected in smears from lesions by dark-ground microscopy

2. Serological tests
   a. *Screening tests*
   Antibodies of uncertain origin that bind to a phospholipid (cardiolipin): these are detected in Wasserman and VDRL (Venereal Diseases Reference Laboratory) tests.
   b. *Specific diagnostic tests*
   Specific anti-treponemal antibodies: these are detected in Treponema immobilisation, haemagglutination and fluorescent antibody tests.

VIRUS INFECTIONS

VIRUS INFECTIONS

Viruses are obligate intracellular pathogens that can replicate only by utilising the resources of the infected cell. The virus particle, or *virion*, consists of a central core of genetic material, either RNA or DNA, surrounded by a protein coat (*capsid*). In addition there may be a membranous *envelope* containing host and viral lipids.

The diagram shows DNA virus using the host cell for replication: at the same time causing cell death.

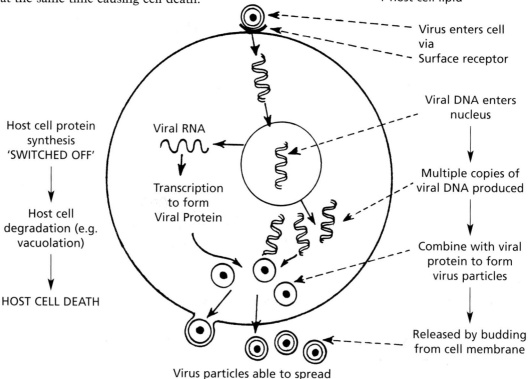

Central core DNA or RNA

Capsid
– virus protein
+ host cell lipid

Envelope

Virus enters cell via
Surface receptor

Viral DNA enters nucleus

Multiple copies of viral DNA produced

Combine with viral protein to form virus particles

Released by budding from cell membrane

Host cell protein synthesis 'SWITCHED OFF'

Host cell degradation (e.g. vacuolation)

HOST CELL DEATH

Viral RNA

Transcription to form Viral Protein

Virus particles able to spread and infect new cells

In addition to this direct cytopathic effect of the virus, damage to host may also be caused by:
(i) Side effects of the immune response,
(ii) Incorporation of virus into the cell genome severely affecting the intracellular metabolism.

RETROVIRUSES

An important variation occurs in a small group of RNA viruses. These contain an enzyme – **reverse transcriptase** – which, within the cell cytoplasm, is able (using the virus RNA as the template) to synthesise virus DNA which is then incorporated into the nuclear genetic material (note that messenger RNA is not required).

The virus DNA may remain there inactive for long periods. When activity is resumed, replication and cytopathic changes are effected as indicated in the diagram.

Retroviruses are important agents in carcinogenesis and AIDS (see p.105).

VIRUS INFECTIONS

ACUTE VIRUS INFECTION

The evolution of a typical acute virus infection can be understood in terms of virus replication, release and spread within the body, and of the host's reaction.

Typical evolution

Incubation period

Local lesion

Penetration of cells at site of infection
↓
Replication of VIRUS within
CELLS LOCALLY
↓
CELL DEATH
liberation of virus
↓
Virus spread to
LOCAL LYMPH NODES
↓
Further replication of virus
Cell death

Local symptoms.
The common cold,
Influenza,
Enteritis (due to
enterovirus)
illustrate diseases
of this type

- -

Overt disease

Primary viraemia

Liberation of virus into blood stream
↓
VIRUS spread by blood to
LYMPHOID TISSUES GENERALLY
↓
Further replication of virus

General malaise and
fever with lymph node
enlargement

↓
CELL DEATH
Liberation of virus into blood stream
↓

Secondary viraemia

Virus spread, GENERALLY
throughout the body with
effects seen particularly in
organs and tissues which
possess specific receptors
for particular viruses

Specific symptoms
referable to organ
or tissue damage,
e.g. poliomyelitis –
nerve cells, infective
hepatitis – liver cells,
small pox – skin cells.

This typical evolution is produced by successive waves of virus. However, the great majority of virus infections are clinically latent or mild because virus replication and spread are prevented by the body's defence mechanisms. Severe overt disease occurs when there is a specially virulent virus or when the body's resistance is inadequate, especially in a primary infection.

Not all virus infections cause disease in this way, 2 important variations are:

    (1) LATENT   (2) ONCOGENIC

VIRUS INFECTIONS

LATENT VIRUS INFECTION

A good example is the common 'cold sores' of the lips and face caused by the virus Herpes simplex (an enveloped DNA virus).

Initial infection   **Reactivation**

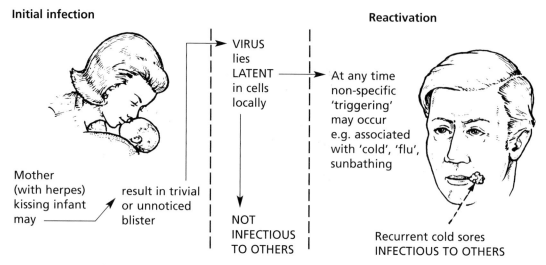

Mother (with herpes) kissing infant may —— result in trivial or unnoticed blister

VIRUS lies LATENT in cells locally

NOT INFECTIOUS TO OTHERS

At any time non-specific 'triggering' may occur e.g. associated with 'cold', 'flu', sunbathing

Recurrent cold sores INFECTIOUS TO OTHERS

Another example is **herpes zoster (shingles).**

This is a painful affection of segmental sensory nerves and root ganglia due to infection by CHICKEN POX VIRUS **Varicella.**

Initial infection in childhood

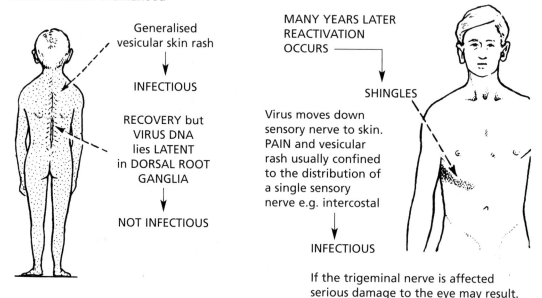

Generalised vesicular skin rash

↓

INFECTIOUS

RECOVERY but VIRUS DNA lies LATENT in DORSAL ROOT GANGLIA

↓

NOT INFECTIOUS

MANY YEARS LATER REACTIVATION OCCURS

SHINGLES

Virus moves down sensory nerve to skin. PAIN and vesicular rash usually confined to the distribution of a single sensory nerve e.g. intercostal

↓

INFECTIOUS

If the trigeminal nerve is affected serious damage to the eye may result.

VIRUS INFECTIONS

ONCOGENIC VIRUS INFECTION

Several DNA viruses and retroviruses of the RNA family can give rise to tumours (see also p.149).

Examples include the following:

(a) Human Papilloma Virus (HPV) – HPV-16 and 18, strains of the common wart virus, are implicated in the aetiology of cervical carcinoma.

(b) Hepatitis Virus – both hepatatis B and C viruses are firmly associated with hepatocellular carcinoma.

(c) Epstein-Barr Virus (EBV) – a member of the herpes group causes glandular fever (infectious mononucleosis – a non-malignant condition) in young adult in Western societies. This virus is also closely associated with Burkitt's lymphoma (a malignant tumour) found in young Africans living in malarial areas, nasopharyngeal carcinoma particularly in the Far East and with Hodgkin's disease.

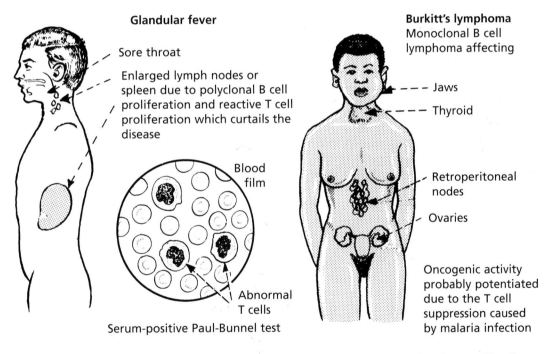

Glandular fever

Sore throat

Enlarged lymph nodes or spleen due to polyclonal B cell proliferation and reactive T cell proliferation which curtails the disease

Blood film

Abnormal T cells

Serum-positive Paul-Bunnel test

Burkitt's lymphoma
Monoclonal B cell lymphoma affecting

– – – Jaws

– – – Thyroid

Retroperitoneal nodes

Ovaries

Oncogenic activity probably potentiated due to the T cell suppression caused by malaria infection

(d) Retroviruses – T-cell leukaemias are caused by specific retroviruses i.e. human T cell Leukaemia-Lymphoma Virus (HTLV). HTLV-1 is endemic in Japan, the West Indies and central belts of Africa.

The mechanisms by which viruses cause tumours are illustrated on page 149.

HOST/VIRUS INTERACTION

The reactions occurring in the host are important.

1. **Changes in the infected cells**

(a) Cell degeneration
   (with loss of function)
   leading to cell death.

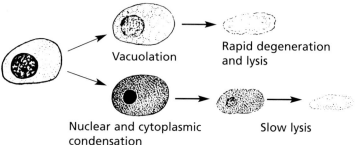

Vacuolation

Rapid degeneration
and lysis

Nuclear and cytoplasmic
condensation

Slow lysis

(b) Fusion of adjacent infected
   cells – giant cell formation,
   e.g. the Warthin-Finkeldy
   cell of measles

Lymphocytes

(c) Cell proliferation
   e.g. common wart
   of HPV infection.

Proliferation of skin
epithelial cells causing
a warty growth

(d) Formation of 'inclusion'
   bodies within cytoplasm
   or nucleus: they consist
   of aggregates of virus
   and/or products of cell
   degeneration.

Diagnostic eosinophilic
intracytoplasmic Negri
bodies in nerve cells of
the hippocampus in
RABIES

Nuclear and
cytoplasmic
inclusion in
cytomegalic virus
infection of
salivary ducts

(e) No apparent change in cell but virus remains latent – reactivation later with continuous
   and slow release associated with gradually progressive disease.

(f) No apparent change but later malignant proliferation occurs, i.e. oncogenic infection.

HOST/VIRUS INTERACTION

Reactions in host *(continued)*

2. **Interferon production** by the infected cells and specifically activated T lymphocytes. Interferons are a group of protein molecules – not antibodies. They represent the first and very important line of defence by interfering with the synthesis of viral protein and thus protect healthy cells.

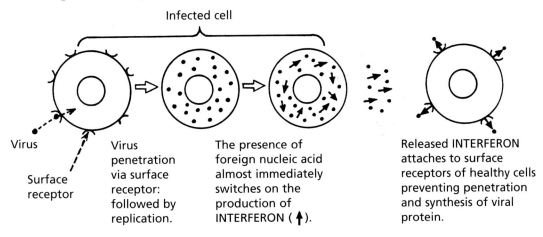

Infected cell

Virus

Surface
receptor

Virus
penetration
via surface
receptor:
followed by
replication.

The presence of
foreign nucleic acid
almost immediately
switches on the
production of
INTERFERON (↑).

Released INTERFERON
attaches to surface
receptors of healthy cells
preventing penetration
and synthesis of viral
protein.

3. **The immune response** (see p.89) begins 4–7 days after initial infection.
    (a) Antibodies to virus ⎱ limit initial infection but are very
    (b) Cell-mediated immunity ⎰ important in protecting against RE-INFECTION.
    (c) Occasionally virus antibody complexes cause special types of reaction in the host, e.g. inflammatory necrosis of arteries (arteritis), some forms of kidney damage, and the skin rashes of childhood viral infections.

4. **The inflammatory response**
    The vascular and exudative elements follow the usual pattern; **neutrophils** are **not** a feature unless there is considerable tissue necrosis or secondary bacterial infection. However, **macrophage** phagocytic activity is important in the defence against viral infection. There is often a relative **lymphocytosis**.

OPPORTUNISTIC INFECTIONS

This term is used for infections caused by organisms which are often nonpathogenic or of low grade virulence, occurring in individuals whose resistance to infection is impaired. They are occurring more frequently in modern medical practice because of the increasing use of powerful immunosuppressive drugs.

CAUSES OF LOWERED RESISTANCE

1. Congenital immunological deficiencies (rare).
2. Acquired
   (a) *the result of disease:* HIV infection (AIDS); uraemia; liver disease; malignant tumours, particularly Hodgkin's disease and leukaemias;
   (b) *the result of therapy:*
      e.g. immunosuppression in transplant surgery; immunosuppression – a side effect of tumour therapy; antibiotics – changing commensal populations;
   (c) *introduction of foreign material:* e.g. heart valve prostheses; I.V. long lines in intensive care; tracheostomy.

Examples of infecting organisms

Bacteria → *Acinetobacter* wound infections: septicaemia

Staph. epidermidis on heart valves; low grade septicaemia

Vegetations on artificial heart valve

Protozoa

Toxoplasma gondii reactivation of latent infection causes encephalitis (particularly in AIDS patients)

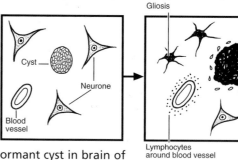

Dormant cyst in brain of immunocompromised patient

Reactivation in immuno-suppressed patient

Virus
Cytomegalovirus pneumonia

Fungi

Pneumocystis carinii: a severe pneumonia (seen in AIDS cases particularly)

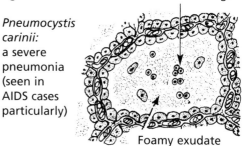

Clusters of organisms

Foamy exudate

INFECTION – GENERAL EFFECTS

The more general body reactions in infection are: FEVER and CHANGES IN METABOLISM.

FEVER (PYREXIA)
The body temperature rises above normal initially due partly to an imbalance between heat production and loss, but mainly due to a resetting at a higher level of the 'thermostat' mechanism in the hypothalamus. This results in:

1. Increased HEAT PRODUCTION due to INCREASED METABOLISM

2. Increased HEAT LOSS

Heat-sensitive nerve endings in skin

Muscle

Skin blood vessels dilate

Sweat glands secrete

WARM MOIST SKIN

In early stages, when the temperature is rising internally, there may be a paradoxical feeling of cold with shivering (rigor).

Thermostat set at higher level due to pyrogens derived from (a) infecting organisms or (b) endogenous, derived from macrophages (e.g. interleukin-1) and polymorphs: the change is mediated by prostaglandin-E.

These changes are associated with an INCREASED PULSE RATE and a tendency to DEHYDRATION.

Pyrexia also occurs when there is:

(a) Considerable tissue necrosis, e.g. infarction and tumours

(b) Cerebral disease – especially in the region of the pons.

(c) Heat-stroke – where the environmental temperature and humidity are high and there is excessive water and salt loss.

Hyperpyrexia [when the temperature exceeds 41°C (106°F)] is extremely dangerous because of damage to the nerve cells in the brain.

INFECTION – GENERAL EFFECTS

CHANGES in METABOLISM
Tissue breakdown is greatly increased, and in some infectious fevers there is a marked loss of body weight.

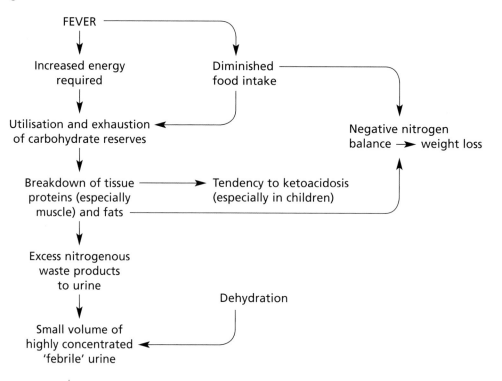

CHANGES in the BLOOD

(a) (i) **Neutrophil leukocytosis** – in acute bacterial infections.

(ii) **Lymphocytosis** – often in viral infections.

(iii) **Lymphopenia** – in typhoid fever and chronic debilitating infections.

(b) **Biochemical changes**

(i) **Non-specific** changes in plasma proteins → cause a rise in the **Erythrocyte Sedimentation Rate (ESR).**

(ii) Specific antibodies are present in both bacterial and viral infections (See next chapter).

(iii) Acute Phase Reactants – a group of serum proteins which rise in response to inflammation: examples are C-reactive protein (used in diagnosis): complement components: and serum amyloid A protein: in long-standing chronic inflammation AMYLOIDOSIS may be a complication (see p.24).

(iv) Other chemical changes are listed on page 36.

IMMUNITY

IMMUNITY

The immune system protects us from invading pathogenic microorganisms and cancer. Immunity – the state of protection from infectious disease – has both a less specific or INNATE and a more specific or ADAPTIVE component.

INNATE IMMUNITY

This provides the first line of defence against infection and is not specific to a particular pathogen. It consists of four types of defensive barriers, some of which have been mentioned previously.

INNATE IMMUNITY

PHYSICAL BARRIERS
e.g. skin, mucous membranes

INFLAMMATORY BARRIERS
e.g. leakage of fluid containing chemical mediators

CHEMICAL BARRIERS
e.g. lysozyme, complement, interferon, toll-like receptors – these are cell surface receptors with the property of pattern recognition, e.g. TLR2 recognizes LPS on Gram-negative bacteria

PHAGOCYTE BARRIERS e.g. neutrophils, macrophages

ADAPTIVE IMMUNITY

This provides a specific immune response directed at an invading pathogen. Following exposure to a foreign organism there is an initial EFFECTOR RESPONSE that eliminates or neutralizes a pathogen. Later re-exposure to the same foreign organism induces a MEMORY RESPONSE with a more rapid immune reaction that eliminates the pathogen and prevents disease.

It has been known from historical times that a person who has recovered from an infectious disease, e.g. smallpox, is most unlikely to suffer from it again – even when exposed maximally – although he would remain susceptible to other infections.

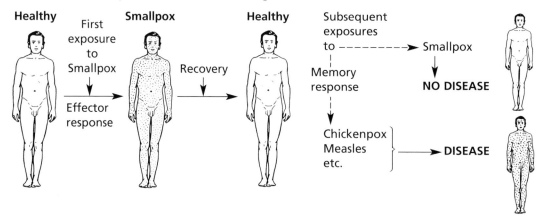

That is, during the recovery period he has ACQUIRED SPECIFIC IMMUNITY to smallpox but not to other unrelated infections.

Note: This immunity may extend to related infections: the use of the immunity against smallpox conferred by world-wide vaccination with cowpox (pioneered by Jenner in the 18th century) has completely eliminated smallpox throughout the world.

THE ADAPTIVE IMMUNE RESPONSE

The sequence of events in an infection is as follows:

Substances that can be recognised by the immunoglobulin receptor of B cells, or the T-cell receptor when complexed with MHC, are called ANTIGENS. Antigens are usually part of infectious agents such as bacteria and some viruses, but other substances foreign to the human body will stimulate an immune response. Most antigens are proteins but complex chemical substances such as some large carbohydrate molecules, lipoproteins and lipopolysaccharides will induce antibody formation. EPITOPES are the immunologically active regions of an antigen that bind to specific membrane receptors on lymphocytes or to secreted antibodies. B and T cells recognise different epitopes on the same antigenic molecule. B cells usually recognise soluble antigen (exogenous). Epitopes recognised by T cells are often internal peptides that are exposed by processing within antigen-presenting cells (endogenous).

CELLULAR BASIS OF THE IMMUNE RESPONSE

The process is essentially an activity of the small lymphocytes of which there are two main types. They are indistinguishable by light microscopy using conventional stains but can be separated by the presence of different surface proteins on T and B cells.

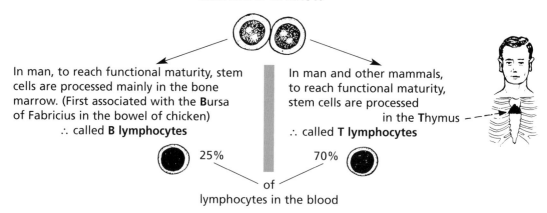

Stem cells in MARROW

In man, to reach functional maturity, stem cells are processed mainly in the bone marrow. (First associated with the **B**ursa of Fabricius in the bowel of chicken)
∴ called **B lymphocytes**

In man and other mammals, to reach functional maturity, stem cells are processed in the **T**hymus --
∴ called **T lymphocytes**

25%   70%

of lymphocytes in the blood

The introduction of an antigen results in activation and proliferation of these two lymphocyte populations. This activity takes place in the lymphoid tissues.

'Resting' B cell   **ANTIGENIC STIMULATION**   'Resting' T cell

In germinal centre (not in blood)

In paracortical area and blood

Antigen

Activation

Transformation

Blast cells

Enlargement

Blast cells

Division (Clonal proliferation)

Memory cells

Maturation

Memory cell

PLASMA CELLS
(i) Synthesis of specific antibody (Ig) within the cell

(ii) Cell surface Ig

(iii) Secretion of Ig into tissue fluids and blood

The end result of the B cell response is the formation of humoral antibodies or **HUMORAL IMMUNITY**
– protection against extracellular infection.

SPECIFICALLY SENSITISED LYMPHOCYTES
(i) Cytotoxic activity.
(ii) Production of messenger mediators (cytokines).

The end result of the T cell response is the formation of **CELL-MEDIATED IMMUNITY**
– protection against intracellular organisms e.g. viruses and some bacteria (e.g.T.B.).

GENETIC INFLUENCES ON THE IMMUNE RESPONSE

The MAJOR HISTOCOMPATIBILITY complex, also known as the human leucocyte antigen (HLA), has an important role in the IMMUNE RESPONSE and DISEASE.

The genes controlling the system are in 2 major groups (Class I and Class II) on CHROMOSOME 6: each group has 3 genes which are highly polymorphic (i.e. show great variation within individual members of the same animal species). The multiple alleles of each gene encode for surface membrane glycoproteins.

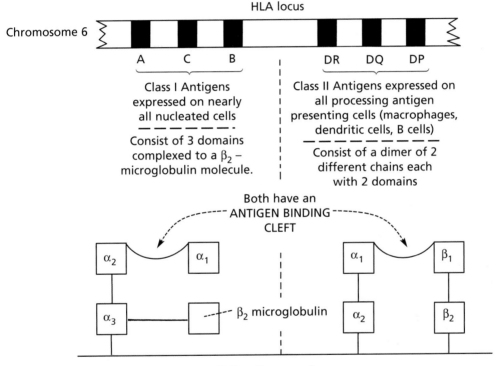

The important roles of HLA are:
(i)   Presentation of peptides from foreign antigens to T lymphocytes
          Class I antigens to cytotoxic T cells (normally CD8 +ve)
          Class II antigens to helper T cells (normally CD4 +ve).
(ii) They are the main stimulus to **graft rejection** in incompatible hosts. (The better the HLA match, the better the chance of graft survival.)
(iii) There is a strong association with diseases – especially **auto-immune** disorders (p.107).
      The most striking example is **ankylosing spondylitis** where >90% of patients carry the allele HLA B27.

CELL-MEDIATED IMMUNITY

Activation of T cells requires the involvement of ANTIGEN PRESENTING CELLS. Within these cells, foreign antigen is proteolytically digested to short peptides and then presented with HLA molecules to the T cell which possesses a specific receptor for that antigen.

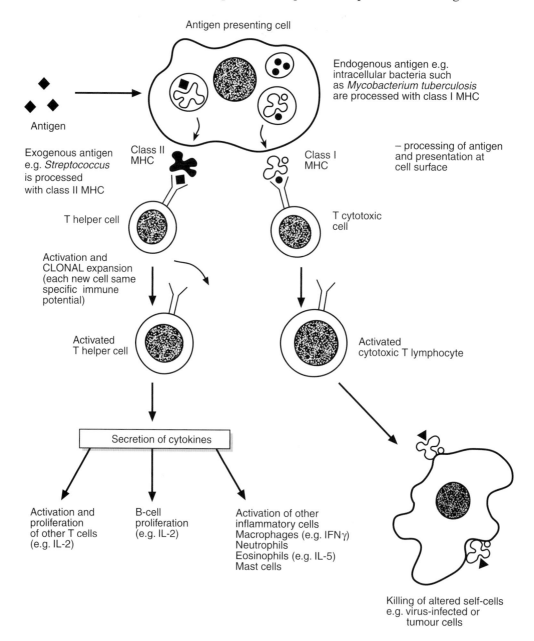

Antigen presenting cell

Endogenous antigen e.g. intracellular bacteria such as *Mycobacterium tuberculosis* are processed with class I MHC

Antigen

– processing of antigen and presentation at cell surface

Exogenous antigen e.g. *Streptococcus* is processed with class II MHC

Class II MHC

Class I MHC

T helper cell

T cytotoxic cell

Activation and CLONAL expansion (each new cell same specific immune potential)

Activated T helper cell

Activated cytotoxic T lymphocyte

Secretion of cytokines

Activation and proliferation of other T cells (e.g. IL-2)

B-cell proliferation (e.g. IL-2)

Activation of other inflammatory cells Macrophages (e.g. IFNγ) Neutrophils Eosinophils (e.g. IL-5) Mast cells

Killing of altered self-cells e.g. virus-infected or tumour cells

CYTOKINES

Cytokines are a group of small protein molecules that mediate the complex interactions between inflammatory cell, lymphoid cells and cells in the surrounding tissues.

CYTOKINES INVOLVED IN INNATE IMMUNITY

CYTOKINES INVOLVED IN ADAPTIVE IMMUNITY

The immune response to a particular pathogen must induce an appropriate set of effector functions that can eliminate the pathogen from the host. Differences in cytokine secretion patterns among T helper cells are determinants of the type of immune response made to a particular antigenic challenge. Accordingly the cytokine secreting T helper cells are divided into 2 subsets:

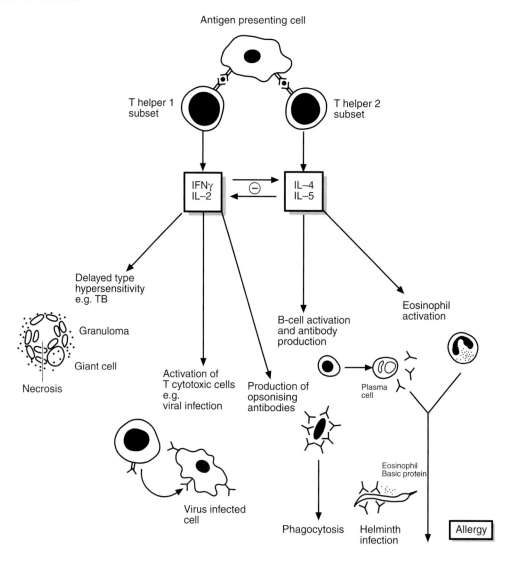

The balance between the two subsets determines disease outcome, e.g. tuberculoid leprosy is characterised by a TH1 response (destructive granulomas, few parasites). In lepromatous leprosy there is a TH2 response (disseminated disease, many parasites).

HUMORAL IMMUNITY

BASIC STRUCTURE OF IMMUNOGLOBULIN

The basic immunoglobulin is a protein molecule consisting of 2 identical LIGHT chains and two identical HEAVY chains. Each light chain is bound to a heavy chain by a disulphide bond. Similarly disulphide bridges link the two heavy and light chain combinations to form the basic four chain structure.

1 and 2 are heavy chains. Differences in structure allow separation of five main Ig classes – IgG; A; M; D; E. 3 and 4 are light chains. They exist in two forms – Kappa (κ) and Lambda (λ). In any one molecule both chains are either κ or λ.

Fc is the constant part of the molecule and does not participate in antigen binding. Secondary effects after antigen binding has occurred include:
  – complement activation
  – chemotaxis
  – opsonisation.

Fab are the variable parts of the molecule and are the site of antigen binding, the variation in amino acid content allowing a wide range of specific activity.

ANTIBODY MEDIATED EFFECTOR FUNCTIONS

(1) **Opsonisation**
   Fc receptors on macrophages and neutrophils can bind the Fc of Ig molecule resulting in phagocytosis of the antigen-antibody complex.

(2) **Complement Activation**
   IgM and IgG subclasses can activate the complement system

(3) **Antibody-Dependent Cell-Mediated Cytotoxicity (ADCC)**
   The linking of antibody bound to target cells (e.g. virus infected cells) with the Fc receptors of natural killer (NK) cells, enables the NK cell to recognise and kill the target cell.

(4) **Crossing of Epithelium (Transcytosis)**
   The delivery of antibody to the mucosal surfaces of the eyes, nose, mouth, bronchi and gut, as well as transport to breast milk, requires the movement of immunoglobulin across epithelium, a process called transcytosis.

(5) **Activation of Mast Cells, Eosinophils, Basophils**
   This is unique to IgE (see p.102)

IMMUNOGLOBULINS

ANTIBODY CLASSES AND ACTIVITIES

These groups are named according to the composition of the heavy chains.

IgM

IgM (heavy chain = μ) is a polymer, joined by J chains, of five identical Ig molecules, therefore called macroglobulin. Although in low concentration in the blood, 0.5–2 mg/ml, it is the main Ig on the surface of B lymphocytes (before conversion to plasma cells). It is the first immunoglobulin class produced and is active in the primary response. It neutralises viruses. In combination with complement, it is actively bactericidal and is especially effective in bacteraemia.

Note: The numerous (10) antigen-binding sites increase its efficiency.

The natural blood group antibodies, anti-A and anti-B are M globulins.

IgG

IgG (heavy chain = γ) is a single molecule with two antigen binding sites.

This is the most abundant class of immunoglobulin, with a concentration in blood of 8–16 mg/ml. There are 4 subclasses IgG1, IgG2, IgG3 and IgG4. Of its several activities the important ones are:

(1) Passive transfer of IgG (IgG1, IgG3, and IgG4) from mother to baby occurs via the placenta and colostrum. The immunity only lasts a few months.

Transplacental passage of IgG

Colostrum, rich in IgG, absorbed from alimentary tract into the blood stream of the neonate.

(2) Neutralisation of virus and toxins

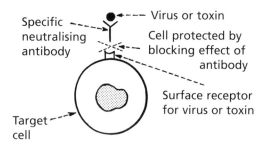

Specific neutralising antibody — Virus or toxin — Cell protected by blocking effect of antibody — Surface receptor for virus or toxin — Target cell

(3) Opsonisation (IgG1 and IgG3) See page 36

(4) Complement Activation (IgG3, IgG1 and IgG2) See page 99.

IMMUNOGLOBULINS

IgA

α   α

IgA (heavy chain = α) occurs in the blood (1.5–4 mg/ml) where its function is unknown.

It is the predominant immunoglobulin in secretions of eyes, nose, mouth, bronchi and gut. Its function is to protect mucous surfaces from antigenic attack and prevent access of foreign substances to the circulation and general immune system. It may neutralise toxins and prevent binding to mucous surfaces. IgA is a single molecule in the serum.

The diagram illustrates the local production of IgA in the gut.

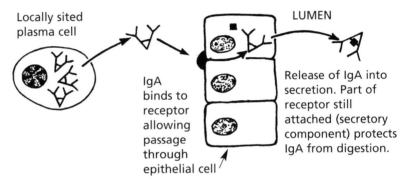

In secretions, the IgA molecule is a dimer of 2 identical molecules linked by a J (joining) chain.

Locally sited plasma cell

IgA binds to receptor allowing passage through epithelial cell

LUMEN

Release of IgA into secretion. Part of receptor still attached (secretory component) protects IgA from digestion.

IgD (heavy chain Δ) of uncertain function: concentration in blood very low. Like IgM it is present on the surface of B lymphocytes prior to transformation.

IgE (heavy chain ε) – a single molecule similar to IgG and IgA.
It is sometimes called REAGIN: concentration in blood is low (20–500 ng/ml). The serum level is raised in worm infestation and is probably protective. Its main activity is mediated by MAST CELLS (or BASOPHILS); it is the principal mediator of atopic and anaphylactic disease.

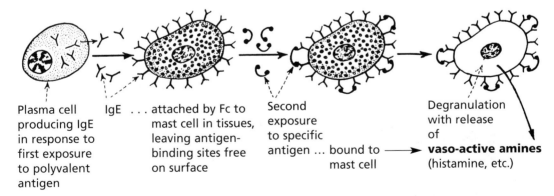

Plasma cell producing IgE in response to first exposure to polyvalent antigen

IgE ... attached by Fc to mast cell in tissues, leaving antigen-binding sites free on surface

Second exposure to specific antigen ... bound to → mast cell

Degranulation with release of **vaso-active amines** (histamine, etc.)

The range of antibodies is immense. B cells produce this vast number by rearranging the genes from the immunoglobulin light and heavy chains. The appropriate clone of plasma cells is stimulated by binding of antigen to the cell surface receptor (so-called clonal selection).

IMMUNE REACTIONS

ANTIGEN-ANTIBODY INTERACTIONS

When an antigen (Ag) binds with an antibody (Ab) an Ag/Ab complex is formed. This reaction is reversible in varying degrees and depends on the **affinity** of the antibody for an individual antigen and the **avidity** (strength when multiple epitopes on an antigen interact with multiple binding sites).

The consequences of Ag/Ab interaction include:

1. **PRECIPITATION**

A soluble antigen is rendered insoluble by aggregation of the Ag/Ab complexes into a lattice.

Antigen in solution + Antibody in solution

Aggregation leads to

PRECIPITATION

This reaction is the basis of immunoelectrophoresis, used e.g. to identify a monoclonal band in myeloma.

2. **AGGLUTINATION**

Particulate antigen, e.g. bacteria and red blood cells, are aggregated in the same way as in the precipitation reaction and the process is called AGGLUTINATION. Agglutination reactions are routinely performed to type red cells (ABO typing).

3. **CROSS-REACTIVITY**

In some cases antibody elicited by one antigen can cross-react with an unrelated antigen usually because they share a similar epitope.
e.g. Streptococcus pyogenes

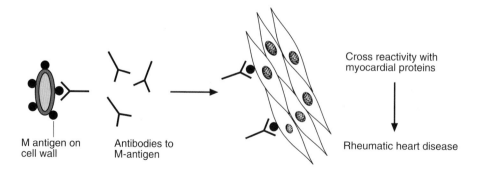

M antigen on cell wall

Antibodies to M-antigen

Cross reactivity with myocardial proteins

Rheumatic heart disease

IMMUNE REACTIONS

COMPLEMENT SYSTEM

Complement consists of nine main protein components present in inactive form in the blood. There are 3 pathways of complement activation. Activation results in the formation of multi-molecular enzymes that activate further components in a cascade ultimately generating a membrane attack complex that is capable of causing cell lysis.

The lectin and alternative pathways do not require antibody for activation and are therefore a component of the **innate** immune system.

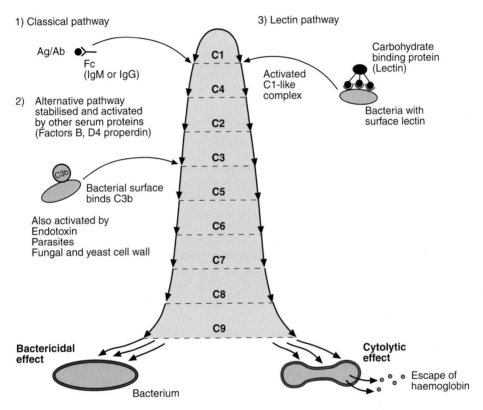

Activation of C by Ag/Ab complex is called **fixation of complement.** Using red cells as markers, this fixation can detect the presence of antigen or antibody in serum.

E.g. Test serum + antigen + C.
  If serum contains antibody, C is fixed, otherwise it remains free.
  Add sensitised RBC (coated with Ab).
  Lysis of RBC = complement still free ∴ no Ab in original serum.
  No lysis = C was fixed by Ab in test serum.

TOLERANCE

Humoral and cell-mediated immunity are specific active immune responses with a protective function.

In certain circumstances an antigen does not evoke these active responses. This is because the lymphocytes, although recognising the antigen, do not react – this is TOLERANCE.

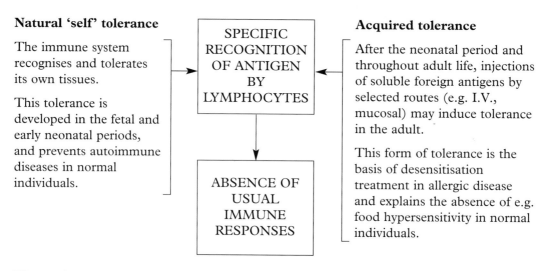

Natural 'self' tolerance

The immune system recognises and tolerates its own tissues.

This tolerance is developed in the fetal and early neonatal periods, and prevents autoimmune diseases in normal individuals.

SPECIFIC RECOGNITION OF ANTIGEN BY LYMPHOCYTES

ABSENCE OF USUAL IMMUNE RESPONSES

Acquired tolerance

After the neonatal period and throughout adult life, injections of soluble foreign antigens by selected routes (e.g. I.V., mucosal) may induce tolerance in the adult.

This form of tolerance is the basis of desensitisation treatment in allergic disease and explains the absence of e.g. food hypersensitivity in normal individuals.

The mechanisms of inducing tolerance are not yet completely understood: main candidates are:

(1) **Clonal deletion** – in fetal life all lymphoid cells which recognise 'self' antigens are permanently eliminated by apoptosis. This mainly affects T cells and occurs in the **thymus.**

(2) **Clonal anergy** – T and B cells which recognise 'self' antigens in the periphery during development are 'switched off' but remain present in the body. This occurs during development and in adult life.

(3) **Peripheral tolerance** – For activation of T cells two signals are required. The first is the interaction of antigen with the T cell receptor. The second signal is known as CO-STIMULATION. If this second signal is absent then tolerance is induced.

Tolerance is an important protective mechanism. When it breaks down, the serious effects give rise to **autoimmune disease** (see p.107).

IMMUNOPATHOLOGY

The complicated and delicately balanced immune mechanisms clearly have been developed to protect against antigens, particularly infections. When these immune reactions are upset, the protective mechanism can itself be a source of disease states.

There are three main categories: (1) hypersensitivity states, (2) immune deficiency states and (3) autoimmune diseases.

HYPERSENSITIVITY REACTIONS

Basically these consist of an inappropriate response by an individual to an antigen, following a previous exposure. Depending on the main type of immune response concerned, these are classified as follows:

(a) Those associated with
HUMORAL ANTIBODIES
∴ immediate – types I, II, III

(b) Those associated with
CELL-MEDIATED IMMUNITY
∴ delayed (24–72 hours) – type IV.

This classification is to some extent artificial. Hypersensitivity may start as an immediate humoral reaction but end in a mixed state with both humoral and cell-mediated activities.

Type 1 Anaphylaxis, atopy, allergy

This occurs within 20–60 minutes of exposure to antigen and is often referred to as 'immediate type hypersensitivity'.

All 3 terms have been used for this reaction. The basic mechanism is as follows.

First exposure to Ag → Formation of IgE (Y) → Fixation of IgE to MAST CELLS and basophils by Fc fragment

Second exposure to Ag (●) → Ag/Ab reaction on surface of mast cell → DEGRANULATION of mast cell → Release of mediators and vasoactive substances – IMMEDIATE SYMPTOMS (within minutes)

Antigens and 'allergens'

The most potent allergens are usually large molecules with molecular weights up to 40 000. Examples of common 'allergens' are pollen, house mite dust, cat fur and penicillin. Food allergy, e.g. to peanuts and milk, is uncommon.

Antibody

This is IgE. Plasma cells forming IgE are not normally found in the internal secretory surfaces of the body – tonsils, bronchi, gastrointestinal tract – but are present in large numbers in cases of allergy (and in defence against parasitic infections).

HYPERSENSITIVITY STATES

Mast cells

These have a wide distribution but are prominent in the same areas as the IgE-producing plasma cells, plus skin, bladder and synovial membranes. This explains the frequently used term 'target organs' when discussing hypersensitivity.

Clinical examples of Type I reaction

ANAPHYLACTIC SHOCK

1st injection of antigen e.g. penicillin or a bee sting
→ General sensitisation

- - - - - - - - - - - - - - - - -

2nd injection of above →
Acute collapse: bronchial constriction; vomiting; diarrhoea; perhaps a skin rash. May be fatal. Note that the antigens are injected – enter blood stream
→ basophils affected
→ widespread reaction

HAY FEVER

1st contact with grass pollen → Local sensitisation of conjunctiva and nasal passages

- - - - - - - - - - - - - - - -

2nd contact with above
→ Irritation or swelling of conjunctiva with excessive watery secretion

ASTHMA

1st contact with house mite dust or animal dander → Local sensitisation of bronchi

- - - - - - - - - - - - - - - -

2nd contact with above
→ Bronchial constriction and secretion of thick mucus cause dyspnoea (difficult breathing)

Chronic asthma may involve cell-mediated immunity with tissue destruction.

Eosinophils are a common finding in the tissues of patients with allergies, attracted by eosinophil chemotactic factor released by mast cells. Allergic conditions are often familial with a genetic basis. Several candidate loci have been proposed including loci linked to cytokine genes and a gene for the IgE receptor on mast cells.

Type II – Cytotoxic type

The antigen is on the cell surface --- Specific antibody combination produces

NK cells, macrophages, monocytes, neutrophils or eosinophils bind Fc region via specific receptors

Complement activation, via classical pathway

Increased phagocytic activity (opsonic effect)

Antibody dependent cell mediated cytotoxicity

DESTRUCTION OF CELL

This cytotoxic reaction causes some forms of haemolytic anaemia [e.g. autoimmune HA (p.396): Rhesus incompatibility (p.397)] and some blood transfusion reactions.

In some auto-immune disorders antibodies of this type are directed against specialised cell surface receptors, e.g. Graves' disease or myasthenia gravis (see p.109).

HYPERSENSITIVITY STATES

Type III – Immune complex (Arthus) type

The reaction is due to the consequences of specific direct antigen/antibody combination – particularly complement activation (p.99) and platelet aggregation. The antibodies involved are IgG or IgM.

Ag/Ab (immune complex) → Complement activation → Vasoactive amines (anaphylatoxin) → Effects on vessel wall

Neutrophils (chemotaxis)

Platelet aggregation → Thrombosis (especially in venules)

In most cases where there is Ag/Ab reaction, the immune complexes are removed from the circulation and hypersensitivity does not develop. Type III hypersensitivity may be a localised reaction e.g. at the site of an insect bite or the development of farmer's lung following inhalation of fungal antigens (see p.272). When large amounts of circulating antigen enter the bloodstream and bind to antibody, circulating immune complexes are formed. Historically serum sickness occurred in some individuals following administration of antitoxin in foreign serum. Damage occurs particularly in the kidney when immune complexes aggregate in small vessels. Circulating immune complexes are important in the pathogenesis of systemic lupus erythematosus (SLE) and rheumatoid arthritis (see p.620).

Type IV – (delayed) type

This reaction is an antigen elicited cell mediated immune response which produces tissue injury independently of the presence of antibody. The reaction is usually delayed taking 24–72 hours to develop. Classic examples include the tubercle follicle, graft rejection and contact dermatitis.

Antigen → Sensitised T_h cell → Release of cytokines → T_C cell activation → Tissue damage

Macrophage activation

e.g. Contact dermatitis

Normal skin

Antigen presented by Langerhans cell

First application of chemical

Subsequent application

Epidermal oedema and lymphocytic infiltration

Perivascular lymphocytes in dermis

Chemical + tissue protein = 'foreign' antigen → cell-mediated immunity → inflammation

IMMUNE DEFICIENCY STATES

The systems involved are:

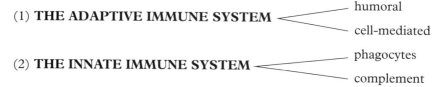

(1) **THE ADAPTIVE IMMUNE SYSTEM** — humoral / cell-mediated

(2) **THE INNATE IMMUNE SYSTEM** — phagocytes / complement

Failure in any one alters the immune response. The deficiencies may be of a primary nature, commonly genetic in origin, or secondary to some other disease or circumstance. Equally, the alteration in any system may be quantitative or qualitative. In many of these deficiencies there is a failure in more than one system.

Primary (inherited) deficiencies of the specific system are rare. They include B cell, T cell and combined B and T cell deficits. B cell deficiency leads to infection by pyogenic bacteria. T cell deficits lead to infection by viruses, fungi and intracellular bacteria.

Secondary deficiencies of the specific system are common. Usually T cell activity is affected, resulting in deficient cell-mediated immunity and, later, B cell deficit occurs.

The acquired immunodeficiency syndrome (AIDS) is now a major world-wide public health problem. Other predisposing conditions and diseases include:

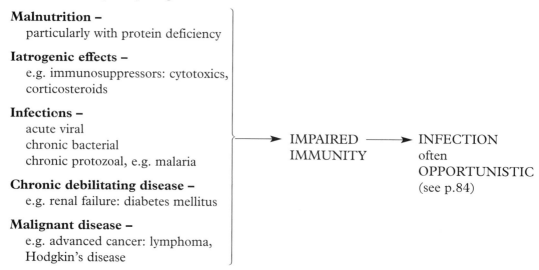

Malnutrition –
  particularly with protein deficiency

Iatrogenic effects –
  e.g. immunosuppressors: cytotoxics, corticosteroids

Infections –
  acute viral
  chronic bacterial
  chronic protozoal, e.g. malaria

Chronic debilitating disease –
  e.g. renal failure: diabetes mellitus

Malignant disease –
  e.g. advanced cancer: lymphoma, Hodgkin's disease

IMPAIRED IMMUNITY → INFECTION often OPPORTUNISTIC (see p.84)

Deficiencies of the innate immune system are rare. The disorders of neutrophil function are described on page 413.

IMMUNE DEFICIENCY STATES – AIDS

The acquired immune deficiency syndrome (AIDS) is a world-wide epidemic with large numbers of cases in sub-Saharan Africa and South East Asia. Globally, an estimated 40 million people are infected with the virus.

The virus [human immunodeficiency virus (HIV)] is of the retrovirus group: it infects and destroys CD4 T-lymphocytes (macrophages are also infected).

The disease is slowly progressive and is usually ultimately fatal. Recently highly active antiretroviral therapy (HAART), usually a combination of drugs such as nucleoside analogues and proteases, has been shown to reduce viral load to undetectable levels and has decreased the incidence of opportunistic infections and the death rate in the USA. However these drugs are expensive and have significant side effects.

Infection	**Latent period**	**AIDS**
CD4 > 500 × 10⁶. Asymptomatic or a short febrile illness. Although the patient's cells contain HIV, tests for antibodies may be negative for up to several months.	CD4 – 200–500 × 10⁶. Virus present in lymphocytes: may be persistent lymph node enlargement and fever.	CD4 < 200 × 10⁶ Infections and tumours

Infection — opportunistic, others
Tumours — Kaposi sarcoma, lymphomas

The whole range of opportunistic infection (see p.84), including disseminated virus infection (e.g. herpes simplex and cytomegalovirus), occurs.

The diagram shows the more common AIDS-associated diseases and sites:

Brain
  Tumours – especially lymphomas
  Inflammation – encephalitis
  Dementia
Mouth, Trachea, Oesophagus
  Candidiasis

Lungs
  Pneumocystis carinii infection
  Other fungal infections, Tuberculosis
Intestines
  Protozoal, Salmonella infections

Skin
  Kaposi's sarcoma, Fungal infections, Herpes zoster

Blood Changes

Antibodies – Specific antibodies appear up to 6 months after infection and form the basis of the diagnostic test for HIV. The antibody titre may fall greatly late in the disease.

Immunoglobulins are usually elevated in the early stages.

CD4 lymphocytes may be severely reduced, producing a lymphopenia (see above).

Corrections to scientific notation: CD4 > 500×10^6, CD4 – 200–500×10^6, CD4 < 200×10^6.

IMMUNE DEFICIENCY STATES – AIDS

EPIDEMIOLOGY AND TRANSMISSION

Although the virus may be present in many body fluids and secretions, transmission is by the parenteral route, usually by (1) **sexual contact,** (2) **infected blood** or (3) **from mother to infant**.

Transmission does not occur with normal social contact and there is a very low risk to medical or nursing personnel using normal procedures.

(1) **Sexual contact:** HIV is present in semen and vaginal fluid. Transmission may occur by homosexual intercourse. The risk of transmission is increased where there is genital ulceration or abrasion.

(2) **Infected blood:** the risk from blood transfusion and blood products has now been virtually eliminated by screening and sterilisation procedures (in the past many haemophiliacs were infected). The communal use of contaminated syringes and needles is important among drug addicts.

(3) **Mother to infant:** around half a million infants become infected with HIV each year. The majority of these infections result from transmission of virus from HIV infected mothers during childbirth or by transfer of virus in milk during breastfeeding. Maternal antiretroviral therapy can reduce the incidence of transmission.

Cellular mechanisms

HIV virus

Envelope
gp120–surface glycoprotein
host protein including MHCI + II molecules

Nucleocapsid

Viral genome
2 copies of single stranded RNA
2 molecules of reverse transcriptase

a) Infection of cells

1) HIV gp120 attaches to CD4
and the chemokine receptor CCR5

2) Nucleocapsid containing viral genome enters cell

3) Viral genome released

4) Reverse transcription yielding HIV dsDNA

5) Translocation to nucleus and integration into host DNA

b) Effects

1) Transcription of viral DNA to genomic ssRNA

2) Synthesis of viral proteins on ribosomes

3) Budding of membrane forming viral envelope

4) Virions that can infect other cells
Infected cells have a half-life of around 15 days

Note: Individuals with certain mutations in the CCR5 receptor are resistant to HIV. These mutations are more prevalent in Caucasian populations compared with African populations.

106

AUTOIMMUNE DISEASES

Autoimmune diseases result from, or are associated with, an immune response against the individual's own cells, or in some cases cell products. Although both humoral and cell mediated immunity are involved, it is thought that changes in the latter are of primary importance.

Aetiology

The aetiology of autoimmune diseases is not established, but clues to their genesis are available.

An increased FAMILIAL incidence of autoimmune diseases in general and of particular individual diseases	The overlapping of the incidence of antibodies and of the types of damage produced

suggest
an INBORN INSTABILITY OF IMMUNE TOLERANCE
particularly associated with inheritance of specific class II HLA antigens

The reasons for the breakdown of tolerance involve:

1. Antigenic abnormality and 2. Dysregulation of the immune response
(particularly T cell activity).

(1) **Antigenic abnormality**

(a) Cell surface antigens modified by drugs or chemicals.
(b) Cell antigens modified by proteolysis associated with disease processes, particularly inflammation, when 'new' antigens are formed.
(c) Microbial cross-reacting antigens

(2) **Immune dysregulation**

Abnormal presence/activity of auto-reactive T cells +/- failure of regulatory cells

CD4 cell activity INCREASED

B cell activity

Auto-antibodies

Ag/Ab + complement

Cytotoxic T cells primed

Cytokines (delayed hypersensitivity reactions)

CELL DESTRUCTION

AUTOIMMUNE DISEASES

	Antibody or cell mediated reaction to	Target Organ	Associated Diseases
ORGAN-SPECIFIC	(a) Thyroid cells and hormones, or (b) TSH receptor	Thyroid	Primary myxoedema Hashimoto's disease Thyrotoxicosis (Graves' disease)
	Parietal cells Intrinsic factor Intrinsic factor/ B12 complex	Stomach	Pernicious anaemia
	Red blood cells	Red blood cells	Haemolytic anaemia
	Pancreatic islet beta cells	Pancreas	Type 1 diabetes
	Adrenal cortical cells ACTH receptor	Adrenal	Addison's disease
	Parathyroid cells	Parathyroid	Primary hypoparathyroidism
	Acetylcholine receptor	Voluntary muscle	Myasthenia gravis

	Antibody to	Target Organ	Associated Diseases
NON-ORGAN-SPECIFIC	Mitochondria	Liver	Primary biliary cirrhosis
	Smooth muscle	Liver	Autoimmune chronic hepatitis

	Nuclear constituents – e.g. DNA	Skin and muscles	The connective tissue diseases
			    Dermatomyositis
			    Rheumatoid arthritis
			    Systemic lupus erythematosus (SLE)
			    Progressive systemic sclerosis

	IgG		
	Many other body proteins	Skin, kidney endocardium, blood vessels, joints	

AUTOIMMUNE DISEASES

Primary thyrotoxicosis (Graves' disease) and myasthenia gravis are of particular interest. In these diseases specific autoimmune antibodies combine with antigen on the cell surface and either stimulate or block the action of the physiological agent which would normally turn on the activity of the cell.

Stimulatory effect

In Graves' disease, excessive amounts of thyroid hormone are produced. LATS (long acting thyroid stimulator), an IgG auto-antibody, combines with antigen on the thyroid cell surface and produces changes mimicking those produced by TSH (thyroid stimulating hormone) – physiologically manufactured by the pituitary.

Normal production of thyroid hormone

TSH from pituitary

Receptor site on thyroid cell surface

GRAVES' DISEASE

LATS (IgG antibody)

Antigen

Receptor site activated by Ag/Ab combination

Message to nucleus activates cell – thyroid hormone produced

See also page 634.

Blocking effect

In myasthenia gravis, the acetylcholine formed at the motor nerve endings is prevented from stimulating the muscle motor end plate due to the antibody blocking the specific acetylcholine receptors. The end plate is also damaged (Ag/Ab + complement).

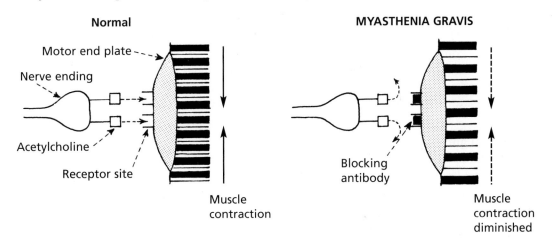

Normal

Motor end plate

Nerve ending

Acetylcholine

Receptor site

Muscle contraction

MYASTHENIA GRAVIS

Blocking antibody

Muscle contraction diminished

APPLIED IMMUNOLOGY

Immunohistochemical identification

Immunohistochemistry is now well established and allows identification of specific substances in histological sections.

Example:

(1) Monoclonal antibody to antigen (e.g. cytokeratin)

(2) Enzyme converts substrate to coloured reaction product

Slide containing cells with antigen.

Only cells containing cytokeratin contain coloured product e.g. Carcinoma cells.

This or similar techniques are used to identify a wide range of substances.

Flow cytometry

In this technique, cells in suspension are labelled by fluorescent markers, excited by a laser and counted electronically by passing them through a flow cytometer. This is the technique employed, among others, for monitoring $CD4^+$ counts in HIV.

Prophylaxis and treatment of infections

1. **Passive immunisation** is the term used when antibody formed in one individual is given to another individual who is at risk of infection — the protection is temporary. Examples include:

   Pooled human γ-globulin → general protection → particularly useful in cases of immune deficiency in agammaglobulinaemia.

2. **Active immunisation** is the term used when the infective agent is modified in some way to eliminate its harmful effects without loss of antigenicity. The subject's own immune response is activated. Examples include:

   TOXOID – e.g. tetanus toxin modified chemically.
   KILLED ORGANISMS – e.g. TAB (typhoid, paratyphoid A and B) vaccine.
   ATTENUATED ORGANISMS – e.g. viruses; cowpox, polio, measles.
   GENETICALLY ENGINEERED – e.g. hepatitis B where recombinant DNA
       technology is used to manufacture specific HBV proteins

Monoclonal antibodies

These are formed by immortalising a single clone of plasma cells, by fusion with myeloma cells, so that a large amount of identical antibody is produced.

Plasma cell   +   Myeloma cell   →   Immortal plasma cell clone

Note: Monoclonal antibodies can now be constructed from Ig gene libraries.

APPLIED IMMUNOLOGY – TISSUE TRANSPLANTATION

In the past, allografting (transplanting of tissues or organs from one individual to another of the same species) inevitably led to rejection of the graft by the host. Understanding of the mechanisms has allowed intervention so that nowadays successful survival of grafts is usual (e.g. 90% survival of renal transplants after 1 year).

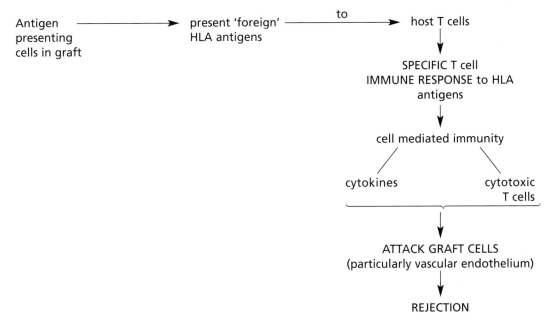

Rejection may also occur, very rapidly, if pre-existing antibodies are present (e.g. due to previous incompatible blood transfusion or pregnancy) – leading to activation of complement with haemolysis.

Usually rejection takes weeks while the cell mediated immune response is building up.

The remarkable improvement in transplant prognosis is due to:

    (a) careful matching of HLA compatibility between donor and recipient,
    (b) use of immuno-suppressive agents (particularly cyclosporin A),
    (c) screening for the presence of pre-existing HLA and cytotoxic antibodies.

Paradoxically the pre-transplant transfusion of compatible blood improves the chances of graft survival.

GRAFT versus HOST DISEASE (GvHD)

When immunosuppressed individuals (e.g. leukaemia patients) undergo bone marrow transplantation, T cells from the graft proliferate in the recipient (host) and establish an immune response against the host tissues: the main target organs are the skin, the liver and the alimentary tract.

NEOPLASIA

NEOPLASIA

Cancer as a cause of death in the Western world (25%) is second only to heart disease. Knowledge of non-neoplastic proliferation is helpful in understanding neoplasia.

Physiological proliferation occurs

1. in somatic growth during fetal development

   'explosive'

throughout CHILDHOOD → gradually diminishing → till ADULT MATURITY

2. in tissues where constant proliferation is needed in RAPID CELL TURNOVER e.g. in

   (a) bone marrow   (b) gut epithelium   (c) skin

Constant supply of cells to blood

Cell loss on surface

Proliferation at base

3. Proliferation at a much slower rate occurs in tissues where cell turnover is low e.g. LIVER, but will increase rapidly following injury.

Pathological proliferation is seen especially following tissue damage.

ENLARGEMENT of an organ due to increase in the parenchymal cell mass may be due to:

    (1) an increase in the size and functional capacity of the individual cells – hypertrophy

or (2) an increase in the number of cells – hyperplasia

or (3) commonly a combination of (1) and (2).

The stimuli responsible are: (a) increase in functional demand

                           (b) increased trophic hormonal activity.

Physiological enlargement of organs is common and well illustrated by the increase in muscle bulk consequent upon training and the enlargement of uterus and breasts in pregnancy.

Pathological enlargement is the result of disease processes.

HYPERTROPHY (pathological)

Enlargement of the heart as a result of hypertension is a good example of hypertrophy: the result of the increased functional demands to maintain the high blood pressure is an increase in the size of the myocardial cells.

Left ventricle   **Normal**   **Hypertension**   Left ventricle

Heart weight: up to 350g   Heart weight: 400–650g due to hypertrophy of left ventricle

Note: The process of hypertrophy per se does not involve proliferation, but there is often co-existent hyperplasia.

NON-NEOPLASTIC PROLIFERATION

HYPERPLASIA (pathological)

The two main causes are:

(a) *Chronic irritation* (and inflammation) e.g. in the skin, increased thickness results.

Hyperplastic epithelium

Normal epithelium

Chronic inflammation

(b) *Imbalance of hormonal activity*, e.g. the irregular enlargement of the prostate in old age is due to hyperplasia of the component tissues.

Normal prostate

Nodular hyperplasia of prostate

Hypertrophied muscle of bladder

Hyperplastic middle lobe

Distorted, partially occluded urethra

Note: If the abnormal stimulus is removed, the affected organ can return to normal.

METAPLASIA

This is a change from one type of differentiated tissue to another, usually of the same broad class but often less well specialised. The change is commonly seen in lining epithelia but occurs also in connective tissues. There is frequently an associated hyperplasia.

e.g. (a) Change from mucus-secreting epithelium to stratified squamous epithelium as in the bronchial irritation associated with smoking.

(b) Formation of bone in fibrous tissue – sometimes in healing process, e.g. prostatectomy scars.

Chronic inflammation

Bone

Reflux of acid results in metaplasia of the squamous epithelium of the lower oesophagus to glandular mucosa (Barrett's oesophagus p.293)

DYSPLASIA

This term refers to disordered growth which is frequently the precursor of malignancy. It is described on page 144.

115

NEOPLASTIC PROLIFERATION

A tumour is a proliferation of cells which persists after the stimulus which initiated it has been withdrawn. It is:

1. **Progressive**

e.g. Tumour of bone

2. **Purposeless**

e.g. Tumour of fibrous tissue

The fibres of a tumour of fibrous tissue have no regular arrangement and serve no useful purpose.

In normal fibrous tissue, the strands have a definite arrangement, supporting some structure such as an epithelial surface.

Note: Individual cells of a tumour may exhibit function – the fibroblasts form collagen – but it has no purpose.

3. **Regardless of surrounding tissue**

e.g. Smooth muscle tumour of uterus compresses normal tissues and distorts uterine cavity

4. **Not related to needs of the body**

e.g. Certain tumours of bone-marrow cells produce, needlessly, enormous numbers of leucocytes which fill the marrow, and then enter the blood stream

Normal marrow

5. **Parasitic**

The tumour draws its nourishment from the body while contributing nothing to its function. It induces the body to provide a blood supply and, in the case of epithelial tumours, a supporting stroma.

Since the development of a neoplasm is independent of the normal processes in the body it is *autonomous* although its growth may to some extent be influenced by these processes.

NEOPLASMS – CLASSIFICATION

Tumours may be classified in two ways: (1) clinical and (2) histological origin.

1. CLINICAL

The tumour is classified according to its morbid anatomy and behaviour. Two main groups are recognised – *benign* (simple) and *malignant*. The contrast between these two groups is as follows:

	BENIGN	MALIGNANT
Spread (the most important feature)	Remains localised	Cells transferred via lymphatics, blood vessels, tissue planes and serous cavities to set up satellite tumours (metastases)
Rate of Growth	Usually slow	Usually rapid
Boundaries	Circumscribed, often encapsulated	Irregular, ill-defined and non-encapsulated
Relationship to surrounding tissues	Merely compresses normal tissue	Invades and destroys normal tissues
Effects	Produced by pressure on vessels, tubes, nerves, organs, and by excess production of substances e.g. hormones. Removal will alleviate.	Destroys structures

In practice, there is a spectrum of malignancy. Some tumours may grow locally and destroy normal tissues but never produce metastases. Others will produce metastases only after a very considerable time while, at the other end of the spectrum, there are tumours which metastasise very early in their development.

2. HISTOLOGICAL ORIGIN

Although tumours may arise from any tissue in the body, they can be conveniently accommodated in five groups.

1. Epithelia.
2. Mesenchymal tissues including fibrous tissue, bone, cartilage and vessels.
3. Neuroectoderm.
4. Haemopoietic and lymphoid cells.
5. Germ cells.

The commonest tumours arise from tissues which have a rapid turnover of cells and which are exposed to environmental mutagens, e.g. epithelium of mucous membranes, skin, breast and reproductive organs and lymphoid and haemopoietic tissues.

BENIGN TUMOURS – HISTOLOGY

In general, the cells of benign tumours are well differentiated. They:

1. **Mimic the structure of their parent organ.**

e.g. In an adenoma
(simple gland-
forming tumour)
of colon the
cells arrange
themselves in acini.

In a skin
papilloma (wart)
the squamous
epithelium still
forms a covering
for underlying
connective tissue

2. **Resemble the cells of their tissue of origin.**

e.g. The cells of a skin
papilloma are squamous

The cells of a
myoma are
muscle cells

The cells of a
chondroma are
recognisable
cartilage cells

3. As in normal tissue, **show a remarkable
    uniformity in size, shape and nuclear configuration.**

4. **Show evidence of normal function.**

    This may be useless, e.g.

    or

    pathological, e.g. excess secretion
    of parathyroid hormone by a
    parathyroid adenoma.

Mucous secretion in
acinus of an adenoma

5. **Have relatively infrequent
    mitotic figures:** these are
    of normal type.

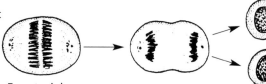

Equatorial
chromosomes

Division
into two
identical
daughter
cells

MALIGNANT TUMOURS – HISTOLOGY

The cells of malignant tumours tend to be less well-differentiated than those of benign tumours.

They:

1. **Generally show a haphazard arrangement.** ——————→ e.g. Carcinoma of breast

2. **Bear little resemblance to the cells of origin.**

3. **Tend to vary widely in size, shape and nuclear configuration, reflecting an increase in chromosomal number and DNA content (aneuploidy).** ——————→ e.g. Pleomorphic sarcoma

4. **Provide little evidence of normal function.** ——————→ e.g. Adeno carcinoma of bowel (Secretory activity very limited)

5. **Show frequent mitoses often of abnormal type.** Three daughter cells

There is a spectrum within malignant neoplasms from slowly growing well differentiated examples to rapidly growing undifferentiated highly malignant tumours.

BENIGN EPITHELIAL TUMOURS

Benign epithelial tumours are essentially of two types: (1) papillomas and (2) adenomas.

PAPILLOMA

Papillomas take origin from an epithelial surface. As the epithelium proliferates it is thrown into folds which become increasingly complex.

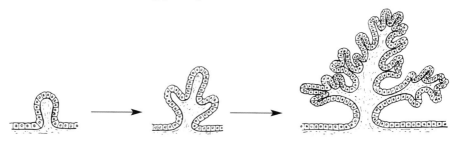

The epithelial proliferation is accompanied by a corresponding growth of supporting connective tissue and blood vessels.

Typical examples are found in the skin, e.g. the common wart.

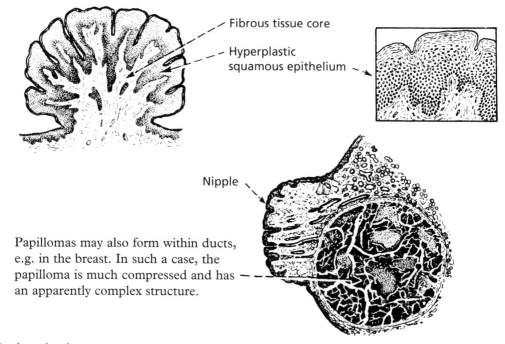

Fibrous tissue core

Hyperplastic squamous epithelium

Nipple

Papillomas may also form within ducts, e.g. in the breast. In such a case, the papilloma is much compressed and has an apparently complex structure.

In these benign tumours:

(a) The normal arrangement of epithelial cells is maintained, e.g. in skin papillomas the surface cells are squamous and proliferation is confined to the deepest layers.
(b) The relationship of epithelium to connective tissue is normal.
(c) Blood vessels are well formed.

BENIGN EPITHELIAL TUMOURS

ADENOMA

Adenomas are derived from the ducts and acini of glands, although the name is also used to cover simple tumours arising in solid epithelial organs.

Again the proliferation of epithelium of a gland causes the formation of tubules which ramify and become compound. The original communication with the parent gland duct or acinus tends to become lost.

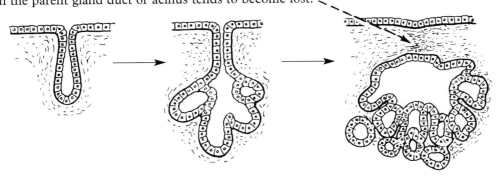

In the case of a hollow viscus, such as the intestine, the adenomatous proliferation, instead of growing down into the subjacent connective tissue, is usually pushed upwards into the lumen of the viscus.

The growth therefore combines the features of a papilloma and an adenoma. The term adenomatous polyp is often applied in such a case.

BENIGN EPITHELIAL TUMOURS

ADENOMA *(continued)*

In the type which grows into the subjacent connective tissue, the progressive budding of the epithelium results in new acini which become nipped off from the parent acini.

In cases in which retention of secretion is marked, a cyst forms and the tumour is then called a **CYSTADENOMA** which may reach an enormous size, e.g. some cystadenomas of the ovary may be 30–40 cm in diameter, particularly those which secrete mucus.

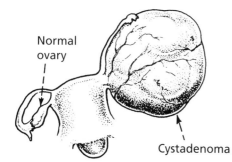

Normal ovary

Cystadenoma   Cut surface

Tall mucus-secreting cells

As in a hollow viscus, the proliferating epithelium may be heaped to form papillomas and the tumour then becomes a **PAPILLARY CYSTADENOMA**. These are also common in the ovary (see p.508).

FIBROADENOMA

In the breast the term is clinically useful for a small nodule consisting of a mixture of acinar elements and prominent supporting fibrous tissue. The histological appearances are variable depending on the distribution of the fibrous tissue (see also p.516).

Small, firm, palpable mobile lump

Well formed acini

Slit-like acini compressed by fibrous tissue

BENIGN CONNECTIVE TISSUE TUMOURS

Benign connective tissue tumours are composed of mature connective tissues – fat, cartilage, bone, nerves and blood vessels. They tend to form encapsulated rounded or lobulated masses which compress the surrounding tissues.

LIPOMA
Circumscribed masses of fat are commonly found in the subcutaneous tissue of the arms, shoulders and buttocks. Less commonly they occur in the deep soft tissues of the limbs or retroperitoneum, but at these sites they must be carefully distinguished from low grade liposarcomas. Lipomas very rarely arise from the viscera.

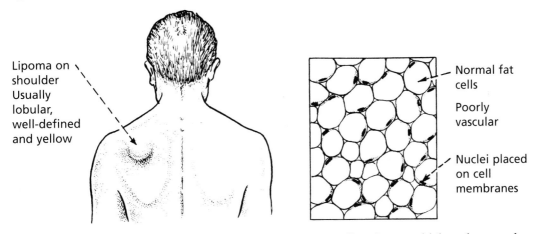

Lipoma on shoulder Usually lobular, well-defined and yellow

Normal fat cells

Poorly vascular

Nuclei placed on cell membranes

Sometimes lipomas may have projections into the surrounding tissues which make complete removal difficult.

CHONDROMA
A chondroma usually arises within the medullary cavity of the tubular bones of the hands and feet; it grows slowly, causing gradual expansion of the bone. Less commonly it occurs in long bones. Rarely multiple enchondromas appear in children and are associated with deformity: they occasionally become malignant.

Firm, bluish white nodule; sometimes flecks of calcification

Shell of expanded cortex

Hyaline, cartilaginous matrix

Regular, rounded, mononuclear cartilage cells often in pairs and quartets

BENIGN CONNECTIVE TISSUE TUMOURS

OSTEOMA

This tumour is mainly found in the bones of the skull, although it may occur in long bones. Osteomas are relatively small but may produce severe symptoms because of their situation.

Osteoma on floor of orbit causing protrusion of eyeball

LEIOMYOMA

Simple tumours of muscle are derived from smooth muscle and the majority occur in the uterus where they are extremely common. They are firm, rounded masses which usually begin in the myometrium. Subsequently, they may move inward to the uterine cavity forming polypi, or towards the serous surface.

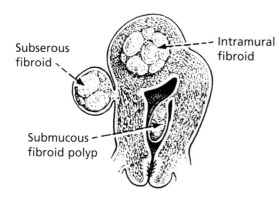

Subserous fibroid

Intramural fibroid

Submucous fibroid polyp

Cells and fibres in parallel bundles which in turn are whorled

TUMOURS OF FIBROUS TISSUE

So-called fibromas are rare but tumour-like growths are fairly common. Examples are FIBROMATOSIS and KELOID (see p.51).

Palmar fibromatosis, at first nodular, causes flexion deformities of fingers (Dupuytren's contracture) due to contraction of fibrous tissue within the palmar fascia. A similar condition may affect the plantar fascia.

Benign tumours of PERIPHERAL NERVE and of VESSELS are described on pages 583 and 584.

MALIGNANT EPITHELIAL TUMOURS

Malignant epithelial tumours are known as
CARCINOMAS (Greek '*karkinos*': a crab),
referring to the typical irregular jagged shape.
This is due to invasion into adjacent normal
tissues (p.135).

Types of CARCINOMA

Like benign epithelial tumours, carcinomas can arise from covering or glandular epithelium.

SQUAMOUS CELL CARCINOMA

This is commonly found on the skin, especially exposed surfaces, but also develops in other
sites covered by stratified squamous epithelium, e.g. lips, tongue, pharynx, oesophagus and
vagina. In addition, it may occur on surfaces covered by glandular type epithelium through
metaplastic transformation as in the bronchus, gall bladder and uterine cervix. It frequently
arises from areas of carcinoma-in-situ (p.144).

(1) It starts as a small papular
mass

(2) The surface breaks down and a
characteristic irregular ulcer is produced.

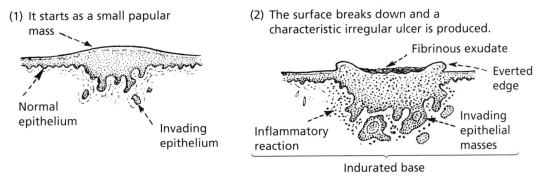

Histologically, it is composed of irregular strands and columns of invading epithelium which
infiltrate the subjacent connective tissue. If well differentiated, the central cells of the
invading masses show conversion into eosinophilic keratinised squames, while the outer layer
consists of young basophilic cells. In cross-section, the appearance is typical.

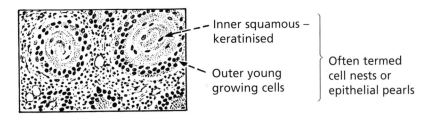

Squamous carcinoma of skin is typically well differentiated and slow growing. In contrast,
uterine cervical carcinomas are poorly differentiated and spread early to draining lymph
nodes.

TYPES OF CARCINOMA

BASAL CELL CARCINOMA (Rodent ulcer)
This tumour may arise in any part of the skin but is most common in the face, near the eyes and nose.

First stage
It starts as a flattened papilloma which slowly enlarges over months or perhaps a year or two.

Second stage
The surface breaks down and a shallow, ragged ulcer with pearly edges is formed.

Usually the malignant tissue spreads slowly but progressively, mainly in a lateral direction. It is composed of cells resembling those of the basal layer of the skin; it has a characteristic histological appearance.

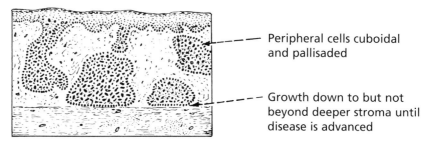

Peripheral cells cuboidal and pallisaded

Growth down to but not beyond deeper stroma until disease is advanced

There are many histological variants. Sometimes they show pseudoglandular structures: melanin deposition occurs in some tumours.

Basal cell carcinoma is a locally invasive growth which can be extremely destructive (hence its name: Rodent ulcer). It almost never metastasises. Thus the two processes of local invasion and distant metastases are not necessarily linked.

TYPES OF CARCINOMA

CARCINOMA of GLANDULAR ORGANS

These may take origin from gland acini, ducts or the glandular epithelium of mucous surfaces. The anatomical structure varies.

(A) On mucous surfaces they may start as a polypoid growth or as a thick plaque.

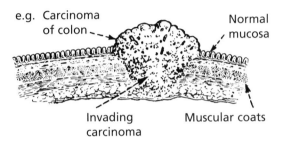

e.g. Carcinoma of colon

Normal mucosa

Invading carcinoma

Muscular coats

Ulceration with the formation of an irregular crater follows.

Everted edge

(B) In compound glands, e.g. the breast, the cancer forms an irregular penetrating mass – the typical crablike appearance.

(C) Some malignant tumours are cystic. Quite commonly the malignant growth originates in a pre-existing benign cyst. This is more likely to occur when there are papillomatous structures within the cyst.

Histologically, carcinomas of glandular tissue have three basic forms.

(1) Adenocarcinoma. In this form the growth shows a varying degree of differentiation with attempts at acinus formation.

(2) The carcinoma may be undifferentiated and take the form of solid masses or columns of pleomorphic cells.

(3) Occasionally a carcinoma will produce large quantities of mucus and merit the term mucoid carcinoma.
The tumours consist of only a few carcinoma cells in large lakes of mucus. They are commonest in organs normally containing large numbers of mucus-secreting cells, e.g. large intestine and stomach, but may also occur in the breast.

MALIGNANT CONNECTIVE TISSUE TUMOURS

Malignant connective tissue tumours are referred to as Sarcomas (Greek *'sarkoma'*: flesh). They arise in soft tissue, in bone and rarely in viscera.

Sarcomas are far less common than carcinomas, but are second in frequency to leukaemias and lymphomas in childhood and early adult life.

Unlike the ill-defined infiltrative carcinomas, sarcomas are large well defined fleshy tumours. Naked eye assessment suggests that they are encapsulated, but histology shows that this is a false impression. Malignant cells do infiltrate between normal tissues at the margin, so that surgical 'shelling out' is almost inevitably followed by local recurrence from aggregates of cells remaining in the tumour bed.

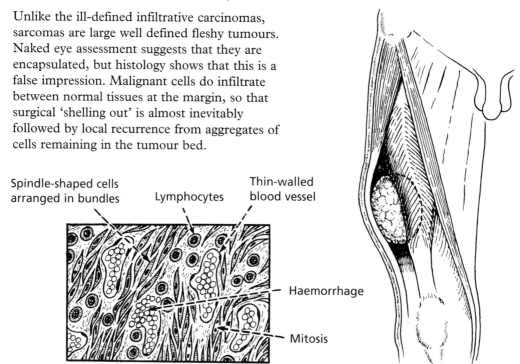

Spindle-shaped cells arranged in bundles

Lymphocytes

Thin-walled blood vessel

Haemorrhage

Mitosis

Most sarcomas consist of spindle shaped cells, although some are of round cell type. They are associated with the formation of many large thin walled blood vessels which are easily invaded by sarcoma cells. Blood borne metastases to lung are common. In contrast, lymph node involvement is rare in most types of sarcoma.

SARCOMAS

Many different histological types of sarcoma have been described. The nomenclature is based on adding the suffix 'sarcoma' to the type of differentiation shown, e.g. chondrosarcoma, liposarcoma, leiomyosarcoma (cartilage, adipose tissue, smooth muscle).

In general, the grade of the tumour is of more prognostic importance than the precise histological type. Some of the commoner forms of sarcoma are described:

Malignant Fibrous Histiocytoma (MFH) is the commonest soft tissue sarcoma of adults. It occurs in the limbs and retroperitoneum and is rapidly growing with a poor prognosis. The histogenesis is uncertain; it is probably a tumour of primitive fibroblasts.

Large multinucleated tumour cells ---

Spindle cells ---

Foamy --- histiocytes (reactive)

A 'storiform' arrangement of spindle cells – mimicking the spokes of a wheel – is an important diagnostic feature.

Liposarcoma

This tumour arises in soft tissues of the limbs and retroperitoneum. A number of sub types are described. Primitive fat containing cells (lipoblasts) are a feature.

Pleomorphic cells with numerous droplets of lipid.

Well differentiated liposarcoma has an excellent prognosis and rarely metastasises. Pleomorphic and round cell liposarcomas are highly aggressive tumours which metastasise early.

SARCOMAS

MYOSARCOMA
There are two varieties:

1. **Leiomyosarcoma**
   These rare tumours arise in the skin, deep
   soft tissues and particularly in the uterus.

Thin-walled blood vessels

Ill-defined margins

Mitoses

2. **Rhabdomyosarcoma**
   This is a rare tumour
   occurring mainly in
   children. It occurs very
   rarely in skeletal muscles.
   More common but still rare
   are polyploid tumours in the
   bladder, uterus and vagina,
   sometimes called sarcoma
   botryoides (grape-like).

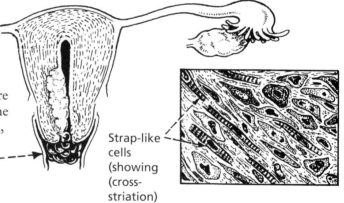

Strap-like
cells
(showing
(cross-
striation)

Pleomorphic or anaplastic sarcoma
Some sarcomas are so
poorly differentiated that
their histogenesis is not
apparent. They are
usually highly malignant.

- - - Bizarre cells and nuclei

Irregular mitotic figures

Absence of matrix

Immunocytochemistry, electron microscopy and cytogenetic analysis (demonstrating typical
chromosome translocations) all help in reaching more specific diagnoses than can be reached
by conventional histology alone.

Sarcomas of bone are described on page 613.

OTHER TUMOUR TYPES

TERATOMA

This is a tumour derived from totipotent germ cells. Most arise in the **ovary** (**usually benign**) and **testis** (**almost always malignant**): they may also occur at any site in the mid-line where germ cells have stopped in their migration to the gonads.

Sites

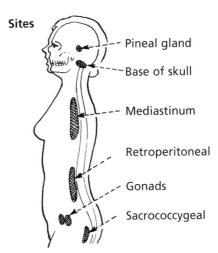

- Pineal gland
- Base of skull
- Mediastinum
- Retroperitoneal
- Gonads
- Sacrococcygeal

For example, **Benign cystic teratoma** is typically seen in the ovary.

It consists mainly of ectodermal structures such as skin and its appendages and neural tissue. Frequently respiratory epithelium, intestinal epithelium, bone and cartilage are present.

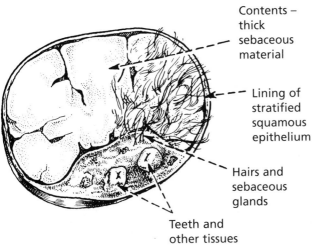

Contents – thick sebaceous material

Lining of stratified squamous epithelium

Hairs and sebaceous glands

Teeth and other tissues

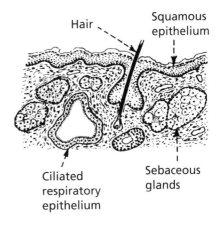

Hair

Squamous epithelium

Ciliated respiratory epithelium

Sebaceous glands

Testicular Teratomas are described on page 526.

MIXED TUMOURS

A number of tumours show differing histological patterns of epithelial and connective tissue components. The commonest is the MIXED PAROTID TUMOUR (PLEOMORPHIC ADENOMA) – presenting as a lobulated, firm, slow growing lump.

The stromal elements arise from metaplasia of myoepithelial cells.

Malignant mesothelioma (p.284), synovial sarcoma (p.623) and the very rare carcino-sarcoma show similar variable patterns.

131

OTHER TUMOUR TYPES

HAMARTOMA

A hamartoma is a tumour-like but non-neoplastic malformation consisting of a mixture of tissues normally found at the particular site.

The commonest forms of hamartoma are those composed of blood vessels and those involving pigment cells of the skin.

Hamartomas are also found involving the peripheral nerves – neurofibromatosis and its variants – the intestinal tract, congenital polyps, and in many other organs. Tuberous sclerosis is a condition in which hamartomas are present in many organs.

Although hamartomas are not neoplastic, true tumour growth may develop from a hamartoma.

Hamartoma	True neoplasm
Developmental abnormality.	New growth.
Present and often visible at birth.	Most occur in adults.
Enlargement continues until physiological growth ceases (i.e. on reaching adulthood).	Growth is progressive, autonomous and not related to stages of body development.
Condition is benign.	May be malignant.

It will be appreciated that the borderline between hamartoma and some types of benign neoplasm is ill-defined and the distinction is often not of practical importance.

HAEMANGIOMA

Two main varieties exist:

1. Capillary angioma

These are common in the skin as 'birth-marks' which vary in size. Occasionally they may be found in internal organs. They are well defined, deep red or purple. A single artery provides a supply separate from the surrounding tissue.

Prominent endothelial cells

Well formed collagen

2. Cavernous angioma

This type is usually confined to internal organs and quite often found in the liver. Like the capillary variety they are well defined and deep purple. Similar tumours are found involving the lymphatic system but less commonly.

OTHER TUMOUR TYPES

BENIGN PIGMENTED NAEVUS (Melanocytic naevus or mole)

Benign pigmented naevus is one of the commonest forms of hamartoma. The term 'naevus' means a birthmark, but most naevi are acquired in childhood and adolescence.

During fetal life melanin-pigment-forming neuroectodermal cells migrate to the skin and are found in small numbers in the basal layer of the skin.

The common congenital pigmented mole is the result of an abnormality in migration, proliferation and maturation of these neuroectodermal cells. A continuous layer of pigmented cells is found adjacent to the basal epidermal cells.

The resulting naevi vary in size and appearance, varying from small flat macular brown areas or smooth papular lesions to warty hairy excrescences. Pigmentation is variable.

Sometimes proliferation of the 'naevus' cells is a striking feature and this varies in degree and extent:

Junctional naevus
In this case proliferation is local and confined to the dermoepidermal junction

Compound naevus
Proliferation is found in the dermis as well as the junctional area.

Intradermal naevus
Proliferation is wholly in the dermis.

Blue naevus is another variation in which melanocytes are arrested in migration in the dermis.

Active proliferative activity may extend into adult life, but the great majority of these lesions undergo a degree of involution. One feature which differentiates them from the malignant change is that the deeper the cells penetrate the dermis the smaller they become and the less active.

OTHER TUMOUR TYPES

MALIGNANT MELANOMA

Malignant proliferation of melanocytes usually arises de novo but some melanomas arise from pre-existing naevi. Exposure to SUNLIGHT (the U.V. component) is the most important aetiological factor.

1. *Chronic* – over many years – especially relevant in the elderly.
2. *Acute* – causing burning. This is particularly important.

Sites

1. Skin of (a) face, soles of feet, palms of hands, nail beds,
      (b) legs (women) and (c) trunk (in men).
2. Mucous membranes of mouth, arms and genitalia – rare.
3. Eye and meninges – rare.

Some growths are amelanotic (non-pigmented). The rate of growth is variable.

Four types of growth may occur:

1. *Lentigo maligna* – an 'in situ' lesion occurring on the face of the elderly. It may spread at one edge and regress at another.

Aberrant melanocytes spread along basal
epidermal layer and round skin appendages.

It may not reach the invasive stage before the patient dies of another disease.

2. *Superficial spreading melanoma* – occurs on female leg, male trunk. It accounts for 50% of all skin melanomas in northern countries.
3. *Acral lentiginous melanoma* – found on palms of hands, soles of feet and mucous membranes.
4. *Nodular malignant melanoma* – usually on trunk. It invades early and ulceration is common.

Types 2, 3 and 4 occur in younger adults, and all can have an in situ stage.

The essential features of malignant melanoma are:

1. Abnormal melanocytes
2. Invasion of epidermis
3. Invasion down into dermis

Breslow thickness

The prognosis depends on depth of invasion, measured as follows:

1.5 mm or less – good prognosis
1.5–3 mm – fair prognosis
3 mm or more – poor prognosis.

SPREAD OF TUMOURS

Tumours spread by several routes.

1. Local invasion.
2. Lymphatic spread.
3. Blood (Haematogenous) spread

4. Transcoelomic spread.
5. Perineural spread.
6. Intraepithelial spread.

LOCAL SPREAD

The proliferating cells break through normal barriers.

Malignant epithelium breaks through basement membrane and subjacent connective tissue

Further spread is by penetration between normal tissues.

Malignant cells permeating spaces

An important principle is that these permeating tumour cells take the line of least physical resistance.

Growth of malignant cells may stimulate the production of new collagen fibres which are sometimes converted into dense fibrous tissue → contracts and fixes the growth to surrounding structures

e.g. Carcinoma of breast ⟶

Retracted nipple

Carcinoma fixed to underlying muscle

Fibrous tissue

The following diagram illustrates the basic mechanisms of cancer cell invasion.

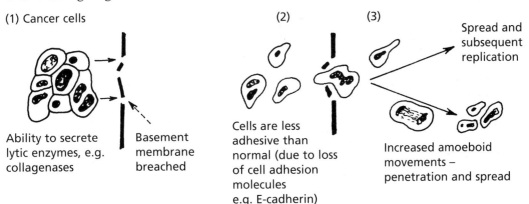

(1) Cancer cells

Ability to secrete lytic enzymes, e.g. collagenases

Basement membrane breached

(2)

Cells are less adhesive than normal (due to loss of cell adhesion molecules e.g. E-cadherin)

(3)

Spread and subsequent replication

Increased amoeboid movements – penetration and spread

LYMPHATIC SPREAD

LYMPHATIC SPREAD

This is the commonest mode of spread of carcinomas and melanomas, but rarely of sarcomas. Malignant cells easily invade lymphatic channels from the tissue spaces.

Groups of cells form emboli in the lymph stream and are carried to the nearest node (the *sentinel node*).

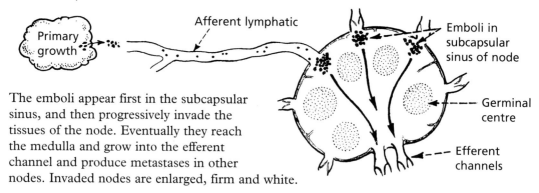

The emboli appear first in the subcapsular sinus, and then progressively invade the tissues of the node. Eventually they reach the medulla and grow into the efferent channel and produce metastases in other nodes. Invaded nodes are enlarged, firm and white.

Growth of carcinoma cells in a node may result in occlusion of afferent and efferent channels. Lymph flow is thus diverted and this has two effects:

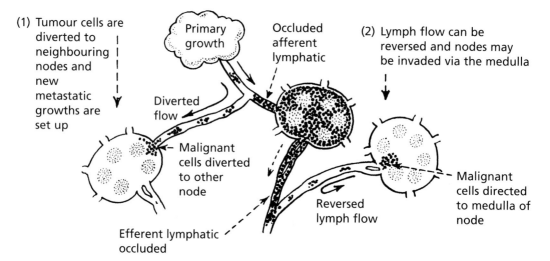

This accounts for the spread of carcinoma in a diverse and often irregular manner.

LYMPHATIC SPREAD

LYMPHATIC SPREAD *(continued)*

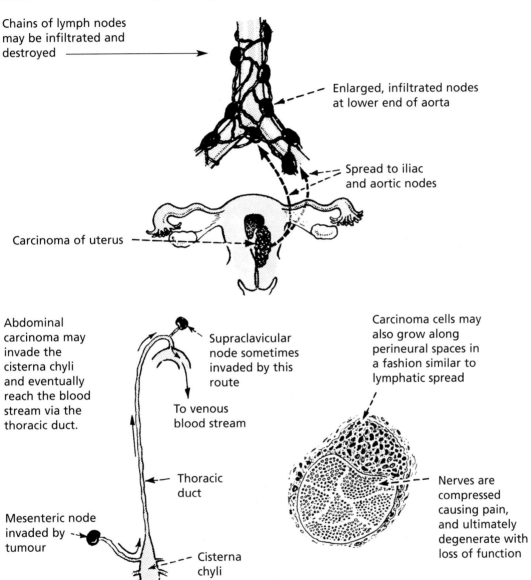

Chains of lymph nodes may be infiltrated and destroyed

Enlarged, infiltrated nodes at lower end of aorta

Spread to iliac and aortic nodes

Carcinoma of uterus

Abdominal carcinoma may invade the cisterna chyli and eventually reach the blood stream via the thoracic duct.

Supraclavicular node sometimes invaded by this route

To venous blood stream

Thoracic duct

Mesenteric node invaded by tumour

Cisterna chyli

Carcinoma cells may also grow along perineural spaces in a fashion similar to lymphatic spread

Nerves are compressed causing pain, and ultimately degenerate with loss of function

Although lymphatic embolism is of major practical importance, tumour cells may also grow along lymphatic channels in continuous solid columns – **lymphatic permeation**.

BLOOD SPREAD

Both carcinomas and sarcomas spread by the blood stream. The entry of malignant cells into the blood is via invasion of VENULES and by lymphatic embolism through the thoracic duct into the subclavian vein.

Carcinoma cells invading the thin wall of the vessel and entering the lumen.

The following are possible sequels:

1. Tumour embolism to lungs (systemic circulation).
2. Embolism to liver (portal circulation).
3. Embolism via pulmonary veins to systemic ARTERIAL circulation. (Primary and secondary lung tumours.)

4. Thrombosis within the lumen: consisting of a mixture of cancer cells and coagulum.

Cancer cells

Fibrin

Subsequent embolism as in 1, 2, 3 above.

VIA LARGER VEINS
Occasionally tumour thrombus is propagated from venules into larger veins. This is classically seen in RENAL CARCINOMA.

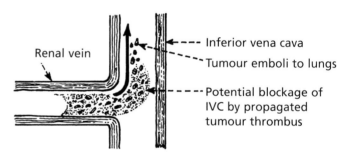

Renal vein

Inferior vena cava

Tumour emboli to lungs

Potential blockage of IVC by propagated tumour thrombus

Larger veins e.g. superior vena cava may suffer compression effects in 2 ways:

(1) Compression by tumour: vein may ultimately be obliterated.

Tumour

Vein

(2) Lumen reduced by growth of fibrous tissue stimulated by the neoplasm.

Fibrous tissue

Vein

Rarely, a malignant process may be complicated by thrombosis of distant veins (thrombophlebitis migrans). This is not due to malignant invasion of the veins but is caused by the action of circulating thromboplastins formed by the tumour.

ARTERIAL SYSTEM
Direct invasion of arteries and arteriolar lumens is very rare because of the physical barrier provided by the thick muscular and elastic walls.

BLOOD SPREAD

DESTINATION OF EMBOLI

This depends on the anatomical drainage of the vessel invaded.

(1) **Portal venous system**
– emboli pass to liver

(2) **Systemic venous system** – emboli pass to lungs. There are exceptions (see 'Retrograde Spread' below).

(3) **Pulmonary venous system** – emboli pass to left heart and general circulation

RETROGRADE VENOUS SPREAD

As in lymphatics, growth of tumour within a vein may cause reversal of blood flow. In addition, reversal of flow is apt to happen in certain areas of the body where veins form a rich plexus and are deficient in valves, e.g. in the pelvis and around vertebrae. Changes in intra-abdominal and intrathoracic pressures easily induce changes in blood flow in these channels. It is for this reason that secondary tumours are relatively common in vertebral bodies.

FATE of CARCINOMATOUS EMBOLI

SEED and SOIL ANALOGY

The distribution of carcinomatous emboli is determined in part by anatomy, but many complex factors both in the 'seed' (the cancer cell) and the 'soil' (the potential metastatic site) are at play in the establishment of metastases at particular sites. They include surface properties of the cancer cells e.g. increased expression of **integrins** and their **receptors** present in the endothelial cells at the metastatic site. Variation in the host IMMUNE RESPONSE is also important

OTHER MODES OF SPREAD OF TUMOURS

TRANSCOELOMIC SPREAD (via SEROUS SACS)

This is an important and frequent route of spread in the peritoneal and pleural cavities. It also takes place in the pericardial sac.

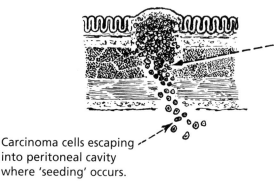

Carcinoma cells penetrate the wall of the stomach and extend to the serous surface.

Carcinoma cells escaping into peritoneal cavity where 'seeding' occurs.

As malignant cells sink in the peritoneal cavity, they will settle in various sites. They may cause an inflammatory reaction with fibrin formation. This can cause adhesions between organs, e.g. loops of bowel.

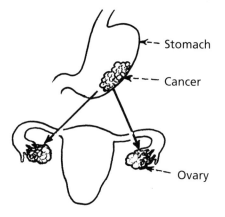

Stomach

Cancer

Ovary

Gastric cancer can spread to both ovaries (so-called KRUKENBERG TUMOUR).

Fibrous adhesions

INTRA-EPITHELIAL SPREAD

This form of spread may occur where carcinoma develops in a gland or its duct, e.g. in the breast. Carcinoma cells spread in the areolar skin. (Paget's disease of the nipple.)

Skin epithelium

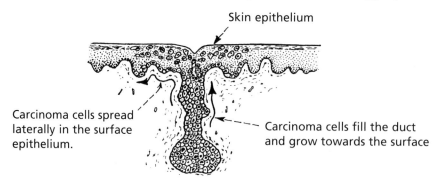

Carcinoma cells spread laterally in the surface epithelium.

Carcinoma cells fill the duct and grow towards the surface

EFFECTS OF TUMOURS

BENIGN TUMOURS

(a) The localised tumour mass may compress neighbouring structures causing loss of function and (b) benign endocrine tumours may produce excess hormones.

A Pituitary Adenoma is illustrative:

Visual fields

Retinae

Optic chiasma

Visual field defects –
BILATERAL TEMPORAL
HEMIANOPIA is the
classic effect.

Tumour produces excess
hormones e.g. growth
hormone → giantism or
acromegaly (see p.630).

PITUITARY ADENOMA
compressing decussation of optic nerve from below.

MALIGNANT TUMOURS

(a) Local effects

A tumour may narrow a hollow viscus e.g causing intestinal obstruction, ulceration and bleeding leading to anaemia.
E.g. 'ring' cancer of colon

(b) Involvement of neighbouring structures

Direct spread compresses adjacent viscera, blood vessels and nerves – LUNG CARCINOMA is illustrative (see p.277–278).

(c) Effects of distant metastases

These are very numerous and variable. Two illustrative examples are given.

1. Metastases to bone cause pain and pathological fracture.

2. Metastases to the brain causing epilepsy, stroke, etc. (see p.579).

NON-METASTATIC COMPLICATIONS

Patients with cancer often have severe weight loss (cachexia), loss of appetite and fever. These are probably due to release of cytokines (e.g. TUMOUR NECROSIS FACTOR) from tumour cells. Other complications include myopathy and neuropathy. Relapsing thrombosis of distant veins (thrombo-phlebitis migrans) is due to release of thromboplastins.

TUMOUR MARKERS

Tumour cells produce substances, many of which are proteins, which are helpful in diagnosis and monitoring of treatment.

(a) Product enters
blood stream
(and/or urine)
where it can
be measured.

Vein

(b) Histological diagnosis is
improved by identifying the
specific product using
immuno-staining in the
cytoplasm of the tumour cells.

Some examples are:

Tumour Marker	Tumour
Human chorionic gonadotrophin (HCG)	Choriocarcinoma, Teratoma of testis
αFeto-protein (αFP)	Hepatocellular carcinoma, Teratoma of testis
Prostate specific antigen, Prostatic acid phosphatase	Prostatic carcinoma
Carcino-embryonic antigen	Gastro-intestinal and other cancers
Calcitonin	Medullary thyroid carcinoma
5-hydroxyindole-acetic acid (5HIAA) in URINE [metabolite of 5-hydroxy-tryptamine (5HT-SEROTONIN)]	Intestinal carcinoid

Monitoring Treatment

Blood levels of tumour markers reflect the effects of treatment.
Example: **Testicular teratoma**

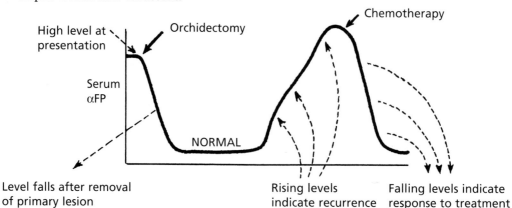

High level at presentation   Orchidectomy   Chemotherapy

Serum αFP

NORMAL

Level falls after removal of primary lesion

Rising levels indicate recurrence

Falling levels indicate response to treatment

PRE-MALIGNANCY

The pathological conditions which are associated with the development of malignancy fall into 3 groups, (1) Benign tumours, (2) Chronic inflammatory conditions and (3) Intraepithelial neoplasia.

1. MALIGNANT TRANSFORMATION OF BENIGN TUMOURS

(a) **Colonic cancer** is a good example in that many arise from a benign adenoma.

DIETARY or genetic factors

◄------------ PROGRESSIVE GENETIC CHANGES ------►

Normal ──► Initiation ──► Adenoma ──────────► Invasive carcinoma

(b) In Familial adenomatous polyposis (Polyposis coli) the transformation to cancer in one or more of the very numerous adenomas is inevitable (p.330).

2. CHRONIC INFLAMMATORY CONDITIONS

The inflammation has to be very long standing and transformation to cancer is RARE. Examples are:

(a) In **Ulcerative colitis**, repeated epithelial damage and repair increase the risk of cancer.

Ulcerated areas

Swollen surviving islands of mucosa forming pseudopolyps

Cancer arising in regenerating area

(b) In **Hashimoto's disease** – an auto-immune thyroiditis – the uniformly enlarged thyroid contains many proliferating lymphoid follicles and lymphocytes.

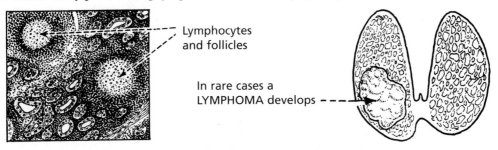

Lymphocytes and follicles

In rare cases a LYMPHOMA develops ------

3. INTRA-EPITHELIAL NEOPLASIA is common and a very important pre-cancerous
condition at several sites.

CARCINOMA IN SITU (INTRAEPITHELIAL NEOPLASIA)

This represents an intermediate stage in the production of a cancer. All the cytological features of malignancy are present, but the cells have not invaded the surrounding tissues. It is frequently found in the cervix uteri at the junction of ecto and endocervix.

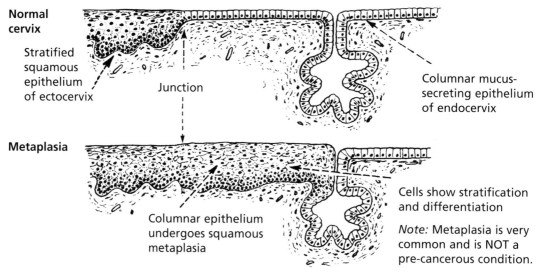

Normal cervix

Stratified squamous epithelium of ectocervix

Junction

Columnar mucus-secreting epithelium of endocervix

Metaplasia

Columnar epithelium undergoes squamous metaplasia

Cells show stratification and differentiation

Note: Metaplasia is very common and is NOT a pre-cancerous condition.

In the cervix, the abbreviation CIN (cervical intraepithelial neoplasia) is used. There are 3 grades of severity.

(1) CIN 1
    (mild dysplasia)

Thickening with moderate loss of polarity and differentiation

(2) CIN 2 – appearances intermediate between Grades 1 and 3,
(3) CIN 3 (Carcinoma-in-situ)

No clear stratification; cells undifferentiated; mitoses

Altered cells filling crypts

These premalignant conditions may revert to normal, but most commonly they become truly malignant and invade the surrounding tissues.

The concept of progressive premalignant proliferation applies equally in other organs (e.g. breast, stomach, oesophagus, bronchus, prostate, mouth, vulva).

CARCINOGENESIS

Malignant tumours are due to UNCONTROLLED PROLIFERATION of cells.
Most tumours are MONOCLONAL i.e. are derived from a single transformed cell.

This concept is well illustrated in MULTIPLE MYELOMA – a malignant tumour of plasma cells.

All the tumour cells produce the same immunoglobulin – including the same light chain.

e.g. all IgGκ

See also page 96.

In contrast, an inflammatory infiltrate of plasma cells is POLYCLONAL...

... producing various immunoglobulins and light chains.

CLONAL EVOLUTION

In time, some cells undergo further mutations which are passed on to their progeny. This is called clonal evolution or progression and explains the morphological variations seen in tumours. Some of the subclones grow more rapidly and metastasise more readily while others are so abnormal that proliferation is not possible and the clone dies out.

Original malignant clone

Continuing proliferation

Subclones

Severe abnormality, loss of proliferation, elimination by apoptosis

Increased proliferation and malignant characteristics increased.

Nuclear morphology and DNA content

In histological sections these abnormalities are indicated by variations in nuclear density (usually increased), size and shape (i.e. PLEOMORPHISM).

The term 'POLYPLOIDY' is used when the nuclear DNA is increased by exact multiples of the normal.

'ANEUPLOIDY' indicates irregular increases in DNA content.→

CARCINOGENESIS

A number of factors, both environmental and genetic, contribute to a cell undergoing malignant change. This should be regarded as a multistep sequence (see p.154).

ENVIRONMENTAL FACTORS

The 3 major environmental factors which induce tumours are 1. Chemical carcinogens, 2. Radiation and 3. Viruses.

CHEMICAL CARCINOGENESIS

Historically, chemical agents were the first to be associated with cancer. Now, many are recognised in (a) industrial processes, (b) social habits and (c) diet.

Industry	Tumour	Chemical Responsible
Aniline dyes	Bladder cancer	Naphthylamine
Insulation e.g. shipbuilding, building	Mesothelioma, lung, laryngeal cancer	Asbestos
Mineral oil and tar	Skin cancers	Benzpyrene and other hydrocarbons
Plastics	Angiosarcomas of liver	Vinyl chloride monomer
Wood dust	Cancer of nose and sinuses	?

Social Habits

Cigarette smoking is strongly associated with the development of many cancers, including lung, mouth, larynx and bladder. Chewing tobacco greatly increases the risk of oral cancer. It is likely that air pollution, e.g. combustion products of petrol and diesel, also contributes to carcinogenesis. Obesity is associated with an increased risk of cancer.

Diet

Chemicals in food may be carcinogenic. Nitrosamines may be formed by the action of bacteria on ingested nitrites. AFLATOXINS are produced by fungi (*Aspergillus flavus*) and by contaminating foodstuffs may cause liver cancer.

Note: Chemical carcinogens may act in 2 ways:
1. Directly at the site of application or portal of entry e.g. skin and lung cancers.
2. After modification, either at the sites of metabolism or excretion e.g. liver and urinary tract tumours.

CARCINOGENESIS

CHEMICAL CARCINOGENESIS *(continued)*

This is a multistep process of long duration.

The stages of **initiation** and **promotion** are important and are exemplified in experimental skin carcinogenesis.

(1) Normal skin

Application of carcinogen e.g. Benzpyrene (a mutagen)

(2) INITIATION Skin appears normal but important changes have occurred in the cell's DNA.

(3) PROMOTION – initiated by co-carcinogens e.g. croton oil, turpentine. (These agents are not mutagenic but act by stimulating cell proliferation.) Visible surface and histological changes are seen.

(a) Keratosis and papilloma formation

(b) Dysplasia i.e. cytological features of malignancy, but no invasion (see p.144).

Proliferation of epithelium

These stages are reversible

(4) Appearance of MALIGNANT TUMOUR – [An irreversible change]

Breach of basement membrane: **INVASION**

The order of application of these agents is important. No tumour follows application of promotor alone, or promotor followed by initiator.

In rodents, these changes take months; in humans the time scale is years and is exemplified in the skin, cervix uteri, bronchus, urinary bladder, colon and breast.

CARCINOGENESIS

RADIANT ENERGY

The potential dangers from irradiation give much cause for concern.

Source of Radiation	Tumours	Type of Radiation
Sunlight	Melanoma, Carcinoma of skin	Ultraviolet (non-ionising)
Nuclear explosions (e.g. atom bombs, Chernobyl)	Leukaemia, carcinomas of lung, breast, thyroid	Ionising
Therapeutic irradiation	Various carcinomas, sarcomas, leukaemia	Ionising
Mining radioactive substances e.g. Uranium	Lung carcinomas	Ionising
X-ray workers (historical)	Skin cancer, leukaemia	X-rays: Ionising

Effects of Irradiation on Cells

The ionising effect of radiation damages the cell's DNA, especially during cell proliferation, ranging from single gene mutation to major chromosome damage, including breaks, deletions and translocations.

Normal chromosomes Dysjunction Random fusion of broken ends Mutation

Proliferating cells are particularly vulnerable. Marrow and gastro-intestinal mucosa are highly sensitive.

Ultraviolet light is of low energy and mainly affects the skin. The 'PYRIMIDINE DIMERS' formed by UV light are normally excised by DNA repair mechanisms. In **xeroderma pigmentosum**, these are deficient leading to numerous skin tumours.

CARCINOGENESIS – VIRUSES

Viruses have long been known to cause cancer in animals (e.g. Rous sarcoma virus and the mouse mammary tumour virus – the Bittner milk factor).

In recent years viruses have been shown to contribute to the development of some human cancers.

Virus	Type	Tumour type
Epstein-Barr (E.B.V.)	DNA	Burkitt's lymphoma, nasopharyngeal cancer, Hodgkin's disease, post-transplantation lymphoma
Human herpes virus 8 (HHV-8)	DNA	Kaposi's sarcoma
Hepatitis 'B'	DNA	Hepatocellular carcinomas
Human papilloma virus (HPV)	DNA	Cervical, penile, anal carcinoma
Human 'T' cell leukaemia virus (HTLV-1)	RNA (Retrovirus)	T-lymphoblastic leukaemia

Mode of action on oncogenic viruses

The essential feature is addition of new DNA to the nucleus of host cells resulting in mutants, but the way in which this is achieved differs in the two types of virus.

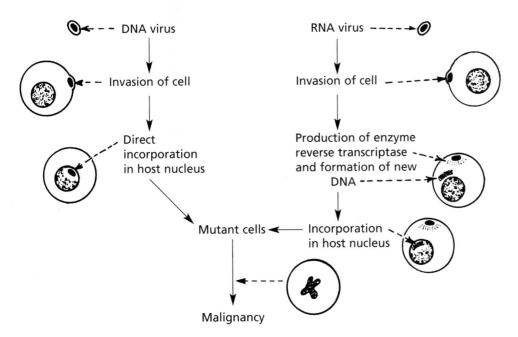

149

CARCINOGENESIS – HEREDITY

The inherited genetic influences in cancer are now well recognised.

1. There is a high risk of cancer in some uncommon syndromes inherited as Mendelian traits. Illustrative examples are:

(a) **Familial adenomatous polyposis coli** (APC). ·--→
An autosomal dominant condition. Numerous polyps occur in the colon in late childhood (10–14 years) and inevitably lead to adenocarcinoma in early middle age (30–45 years). The APC gene responsible lies on chromosome 5.

(b) **Xeroderma pigmentosum.** An autosomal recessive trait where failure of DNA repair mechanism leads to skin cancer.

(c) **Neurofibromatosis** – multiple neurofibromas (NF) – with a 1% risk of sarcoma, is due to a defect of NF-1 gene on chromosome 17.

(d) **Retinoblastoma** – an autosomal dominant (Rb gene on chromosome 13), (p.153).

2. A less well defined, but strong familial tendency, is seen with some common tumours. For some the gene is identified e.g. BRCA-1 gene, chromosome 17, – 60% risk of breast or ovarian cancer by 50 years.

3. In some families, there is a high risk of several types of cancer. In the rare Li-Fraumeni syndrome, childhood sarcomas, breast cancer in young women, and many other cancers are seen. This is due to a germ-line mutation of the p53 gene (p.153).

Illustrative Family Tree:

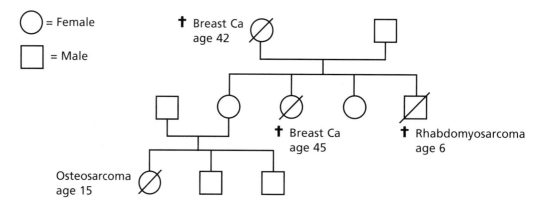

ONCOGENES AND TUMOUR SUPPRESSOR GENES

Cellular proto-oncogenes are NORMAL genes which STIMULATE cell division. Tumour suppressor genes are NORMAL genes which INHIBIT cell division. Their normal activity during somatic growth and in regeneration and repair takes place during the G_0–G_1 phase of the cell cycle and is strictly controlled.

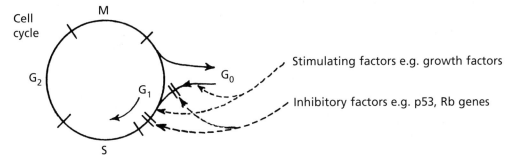

In cancer cells the normal controls are defective so that the balance between factors stimulating and inhibiting cell growth is permanently lost, resulting in increased proliferation.

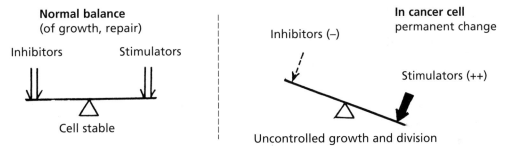

Cellular proto-oncogenes code for a number of proteins involved in cell proliferation:

Binding of GROWTH FACTORS to cell surface
GROWTH FACTOR RECEPTORS sends a signal through the
CYTOPLASM (signal transduction) to the
NUCLEUS, activating
NUCLEAR REGULATING PROTEINS, thus promoting cell growth and cell division.

In the cancer cell, these normal genes are permanently changed to ONCOGENES and proliferation is uncontrolled.

Mutation or overexpression of genes which normally control APOPTOSIS (p.4) are increasingly recognised in many tumours e.g. overexpression of *bcl-2* inhibits apoptosis in follicular lymphoma (p.437).

ONCOGENES

The production and activity of ONCOGENES is complex and there are many ways in which they are activated.

The following are a few illustrative examples.

1. **Production of excess NORMAL protein**

    (a) Gene amplification
    e.g. neuroblastoma
    (*myc* type gene)

    Proto-oncogene   Multiple copies

    (b) Increased mRNA transcription due to chromosomal translocation e.g. in Burkitt's LYMPHOMA chromosomes 8 and 14 are involved.

    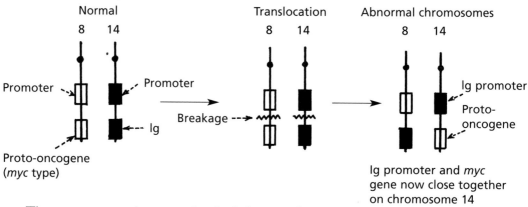

    The *myc* oncogene is now under the influence of the Ig gene control and is permanently switched on.

2. **Production of FUNCTIONALLY ABNORMAL PROTEIN**
    A point mutation of the proto-oncogene produces a protein with an altered function so that over-stimulation occurs.
    Altered **growth factor receptor function** is an example.

    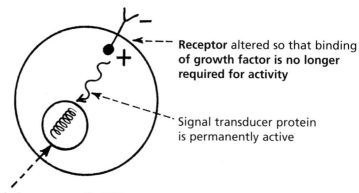

    Receptor altered so that binding of growth factor is no longer required for activity

    Signal transducer protein is permanently active

    Nuclear regulating protein is permanently 'ON'

TUMOUR SUPPRESSOR GENES

Tumour suppressor genes are normal genes which switch off cell proliferation by acting on the cell cycle in G_1. Their biological role is much broader than simply suppressing tumour function, but the name reflects how they have been discovered.

Loss of *both* copies of a tumour suppressor gene is required for cancer to develop. In contrast, only one copy of a given oncogene needs to be activated to cause excess proliferation.

Examples are:

Tumour suppressor gene	Chromosome	Tumours
p53	17	Carcinoma of lung and breast: Sarcomas
Retinoblastoma (Rb)	13	Retinoblastoma, sarcoma: some carcinomas
NF1	17	Neurofibromas, malignant peripheral nerve tumours
APC	5	Colonic carcinoma
WT1	11	Wilms' tumour, bladder cancer, breast cancer: rhabdomyosarcoma

p53 gene: This gene codes for a nuclear phosphoprotein, which is expressed in increased amounts following cellular damage e.g. **irradiation**.

p53 has been called the 'Guardian of the genome'. Abnormalities of p53 are found in at least 30% of all cancers.

Germ line p53 mutation is a feature of the Li-Fraumeni syndrome.

CARCINOGENESIS – SUMMARY

The MULTISTEP STAIRWAY to MALIGNANCY

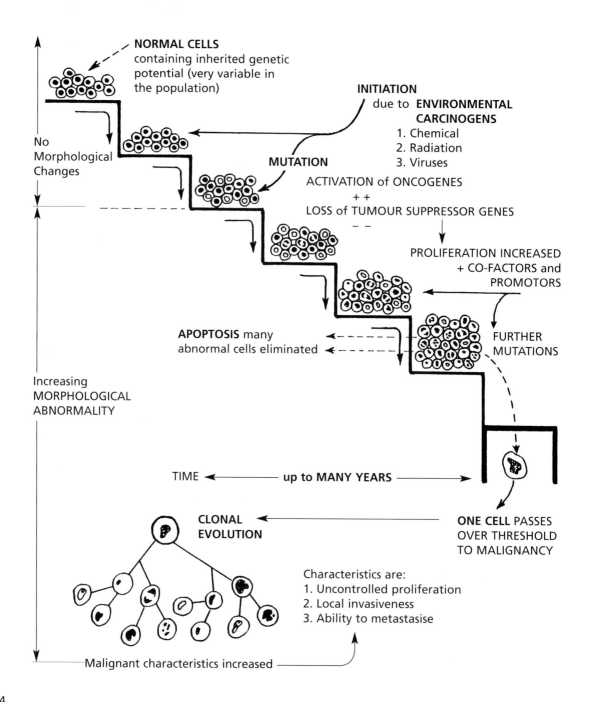

NORMAL CELLS
containing inherited genetic
potential (very variable in
the population)

INITIATION
due to **ENVIRONMENTAL CARCINOGENS**
1. Chemical
2. Radiation
3. Viruses

No Morphological Changes

MUTATION

ACTIVATION of ONCOGENES
+ +
LOSS of TUMOUR SUPPRESSOR GENES

PROLIFERATION INCREASED
+ CO-FACTORS and PROMOTORS

APOPTOSIS many
abnormal cells eliminated

FURTHER MUTATIONS

Increasing MORPHOLOGICAL ABNORMALITY

TIME ← up to **MANY YEARS** →

ONE CELL PASSES OVER THRESHOLD TO MALIGNANCY

CLONAL EVOLUTION

Characteristics are:
1. Uncontrolled proliferation
2. Local invasiveness
3. Ability to metastasise

Malignant characteristics increased

CHAPTER 7

CARDIOVASCULAR DISEASES

GENERAL CONSIDERATIONS

Cardiovascular diseases are the commonest cause of death in Westernised communities. The main forms are:

1. **Ischaemic heart disease.**   2. **Cerebrovascular diseases.**

Some general abnormalities of the circulation require to be discussed first.

THROMBOSIS

A thrombus is a mass formed from blood constituents within a vessel or the heart during life. Blood clotting is a physiological protective mechanism but thrombosis is a pathological process with serious consequences.

MECHANISM OF FORMATION

Platelets adhere to the endothelium and to each other, forming a projecting mass. (1)

The liberation of **thromboplastin** initiates a 'chemical cascade' leading to coagulation.

Release of thromboplastins
↓
Thrombin formation

cleaves | catalyses

Fibrin ← ———— Fibrinogen
strands

If the rate of flow is slow, as in a vein, red cells are entangled so that the lumen is occluded. (2)

Platelet mass
With a slow flow in the joining vessel more fibrin is formed by the platelets at the tip of the thrombus, thus occluding the joining vessel.

In front and behind the platelet mass, the blood stagnates. Further formation of fibrin takes place, resulting in a large solid coagulum.
The thrombus extends in either direction to the nearest junction. At this point more platelets are deposited on the end of the mass. This gives the head of the thrombus a pale tip. (3)

(4) Blood stagnates in the joining vessel and thrombosis extends forward to the next joining vessel. There may be a succession of thrombotic episodes – a propagating thrombus.

156

FACTORS LEADING TO THROMBOSIS

The 3 MAIN factors leading to thrombosis are known as Virchow's triad: they are closely concerned with local changes in the coagulability of the blood (see p.414 et seq.).

1. ALTERATIONS OF BLOOD FLOW

The main effect is to bring platelets into contact with the vessel wall. This results from:
Slowing of blood flow, e.g. in cardiac failure or during bed rest. With slowing, the normal axial stream of blood cells is lost and white cells and platelets fall out of the main stream and accumulate in the peripheral plasma zone.

Clear plasma zone

White cells and platelets

Axial stream of cells

Red cells

Turbulence, e.g. by deformation of vessel wall or around venous valves.

Local increase in lumen, as in varicose veins or aneurysm, causes eddies and platelets and white cells fall out of main stream.

Swelling or compression of vessel wall by disease. Eddies form in front and behind obstruction.

Eddies form around valves if flow slows.

These changes in flow and shear stress cause altered endothelial function with increased production of agents which promote thrombosis (p.158).

FACTORS LEADING TO THROMBOSIS

2. DAMAGE TO ENDOTHELIUM OF VESSEL

This leads to platelet adhesion and aggregation. Common causes are:

(a) Disease in vessel wall e.g. atheroma.

Overlying thrombus

Endothelial loss or dysfunction

Atheroma

(b) Toxins from nearby inflammatory processes.
(c) Local compression of vessels (e.g. during operations).

In **Health**, endothelial cells produce vasodilators and platelet inhibitors to prevent thrombosis.

Thrombosis is provoked by release of vasoconstrictors and platelet activators.

Endothelial cell

Nitric oxide
Prostacyclin
Antithrombin

inhibit

THROMBOSIS

promote

Endothelin
von Willebrand
factor

Thromboxin A

stimulates more platelets

The balance between these processes is usually
AGAINST THROMBOSIS.

3. CHANGES IN COMPOSITION of the BLOOD

(a) INCREASE in platelets, fibrinogen and prothrombin after operations and childbirth: usually after 5–10 days.
(b) INCREASE in platelet adhesiveness – again after surgery.
(c) Rare inherited abnormalities of thrombosis inhibitors – e.g. antithrombin III deficiency: protein C deficiency.
(d) Miscellaneous factors e.g. oral contraceptives, smoking, some cancers.

COMMON SITES AND TYPES OF THROMBUS

ARTERIAL

Thrombi are common in arteries as a complication of **atheroma**. Forming in a rapid circulation, the thrombus consists mainly of PLATELETS (WHITE thrombus).

Common sites include:

BRAIN

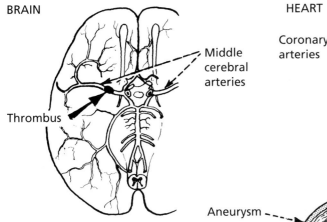

Middle cerebral arteries

Thrombus

HEART

Coronary arteries

Thrombus

Aneurysm

Thrombus formation is common in the walls of **aneurysms**, consisting of layers of red and white thrombus (MIXED or LAMINATED thrombus).

VENOUS

Systemic venous thrombosis is common because of the slow blood flow and lower pressure. It consists of red cells, platelets and fibrin (RED thrombus).

It is most common in the deep veins of the calf and frequently propagates in the femoral and iliac veins – from where it may embolise to the lungs (p.162).

Bed rest, operations and cardiac disease are predisposing conditions.

Portal thrombosis is a rare complication of abdominal disease e.g. hepatic cirrhosis.

Propagation

Thrombus

COMMON SITES AND TYPES OF THROMBUS

CAPILLARY
Thrombi, composed mainly of fused red cells, form when capillaries are damaged, usually in acute inflammatory processes.

Capillaries are occluded by fibrin thrombi in cases of disseminated intravascular coagulation (DIC – see p.419).

CARDIAC
Thrombi may be seen in the ATRIA (especially in the auricles in ATRIAL FIBRILLATION); in the VENTRICLES and on the heart VALVES.

Mural thrombi occur in ventricles, especially the left, usually secondary to INFARCTION of the ventricular wall.

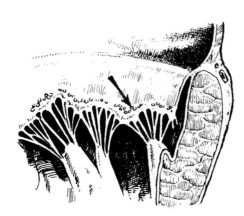

Thrombi of pale variety occur on the heart valves in rheumatic endocarditis.

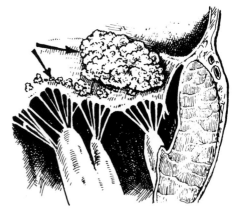

Sometimes infective endocarditis occurs and the thrombi are larger, mixed, friable and contain masses of micro-organisms.

SEQUELS OF THROMBOSIS

1. **FIBRINOLYSIS**
   Many small thrombi are completely removed by the Fibrinolytic System which exists to limit thrombosis.

Fibrin Degradation Products

2. **EMBOLISM**
   Part of the thrombus may be detached and carried along in the blood stream to impact in a distant vessel. This is extremely important clinically.

3. **ORGANISATION**
   Capillaries grow into the point of thrombus attachment within a day or two. Fibroblasts and phagocytic cells accompany the capillaries, and gradually the thrombus material is dissolved and replaced by a fibrovascular tissue. At the same time endothelium covers the ends of the thrombus, thus limiting the thrombotic process.

   Ultimately, the branching capillaries may be converted into one or two larger vessels which may restore the circulation through the vessel – RECANALISATION.

4. **CALCIFICATION**
   In diseased vessels, organisation may not take place. The thrombus shrinks, calcium salts are deposited and convert it into a phlebolith – seen in X-rays.

5. **INCORPORATION**
   A mural thrombus, e.g. in a large artery, may be covered by endothelium and incorporated in the vessel wall. This process may be important in the formation of atheroma.

   PROPHYLAXIS and THERAPY of thrombosis aims at:
   1. Reducing coagulability utilising (a) anticoagulants aimed at specific sites in the coagulation cascade e.g. warfarin derivatives, heparin (see p.420) and (b) inhibiting specific prostaglandin synthesis e.g. aspirin.
   2. Encouraging fibrinolysis, using fibrinolysins.

EMBOLISM

An embolus is any abnormal mass of matter carried in the blood stream and large enough to **occlude some vessel**.

The commonest emboli are derived from material generated within the vascular system e.g. fragments of thrombus or material from atheromatous plaques.

1. **Pulmonary thrombo-embolism**
    Emboli from the systemic veins (especially deep venous thrombosis) pass through the right side of the heart to the pulmonary circulation. The consequences depend on the size of the embolus and the patient's previous health.
    (i) **Massive** embolus → blocks main pulmonary artery trunk → acute total circulatory block → SUDDEN DEATH.
    (ii) **Moderate** embolus
         With a double blood supply – pulmonary and bronchial arteries – and a vast anastomosis, obstruction of a pulmonary artery branch does not necessarily cause infarction. When there is pre-existing circulatory stagnation within the lung, the arrival of an embolus in the pulmonary arterial tree will cause infarction.

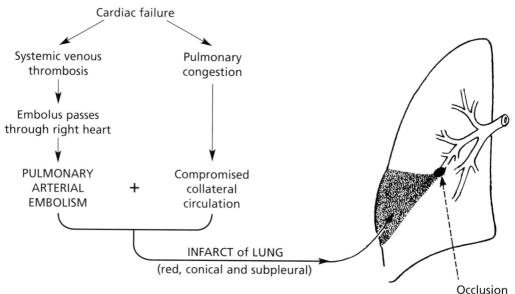

    (iii) **Small** emboli
          Many are removed by the fibrinolytic system and are asymptomatic. However, repeated minor emboli may result in pulmonary hypertension and right heart failure. Repeated small emboli → blockage of peripheral pulmonary arterial branches → **pulmonary hypertension**.

2. **Emboli of the arterial system** are derived from the heart or the larger arteries which have become atheromatous. The results of arterial obstruction are very important.

EMBOLISM

EMBOLISM – Other forms

Matter entering the vascular system may be

(a) *Solid* e.g. tumour cells, bacterial clumps, fat, parasites.
(b) *Gaseous* – air
(c) *Liquid* e.g. amniotic fluid with fetal derived matter.

Fat embolism

This may occur when a long bone is fractured, usually 24–72 hours later. Fat globules enter torn veins and pass to lungs; obstruction of pulmonary blood flow may be sufficient to cause *anoxia*. Cerebral symptoms are common due to anoxia but also to the arrival in the brain of fat particles which have passed through the lung capillaries.

Amniotic fluid embolism

During parturition, amniotic fluid may enter a uterine vein, especially after manipulations. Vernix, hairs and squames enter the circulation. In addition to embolic phenomena, there are also coagulation disorders (p.419).

Ruptured veins in placental bed

Instrument tearing membranes and placenta

Embolism in drug addicts

Lung lesions occur in addicts using intravenous injection due to particulate matter (e.g. talc).

Gas embolism

This occurs mainly in 2 forms:

(a) *Single embolism*
Atmospheric air may enter the blood when a neck or intracranial vein is incised. Inspiration induces a suction effect by causing a negative pressure in the veins. As a result of frothing in the right ventricle, cardiac action is seriously impaired.
(b) *Multiple embolism*, in 'caisson disease'
This occurs in persons working in barometric pressures of several atmospheres, e.g. diving to great depths. The atmospheric gases go into solution in high concentration in the blood and tissues. If decompression occurs too quickly, these gases 'boil' off and appear as bubbles in the circulation. The oxygen is taken up by the tissues but insoluble gases cause widespread 'embolism', especially in the nervous system and bone.

ARTERIAL OBSTRUCTION

Arterial obstruction is usually due to thrombosis or embolism and may be (i) partial or complete, (ii) acute or slowly progressive.

The effects depend on the local anatomy, particularly on the presence of an anastomotic collateral circulation.

Occlusion of end arteries

These may have (a) no collaterals (e.g. splenic artery),

(b) capillary anastomoses (e.g. renal and coronary arteries),

(c) arterial anastomoses which are too small to maintain circulation (e.g. superior mesenteric artery).

Result:

Obstruction → anoxia of tissues → necrosis

INFARCTS

An infarct is an area of necrosis due to ischaemia. It is often found at the periphery of an organ e.g. the kidney.

Blocked
artery

After 12 hours: Area is pale. Degenerative changes already seen with electron microscope or histochemical tests.

After 36 hours: Area shows pallor and swelling due to coagulative necrosis. The surrounding tissues are congested.

Healing

This takes place slowly. Capillaries and fibroblasts replace the necrotic tissue. Collagen is formed, the fibroblasts contract and this results in a depressed scar.

IMPORTANT SITES OF INFARCTION

The HEART, the LUNGS and the BRAIN are the most common sites. Less common are the SMALL INTESTINES (with serious effects) and the kidney and spleen (less serious).

IMPORTANT SITES OF INFARCTION

HEART (p.173)

Infarction is almost always due to coronary arterial thrombosis complicating atheroma.

Cardiac action is immediately upset, eddies form, the endocardium may be damaged and a thrombus forms on the inner surface of the infarcted area. The damage may extend to the external surface causing pericarditis.

If the patient survives, the infarct heals by fibrosis.

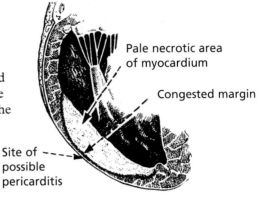

Pale necrotic area of myocardium

Congested margin

Site of possible pericarditis

BRAIN (p.176)

Infarcts are commonly due to thrombosis of diseased vessels or to embolism from the left heart or carotid arteries, e.g. MIDDLE CEREBRAL, posterior cerebral and basilar arteries.

The usual changes of infarction take place, but the necrosis is colliquative – **cerebral softening.**

Infarction may occur without arterial occlusion in severe, prolonged hypotension (shock).

Parts of the brain at the junction of arterial territories are affected (boundary zone or watershed infarcts) (see p.176).

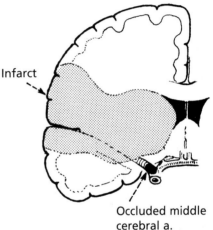

Infarct

Occluded middle cerebral a.

INTESTINE

Infarction may follow thrombosis of or embolisation to the mesenteric arteries. The sequence of changes usually seen in solid organs is altered by the effects of anastomoses and, in the later stages, by **bacterial invasion**.

Occlusion ⟶ Ischaemia ⟶ Collateral congestion ⟶ CONGESTION and HAEMORRHAGE

BACTERIAL INFECTION

GANGRENE

Area of infarction

NORMAL TISSUE FLUID CIRCULATION

There is a continuous interchange of fluid between blood and tissues. Some fluid enters the lymphatics before eventually returning to the blood stream. Two main forces operate pressure gradients controlling the fluid movement.

1. **Hydrostatic pressure**, i.e. capillary blood pressure (BP) encouraging the passage of fluid through the capillary wall, = 35 mm mercury.
2. **Protein osmotic pressure**, (OP), i.e. the plasma proteins encourage the retention of fluid in the capillaries to maintain osmotic equilibrium. This pressure is equivalent to 25 mm mercury.

At the arterial end the blood pressure is greater than the osmotic pressure and fluid is forced out of the capillary. The reverse is true at the venous end and fluid is attracted into the vessel.

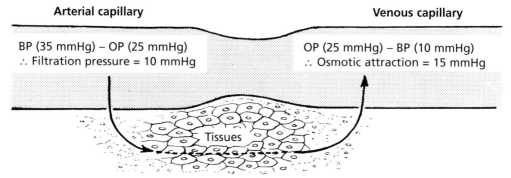

Arterial capillary

BP (35 mmHg) – OP (25 mmHg)
∴ Filtration pressure = 10 mmHg

Venous capillary

OP (25 mmHg) – BP (10 mmHg)
∴ Osmotic attraction = 15 mmHg

Tissues

A small amount of fluid enters lymphatics. This is partly the result of tissue pressure and partly due to osmotic attraction of proteins in the lymphatic system.

In addition to those forces operating at capillary level, there are other mechanisms which influence the movement of fluid within the body in a general manner.

1. **Fluid intake**
   Intake via the gut or parenterally may exceed the ability of the kidneys to eliminate water.
2. **Integrity of the kidneys**
   Damage to the renal parenchyma may diminish the elimination of fluid.
3. **Hormone activity**

ALDOSTERONE

Increases reabsorption of sodium by distal tubule ∴ retention of water

CARDIAC HORMONE [atrial natriuretic peptide (ANP)] antagonises aldosterone when there is any tendency to an increase in intracardiac pressure, e.g. in hypervolaemia. The hormone prevents reabsorption of sodium and therefore increases water excretion.

Increases reabsorption of water by distal and collecting tubules

ANTIDIURETIC HORMONE

OEDEMA

Oedema is an accumulation of excess fluid in the extravascular tissues. It can be local or generalised. A wide variety of causes of oedema can be explained by their effects on the pressure gradients described on the previous page.

DECREASE in blood osmotic pressure
(usually due to HYPOALBUMINAEMIA)

Common causes:
    Liver disease – deficient synthesis.
    Renal disease – protein loss.
    Starvation.

INCREASE in venous pressure
(hydrostatic pressure ↑)

Common causes
    Cardiac failure
    Venous obstruction in lower limbs.

NET INCREASE
in FLOW from CAPILLARY

Arterial capillary — Low albumin — hydrostatic pressure — Venous capillary

INCREASE in vascular permeability
(usual cause – INFLAMMATION
+ passage of albumin)

Loss of osmotic pressure

Causes:

Pressure by tumour

Parasites

LYMPHATIC
OBSTRUCTION
prevents local
lymph flow

More than one factor may apply:

E.g. **Cirrhosis** of liver (p.350)

Hypoalbuminaemia   Portal venous hypertension

Low osmotic pressure   Raised hydrostatic pressure

ASCITES
(oedema of peritoneum)

Cerebral (p.536) and pulmonary (p.186) oedema are life threatening and are dealt with separately.

SHOCK

Shock is a condition in which the vital functions of the body are depressed due to a severe and acute reduction in cardiac output and effective circulating blood volume. There is progressive cardiovascular collapse characterised by hypotension, hyperventilation and clouding of consciousness. Subsequently there is oliguria.

CAUSES

There are many causes, conveniently grouped under 4 main headings:

1. **HYPOVOLAEMIC (i.e. diminished blood volume)**
   Associated with:

   (a) **Trauma**
   (i) Severe haemorrhage – external or internal
   (ii) Severe injury – especially fractures of bones and crushing of tissues
   (iii) Burns – especially where extensive surface damage allows loss of a large amount of exudate.

   (b) **Dehydration** – in cases of severe vomiting, diarrhoea or diabetic ketoacidosis.

2. **CARDIOGENIC**
   Acute diseases of the heart – especially myocardial infarction – in which there is a sudden fall in cardiac output.

3. **SEPTIC** (bacteraemic, endotoxic)
   In serious bacterial infections (especially Gram-negative organisms, e.g. *E. coli*).

4. **ANAPHYLAXIS** – a severe immune hypersensitivity reaction (p.101).

EFFECTS

The loss of effective circulating blood causes tissue and cell damage and, at the same time, initiates reactive changes in the circulation.

These two mechanisms combine to cause the shock syndrome.

The main consequences of shock are:

1. Low cardiac output.
2. Hypotension.
3. Impaired tissue perfusion.
4. Cellular hypoxia.

SHOCK

REACTIVE CHANGES – EARLY STAGE

These changes are concerned with the maintenance of an adequate cerebral and coronary circulation and are effected by a redistribution of the blood in the body as a whole.

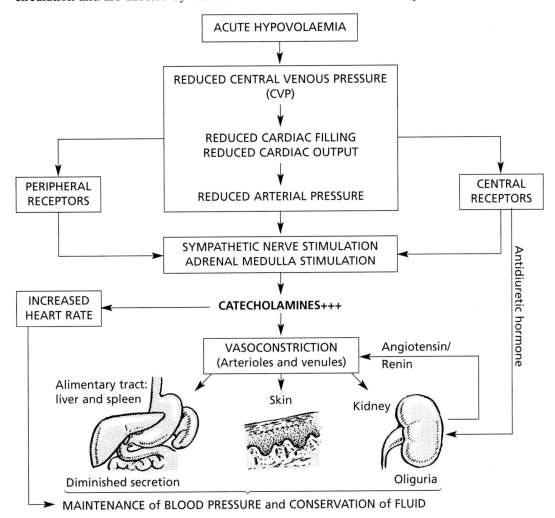

Note: Salt and water are retained due to aldosterone from the adrenal cortex.

At the same time, the circulations in the brain and heart are protected by autoregulatory mechanisms. They are not subject to the generalised vasoconstriction.

Instead:

DILATATION of CEREBRAL and CORONARY ARTERIES — maintains satisfactory flow down to blood pressures of 50–60 mmHg

If the loss of circulating fluid volume is great, the limits of the compensatory mechanism are exceeded and the patient goes into a state of severe shock.

169

SHOCK

ADVANCED STAGE (Decompensation)

The patient is now listless, pale and cold, the face is pinched and the lips blue. The pulse is rapid and weak and the blood pressure is low.

Conditions in Vascular bed

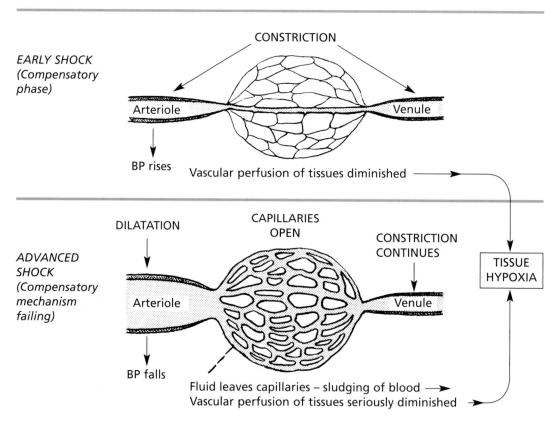

NORMAL

Capillary bed

Arteriole

Venule

Vascular perfusion in tissues in balance

EARLY SHOCK (Compensatory phase)

CONSTRICTION

Arteriole

Venule

BP rises

Vascular perfusion of tissues diminished

ADVANCED SHOCK (Compensatory mechanism failing)

DILATATION

CAPILLARIES OPEN

CONSTRICTION CONTINUES

TISSUE HYPOXIA

Arteriole

Venule

BP falls

Fluid leaves capillaries – sludging of blood

Vascular perfusion of tissues seriously diminished

SHOCK

ADVANCED STAGE *(continued)*

Thus, from the beginning of the shock process, all the body tissues, with the exception of the brain and the heart, suffer from hypoxia. This sets up vicious circles which aggravate the condition:

1.

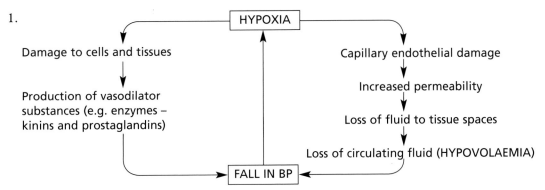

2. When the blood pressure falls below 50–60 mmHg, the autoregulatory control of the cerebral and coronary circulation fails. Serious damage to the brain (p.169) and heart may occur.

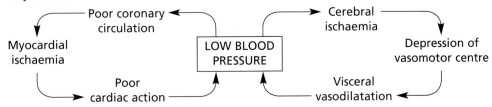

CHANGES IN THE BLOOD AND CELL METABOLISM
As well as these basic circulatory disturbances, important changes in the blood and cellular metabolism occur in shock.

Blood coagulation system

Acute hypoxia → Damaged endothelium → Coagulation cascade triggered → May proceed to formation of FIBRIN → Disseminated intravascular coagulation (DIC) syndrome

Cellular metabolism

Acute hypoxia → Inhibition of respiratory and energy utilisation systems e.g. ↓ATP

Pyruvic and lactic acid build up → METABOLIC ACIDOSIS

Glucose → HYPERGLYCAEMIA

Failure of 'sodium pump' → K+, Water, Na+ → AGGRAVATION of WATER and ELECTROLYTE DISTURBANCE

= SICK CELL SYNDROME

171

SHOCK

BACTERIAL SHOCK (ENDOTOXIC)

Causes

1. *Bacteria* – The GRAM-NEGATIVE BACTERIA, especially the coliform group, are the commonest causes, and the shock is caused by ENDOTOXIN (lipopolysaccharide). Other organisms can also produce shock e.g. staphylococci, streptococci and meningococci.

2. *Associated conditions*

(a) Serious primary bacterial infection e.g. septicaemia, peritonitis – potentiated by deficiency in immune status (p.64) and liver disease where detoxification is impaired.

(b) Bacterial shock may complicate pre-existing shock due to other causes, e.g. burns.

(c) Bacterial shock may complicate relatively trivial surgical procedures, especially in the gastrointestinal and urinary tracts in the presence of infection.

Mechanism

SHOCK in BURNS and SCALDS

Mechanism

1. The immediate reaction is NERVOUS – PAIN, and stimulation of afferent nerves, followed by

2. An INFLAMMATORY RESPONSE evoked by the burned tissues.

Massive exudation and
loss of PROTEIN-RICH fluid ⟶ HYPOVOLAEMIA ⟶ SHOCK
(sludging of blood in capillaries)

The mechanism explains why the SEVERITY of the shock is roughly proportional to the exuding SURFACE AREA and not to the depth of the burn.

Other factors are chemical mediators derived from the burned tissues.

3. Complications which aggravate the shock

(a) Infection: Burned ⟶ Susceptible to infection ⟶ BACTERIAL
tissues   esp. *Staph. aureus*,   SHOCK
             Strep. pyogenes, Gram-neg.   may be superimposed
             bacilli (e.g. Pseudomonas)

(b) Anaemia   Haemolysis of red cells at burned
              site and later if sludging is severe ⟶ ANAEMIA

SHOCK – INDIVIDUAL ORGANS

HEART
There are two main ways in which heart failure may be associated with shock.

1. In hypovolaemic and bacteraemic shock, heart failure is a *COMPLICATION*.

2. In cardiogenic shock, acute heart failure is the *CAUSE* of shock.

Mechanisms

Impaired respiratory function

Poor coronary circulation when BP falls to critical level

HYPOXIA

Chemicals released from damaged tissue (esp. pancreas) → Depresses activity of myocardium

Peripheral vasoconstriction → Increases strain on myocardium

may be focal necrosis

Mechanism

Acute fall in cardiac output

Tissue HYPOXIA

Further cardiac damage

SHOCK reaction

Note: Venous return to heart (CVP) not reduced
Fluid replacement not required

The commonest condition is myocardial infarction

LUNGS
Respiratory function is seriously disturbed in 2 main ways:

Circulatory changes in the lung (especially in septic/traumatic shock). These occur when compensatory mechanisms are failing. There is congestion and oedema, patchy to begin with but becoming confluent. At autopsy the lungs are heavy and wet. This condition is called 'shock lung' or adult respiratory distress syndrome (ARDS).

Early patchy changes throughout the lungs:

Alveoli full of red cells and fluid

Neutrophils are 'sequestered' in alveolar capillaries

SHOCK – INDIVIDUAL ORGANS

Circulatory changes in the lung *(continued)*

The mechanisms initiating and progressively augmenting the damage are complex and interacting:

1.

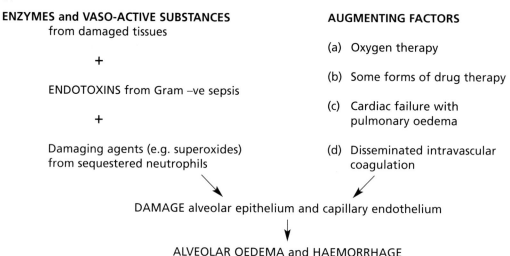

ENZYMES and VASO-ACTIVE SUBSTANCES
from damaged tissues

+

ENDOTOXINS from Gram –ve sepsis

+

Damaging agents (e.g. superoxides)
from sequestered neutrophils

AUGMENTING FACTORS

(a) Oxygen therapy

(b) Some forms of drug therapy

(c) Cardiac failure with
    pulmonary oedema

(d) Disseminated intravascular
    coagulation

DAMAGE alveolar epithelium and capillary endothelium

ALVEOLAR OEDEMA and HAEMORRHAGE

2. There may also be:

   (a) Patchy ALVEOLAR COLLAPSE and
   (b) Formation of HYALINE MEMBRANES

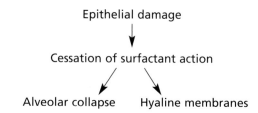

Epithelial damage

Cessation of surfactant action

Alveolar collapse   Hyaline membranes

3. If the patient survives, the organisation is followed by fibrosis: the end result in severe cases may be a combination of fibrosis, emphysema and bronchiolectasis.

SHOCK – INDIVIDUAL ORGANS

KIDNEYS

The excretory function of the kidneys is always disturbed in shock. This is due to the general circulatory collapse and hypotension, but it may be aggravated by the secretion of renin and angiotensin by the kidney, aldosterone by the adrenal and antidiuretic hormone by the posterior pituitary. These hormones are secreted in an attempt to retain fluid and restore the blood volume, but by inducing vasoconstriction they will tend to increase renal damage.

Mechanism

In such cases, at post mortem the kidneys are pale and swollen and the architectural markings are blurred

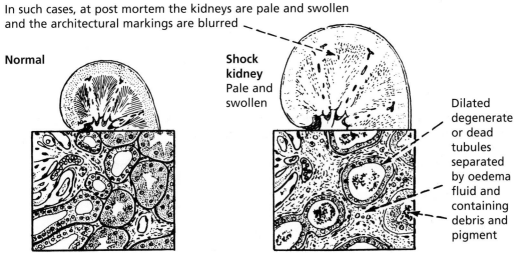

In even more severe shock the entire cortex may become necrotic (acute cortical necrosis).

SHOCK – INDIVIDUAL ORGANS

BRAIN

During the compensated phase of shock, relatively mild cerebral ischaemia is associated with changes in the state of consciousness. When the blood pressure falls to below 50–60 mmHg, the brain suffers serious ischaemic damage which can amount to actual infarction in the 'boundary zones' of the cerebral cortex (and cerebellum).

Boundary zone
(Sluggish circulation)

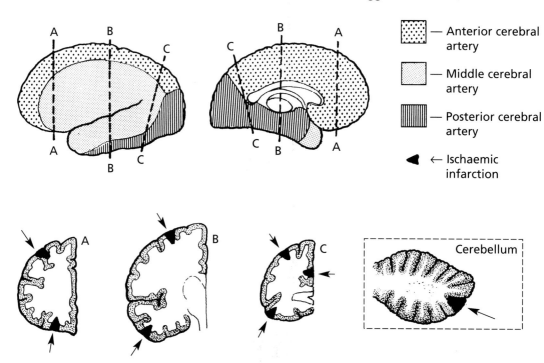

— Anterior cerebral artery

— Middle cerebral artery

— Posterior cerebral artery

◀ ← Ischaemic infarction

Cerebellum

There may also be more diffuse cerebral damage.

ALIMENTARY TRACT

The stomach and duodenum are particularly vulnerable – acute ulceration (Curling's or 'stress' ulcers) which may perforate is a serious complication of shock.

Ischaemia ⟶ necrosis ⟶ ulceration ⟶ perforation.

SHOCK – INDIVIDUAL ORGANS: OUTCOME

LIVER

The liver acinus is supplied by portal venous blood and hepatic arterial blood: in shock, Zone 3 of the hepatic acinus is vulnerable to anoxia (see p.338).

Shock ⟶ reduced arterial blood supply ⟶ ANOXIA.

May proceed to Zone 3 necrosis (i.e. microcirculatory periphery).

Note: In endotoxic shock, damage to cholangioles (cholangiolitis) may lead to cholestatic (obstructive) jaundice.

The OUTCOME of SHOCK

There are 3 possibilities, depending on several factors:

1. RECOVERY
   after convalescence,
   which may be long.

2. SURVIVAL
   with permanent damage
   to various organs.

3. DEATH

Factors favouring recovery	Factors favouring progression of shock
1 AVAILABILITY of EARLY TREATMENT of (a) the INITIATING CAUSE (b) the HYPOVOLAEMIA	1. DELAY in TREATMENT
	2. FAILURE to REMOVE the INITIATING CAUSE
2. Youth	3. Old age
3. Good general health	4. Poor general health
	5. Pre-existing cardiovascular and lung disease
	6. Onset of complications, esp. infection and organ damage

IRREVERSIBLE SHOCK

Theoretically, at some stage in its evolution, shock becomes irreversible due to the severity of vascular impairment and tissue damage. In medical practice, no certain indications are available as to when this point is reached. Measurements of blood pressure and central venous pressure indicate the severity of the vascular disturbance, but many severe cases respond to modern sophisticated treatment. However, the basic essentials remain the early transfusion of fluid and the removal of the original cause of the shock.

CARDIAC FUNCTION

The essential function of the heart is to provide the pumping action in a closed circulation.

Comparison with a simple mechanical system is useful and valid provided that it is appreciated that the animal system is infinitely more sophisticated with delicate built-in controls and balances which influence the inotropic (intrinsic contractility) activity of the heart.

DISTRIBUTION area

Priming chamber (atrium)
Ensures adequate volume for pump

DISTRIBUTION area (capillary bed)

Non-return valves

Pump
(ventricle)

CONTROL valves regulating flow

Electrical CONTROL of pump

Nervous CONTROL of cardiac rhythm and intrinsic conducting system

Many various nervous and hormonal (e.g. natriuretic peptides) controls of flow in capillary bed.

The pump is the essential part of the system: it has to be flexible to accommodate any changes required in the distribution side of the system.

In the animal circulation, very great reserves of ventricular muscle power are available to meet the wide range of metabolic activity required in the distribution area.

HEART FAILURE

Heart failure is very common and occurs when the ***ventricular muscle*** is incapable of maintaining a circulation adequate for the needs of the body (usually assessed in terms of O_2 requirement) – producing symptoms on exercise and at rest.

Although, in the last analysis, heart failure is the result of myocardial failure, it is useful to separate the situations in which heart failure occurs into two main groups:

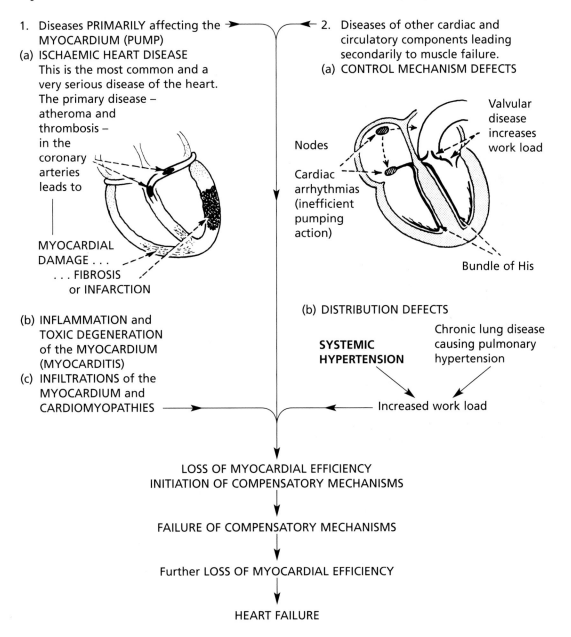

1. Diseases PRIMARILY affecting the MYOCARDIUM (PUMP)
   (a) ISCHAEMIC HEART DISEASE
   This is the most common and a very serious disease of the heart. The primary disease – atheroma and thrombosis – in the coronary arteries leads to

   MYOCARDIAL DAMAGE . . .
   . . . FIBROSIS
   or INFARCTION

   (b) INFLAMMATION and TOXIC DEGENERATION of the MYOCARDIUM (MYOCARDITIS)
   (c) INFILTRATIONS of the MYOCARDIUM and CARDIOMYOPATHIES

2. Diseases of other cardiac and circulatory components leading secondarily to muscle failure.
   (a) CONTROL MECHANISM DEFECTS

   Valvular disease increases work load

   Nodes

   Cardiac arrhythmias (inefficient pumping action)

   Bundle of His

   (b) DISTRIBUTION DEFECTS

   SYSTEMIC HYPERTENSION   Chronic lung disease causing pulmonary hypertension

   Increased work load

LOSS OF MYOCARDIAL EFFICIENCY
INITIATION OF COMPENSATORY MECHANISMS

FAILURE OF COMPENSATORY MECHANISMS

Further LOSS OF MYOCARDIAL EFFICIENCY

HEART FAILURE

HEART FAILURE

ACUTE and CHRONIC

Assignment to a particular category depends on the **suddenness of onset** and **rate of development.**

The causative diseases and the effects are different.

	Acute	Chronic
Time factors	Instantaneous Sudden (Hours – a few days)	Weeks Months
Causal diseases	(a) ACUTE CORONARY ARTERIAL OCCLUSION with infarction or arrhythmia (b) Pulmonary embolism (c) Severe malignant hypertension (d) Acute toxic myocarditis (e) Acute valve rupture	(a) Ischaemic heart disease (b) Hypertension (c) Chronic valvular diseases (d) Chronic lung diseases (e) Chronic severe anaemia
Effects	SUDDEN DEATH May be no time for compensatory mechanisms to be initiated. Acute pulmonary oedema is common. May be acute ischaemic effects in brain and kidneys.	Compensatory mechanisms fully developed – hypertrophy and dilatation. Chronic oedema and chronic venous congestion.

Acute and chronic failure are at opposite ends of a spectrum but may merge into each other in two ways.

HEART FAILURE

LEFT, RIGHT and COMBINED VENTRICULAR FAILURE

Since the initiating causes and symptoms are referable to either the left or right ventricle, from a clinical point of view it is convenient to consider heart failure as affecting one or other side of the heart.

The pulmonary circulation
  A low pressure system
  Systolic arterial pressure = 24 mmHg
  Pressure gradient, artery/vein = 8 mmHg

The systemic circulation
  A high pressure system
  Systolic arterial pressure = 120 mmHg
  Pressure gradient, artery/vein = 90 mmHg

Right ventricular mass and coronary blood supply < Left ventricular mass and coronary blood supply
1:4 (approx.)

MAIN CAUSES OF:

Right ventricular failure

Usually secondary to disease elsewhere, causing obstruction to pulmonary blood flow.

(a) LUNG DISEASE – – – –
    e.g. emphysema, fibrosis

(b) Some forms of cardiac valve disease, esp. MITRAL STENOSIS – – –

(c) Congenital heart disease

(d) As a CONSEQUENCE of LV FAILURE

Left ventricular failure

1. Muscle weakness –
   – – – ISCHAEMIC HEART DISEASE (due to coronary artery disease)

2. Excessive work load –
   – – – SYSTEMIC HYPERTENSION
   Since these causes are so prevalent, LV failure is much more common than RV failure.

Less common causes are:

Aortic valve disease

Mitral incompetence

Congenital heart disease.

However, it should be remembered that in health the function of both ventricles is closely integrated in that they have the same capacity, pump virtually synchronously and are constructed in such a way that layers of muscle fibres pass from one ventricle to the other.

This simplification of a very complex arrangement of muscle fibres shows layers passing between the two ventricles.

Superficial layer   RV ⎫
Deep layer   LV ⎬ ————
Superficial layer   LV ⎫
Deep layer   RV ⎬ - - - -

Thus the action of each ventricle is not isolated; it both influences and is influenced by the action of the other. Therefore, in addition to the combined failure which arises as a consequence of left ventricular failure, cases which begin and progress as combined failure are not uncommon.

HEART FAILURE

COMPENSATORY MECHANISMS

The myocardial reserve is provided by three main mechanisms:

1. **Increased rate of pumping**
2. **Dilatation** of the ventricular chambers ⎫ are designed to meet the normal
   (due to increased muscle stretching) ⎬ physiological reserves
3. **Hypertrophy** is added to these when the pumping load exceeds physiological levels.

In the heart under pathological strain, all three mechanisms are operative and can compensate for considerable derangement.

DILATATION

In physiological conditions, the volume of the ventricular chamber at the end of diastole (pre-load) directly influences the pumping force of the ventricular muscle thus:

The larger the chamber size ⎫
(i.e. the longer the initial fibre length ⎬ the greater the
and the greater the fibre stretch) ⎭ contracting force.

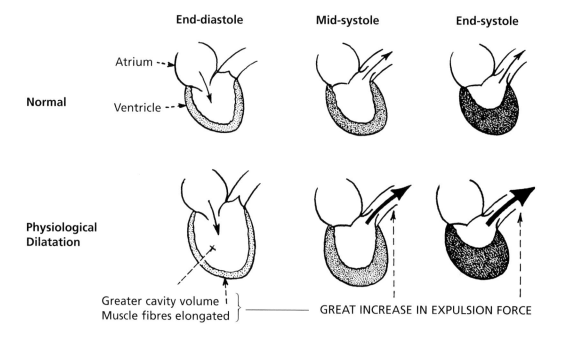

This physiological dilatation also compensates in cardiac disease.

HEART FAILURE

Compensatory Mechanisms – Dilatation *(continued)*

In cardiac disease, particularly in cases of valvular incompetence, dilatation which occurs passively to accommodate the regurgitated blood is an important factor.

Aortic valve incompetence is a good example:

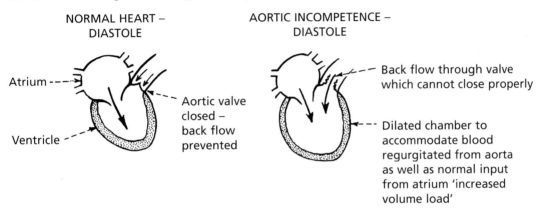

NORMAL HEART – DIASTOLE

Atrium

Ventricle

Aortic valve closed – back flow prevented

AORTIC INCOMPETENCE – DIASTOLE

Back flow through valve which cannot close properly

Dilated chamber to accommodate blood regurgitated from aorta as well as normal input from atrium 'increased volume load'

HYPERTROPHY involves an increase in muscle fibre bulk; the increased muscle mass is able to deal with a greater work load. In its pure form, hypertrophy is seen best in cases of increased pressure load.

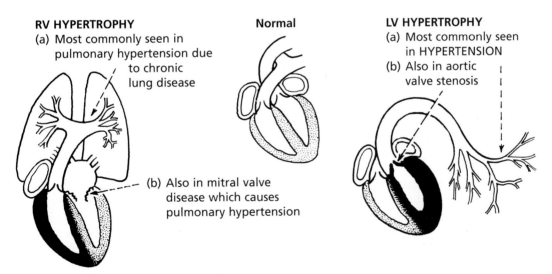

RV HYPERTROPHY
(a) Most commonly seen in pulmonary hypertension due to chronic lung disease

(b) Also in mitral valve disease which causes pulmonary hypertension

Normal

LV HYPERTROPHY
(a) Most commonly seen in HYPERTENSION
(b) Also in aortic valve stenosis

At first the blood supply to the hypertrophied muscle increases to meet the increased metabolic requirements. Later, severe hypertrophy leads to hypoxia and reduced function.

HEART FAILURE

FAILURE of COMPENSATORY MECHANISMS

The increased efficiency derived from all three mechanisms is limited, and beyond this limit serious deficiency ensues – HEART FAILURE.

Beyond the critical limit:

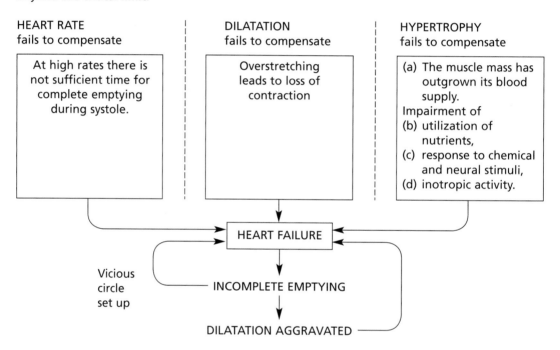

HEART RATE fails to compensate	DILATATION fails to compensate	HYPERTROPHY fails to compensate
At high rates there is not sufficient time for complete emptying during systole.	Overstretching leads to loss of contraction	(a) The muscle mass has outgrown its blood supply. Impairment of (b) utilization of nutrients, (c) response to chemical and neural stimuli, (d) inotropic activity.

HEART FAILURE

Vicious circle set up

INCOMPLETE EMPTYING

DILATATION AGGRAVATED

Thus in most cases of heart failure there is CARDIAC ENLARGEMENT due usually to a combination of hypertrophy and dilatation.

The **effects** and **symptoms** of heart failure are seen in the peripheral organs and are due to HYPOXIA and VENOUS CONGESTION.

(a) In the chronic forms of heart failure, the **weakness and fatigue** which are such common symptoms are probably effects mainly of **hypoxia**, but damage to organs is more difficult to define since the effects of venous congestion and water retention are added.

(b) Venous congestion and oedema are important.
Breathlessness (dyspnoea) is almost a constant concommitant of cardiac failure and is essentially due to venous congestion and fluid retention within the lungs.
In severe failure, particularly when bed rest is obligatory, *hypostatic pneumonia* and *pulmonary embolism* (from leg vein thrombosis) may be serious and terminal complications.

EFFECTS OF HEART FAILURE

Left ventricular failure is the initiating event in most cases of combined failure.

The main effects are the results of:
  (a) low output
  (b) 'backward' pressure

*   INCREASE IN PULMONARY ARTERIAL PRESSURE – partly due to congestion; partly due to reflex nerve action

Dyspnoea is a main symptom

Low output to lungs – not usually significant unless the RV failure is a sequel to LV failure when low output contributes to deficient oxygenation of blood.

Pulmonary oedema

Congestion of pulmonary veins and capillaries

Overfilling of left atrium

RA   LA

RV   LV

RV FAILURE

LV FAILURE

Low output

Overfilling of:
  RIGHT ATRIUM
  SYSTEMIC VEINS and
  CAPILLARIES

CHRONIC VENOUS CONGESTION and OEDEMA

Anoxia in systemic circulation ⟶ Demand for oxygen

Cyanosis is the result of excess reduced haemoglobin in capillaries and venules.

* The increase in pulmonary arterial pressure is important because in most cases of chronic LV failure it eventually leads to RV failure (combined failure).

ACUTE PULMONARY OEDEMA

In **acute left ventricular failure**, accumulation of fluid results in dyspnoea and hypoxaemia.

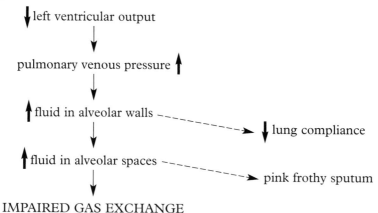

↓left ventricular output

↓

pulmonary venous pressure ↑

↓

↑fluid in alveolar walls - - - - - - - - → ↓lung compliance

↓

↑fluid in alveolar spaces - - - - - - - - → pink frothy sputum

↓

IMPAIRED GAS EXCHANGE

CHRONIC VENOUS CONGESTION of the LUNGS

The results from chronic combined (congestive) failure and/or chronic left ventricular failure:

The lungs are bulky, congested and brownish in colour.

Cardiac failure

Hypoxia

Pulmonary venous engorgement

Hyperventilation

Pulmonary oedema

Alveolar haemorrhage

Breakdown of haemoglobin to haemosiderin and bilirubin

Poorly supported engorged alveolar capillaries

Escape of red cells

Phagocytes ('heart failure cells') full of haemosiderin migrate into the interstitial tissue and to the local lymph glands. This accounts for the firm, tough consistency and brown colour (brown induration).

HEART FAILURE

CHRONIC VENOUS CONGESTION

Congestion of the systemic venous circulation is a result of right heart failure whether secondary to left heart failure or lung disease (cor pulmonale).

The basic mechanism is:

CHRONIC CARDIAC FAILURE

REDUCED left ventricular output
+ MITRAL valve incompetence

chronic | PULMONARY VENOUS CONGESTION

+ increased pulmonary arterial pressure

LUNG DISEASE

increased pulmonary vascular resistance

RIGHT VENTRICULAR FAILURE

TRICUSPID valve incompetence

SYSTEMIC VENOUS CONGESTION

Distension of neck veins

Hepatic congestion

Splenic congestion

Intestinal congestion

Renal congestion

Distension leg veins

Ankle oedema

Pleural effusion is also a common effect (see p.283).

HEART FAILURE

CHRONIC VENOUS CONGESTION *(continued)*

Because of the increase in venous blood, the organs become swollen and purplish. With long continued over-distension, the walls of the venules show reactive thickening and there is mild interstitial fibrosis of the organs, giving them a very firm consistency. These changes are seen typically in the kidney and spleen.

The **liver** shows striking changes: Mechanical distension of the veins causes enlargement of the liver so that it can be felt below the costal margin.

The parenchymal cells furthest from the arterial blood supply, i.e. around the hepatic venules, undergo degeneration with atrophy and ultimately disappear. Cells nearer the arteries show an accumulation of fat.

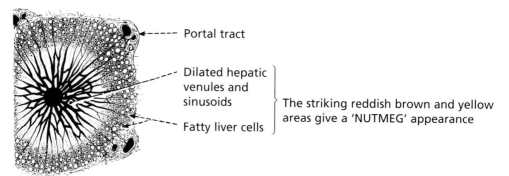

Portal tract

Dilated hepatic venules and sinusoids

Fatty liver cells

The striking reddish brown and yellow areas give a 'NUTMEG' appearance

FLUID RETENTION

This is related to the REDUCED OUTPUT from the LEFT VENTRICLE: the mechanism involves retention of sodium and water.

Reduced LV output ⟶ renin released ⟶ angiotensin is activated

Reduced KIDNEY perfusion | adrenal cortex stimulated

Fall in glomerular filtration | aldosterone secreted

RETENTION of SODIUM and WATER

contributes to OEDEMA – for which there are 2 main mechanisms in heart failure:

(1) **Overfilling of venules**

Increased hydrostatic pressure

(2) **Retention of water and electrolytes**

Increased total body fluid

Oedema of dependent parts where pressure is greatest

Pleural effusion (p.283) and ascites (p.167) are also common effects of fluid retention in congestive cardiac failure.

HIGH OUTPUT CARDIAC FAILURE

LOW and HIGH OUTPUT FAILURE

By definition, in cardiac failure, output is low in respect of body requirements, and in most cases this output is lower than the usual normal output. Such cases are called **Low Output type.**

In a few conditions, the cardiac failure complicates a pre-existing state in which the output before failure was greater than normal. In these cases, the output is not sufficient to meet the body requirements but may still be higher than the normal. Such cases are called **High Output type.**

Low Output Failure

Normal — 5 l/min

Failure — 3 l/min

High Output Failure

Pre-existing high output to meet body requirements — 9 l/min

Failure — 7 l/min

Output still greater than normal

Causes

The common types of failure:

HYPERTENSIVE
ISCHAEMIC HEART DISEASE
VALVULAR HEART DISEASE
MYOCARDITIS

Diseases associated with increased blood volume:

CHRONIC ANAEMIA
ARTERIOVENOUS SHUNTING
HYPERTHYROIDISM
SEVERE ANAEMIA.

In both types of failure, venous overfilling is an important sign, but in high output failure venous overfilling is usually present before failure ensues, reflecting the increased blood volume.

DISEASES OF ARTERIES – ARTERIOSCLEROSIS

Arterial diseases are very common and are important because of their serious effects, especially on the heart and brain.

Normal age related vascular changes:

ARTERIOSCLEROSIS (hardening of the arteries)

This is a generalised degeneration of the specialised muscle and elastic tissue of the media, and replacement by fibrous tissue, proteoglycan and calcium salts. There is also intimal proliferation.

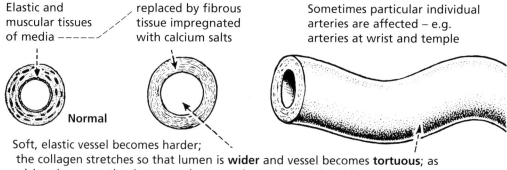

Elastic and muscular tissues of media ----

replaced by fibrous tissue impregnated with calcium salts

Sometimes particular individual arteries are affected – e.g. arteries at wrist and temple

Normal

Soft, elastic vessel becomes harder; the collagen stretches so that lumen is **wider** and vessel becomes **tortuous**; as calcium impregnation increases the artery becomes very hard (pipe stem).

HYALINE ARTERIOLOSCLEROSIS affects the small branches of the arterial system (arterioles) – especially in the kidney.

Muscle replaced by hyaline material in media and intima

The arterioles also become tortuous

Normal

This is due to entry of blood plasma under the endothelium with protein deposition; gradual replacement by collagen occurs. The process is called **plasmatic vasculosis**.

Note that the lumen is usually narrowed so that ischaemia may be an important complication.

Note: Arteriosclerosis is aggravated by HYPERTENSION and DIABETES MELLITUS.

In a variant of arteriosclerosis (Monckeberg), seen in the very elderly, calcium salts are very heavily deposited in the media particularly of the leg arteries. The X-ray appearances are striking but there is no significant loss of lumen unless atheroma co-exists or is superimposed.

ATHEROMA (ATHEROSCLEROSIS)

Atheroma is a common disease in Westernised countries, of gradual onset but progressive. It is commonly seen in the middle aged and elderly but the earliest changes are present in adolescents. It is often asymptomatic but it may cause serious disease or death from complicating thrombosis. The lesions represent patchy deposition of lipid within plaques deep in the intima. The evolution of the disease is described in 3 phases.

(Vessel opened longitudinally)

EARLY PROLIFERATIVE PHASE

Cross section

Microscopic appearances

Intima

Proliferated smooth muscle cells containing lipid droplets

Normal media

Pale yellow streaks slightly raised above surrounding intima

Internal elastic lamina

PROGRESSING PHASE

Cap Core

Hyaline fibrous tissue

Lipid pool part extracellular with CHOLESTEROL crystals: foam cells and lymphocytes

Raised yellow plaques

Reduction of lumen

Atrophic media

Necrotic smooth muscle cells

LATE ULCERATIVE PHASE

Media atrophied and thin and fibrous

Degeneration of elastic lamina

Capillary vessels in fibrous plaque susceptible to rupture and haemorrhage (see p.200).

Raised irregular rough ulcerated plaques. Partly calcified with thrombus material on surface

Branch vessel orifice narrowed and distorted

Lumen narrowed and distorted

Partly calcified lipid.

191

ATHEROMA – COMPLICATIONS

Fibrosis in the intima and media weaken the wall and may lead to aneurysm formation (see p.230), but the most important complication of atheroma is THROMBOSIS.

Local factors at the site of the atheromatous plaque are important:

1. Intimal roughening or distortion with eddying of flow
2. Thin, easily damaged intimal surface
3. Rupture of new capillaries in plaque with haemorrhage into the plaque

In addition, general factors influencing blood coagulability are important, e.g. smoking affecting vessel contractility and platelet function.

Results

(1) Medium and small arteries – coronaries, cerebrals

Usually occlusion by red thrombus

Atheromatous plaque

(2) Larger arteries – aorta, carotids. Lumen usually too large to be completely occluded

Paler platelet thrombus on intimal surface

Small emboli may be detached – esp. to kidney, legs and brain.

The important sites of atheroma and the effects due to complications are:

CEREBRALS (Circle of Willis or branches)
CAROTIDS
— **Acute local ischaemia** – cerebral infarction (stroke). Chronic ischaemia of brain – multi-infarct dementia

CORONARIES ——————— **Acute infarction.**
Chronic ischaemia of myocardium with fibrosis

ABDOMINAL AORTA ——— **Aneurysm** – embolism to legs

RENAL ARTERIES ——— **Chronic ischaemia of kidneys**

Visceral arteries ——————— Acute or chronic ischaemia of bowel

Lower limb arteries ——— With severe atheroma, chronic ischaemia with
(Upper limb arteries claudication occurs and gangrene may develop.
are rarely affected)

In severe cases of atheroma, most of these sites may be affected, but not uncommonly, one particular artery may be much more severely damaged than the others, e.g. coronaries, cerebrals.

ATHEROMA – AETIOLOGY

The cause of atheroma is complex and multifactorial. There are many risk factors, most of which are illustrated in the classical victim – the HEAVY SMOKING, HYPERTENSIVE, OBESE, SEDENTARY MALE.

The various risk factors exponentially increase with AGE. They are considered in 3 groups:

1. ENDOGENOUS
  (a) *SEX* – male > female.
  (b) *HEREDITY*
    (i) Family history of premature heart disease.
    (ii) Familial hyperlipidaemias
  Increased plasma cholesterol is an important risk factor and the ratio of low density lipoprotein (LDL) to high density lipoprotein (HDL) especially, so: LDL↑ risk↑↑
             HDL↑ risk↓

2. ENVIRONMENTAL
  (a) *SMOKING*
  (b) *DIET* – rich in saturated fats and cholesterol and low in fruit and vegetables.
  (c) Lack of exercise
  (d) Low socio-economic group status.

3. DISEASES
  (a) *HYPERTENSION*
  (b) Hyperlipidaemia
  (c) Diabetes Mellitus
  (d) Severe obesity.
  (e) Increased fibrinogen levels.

Modification of some of these risk factors has led to a fall in incidence especially in higher socio-economic groups. Avoiding smoking, dietary improvement and exercise seem most important, while treating raised cholesterol with statins is now widely used.

Endothelial Damage
There is a preferential distribution of lesions, e.g. arch of aorta, coronary arteries, cerebral arteries, carotids, abdominal aorta.
This is determined by local mechanical stresses which potentiate local endothelial damage.

e.g. **Areas of lateral and shearing stresses and turbulence** at acute bends or branching – in aorta, carotids, abdominal aortic branches.

Atheroma

e.g. **Poor support**

Coronary artery

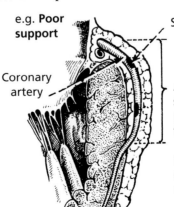

Severe atheroma

Artery poorly supported by pericardial tissues

Similarly in cerebral arteries, mesenterics, etc.

193

ATHEROMA – AETIOLOGY AND PROGRESSION

Atheroma is now regarded as an inflammatory disease of the arterial wall.

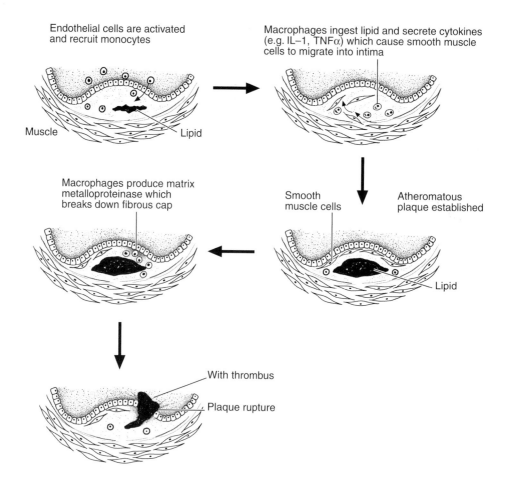

Endothelial cells are activated and recruit monocytes

Muscle

Lipid

Macrophages ingest lipid and secrete cytokines (e.g. IL–1, TNFα) which cause smooth muscle cells to migrate into intima

Smooth muscle cells

Atheromatous plaque established

Lipid

Macrophages produce matrix metalloproteinase which breaks down fibrous cap

With thrombus

Plaque rupture

HYPERTENSION

High blood pressure (BP) is important because it increases the risk of cardiovascular disease, especially:

1. **Left Ventricular Hypertrophy** ⎫ ———————➤ Cardiac failure.
2. **Ischaemic Heart Disease** ⎭ ———————➤ Sudden death.
3. **Stroke** – Cerebral haemorrhage or Infarction.

Blood pressure is a continuous variable within the population. It is determined essentially by 2 variables:

BLOOD PRESSURE = CARDIAC OUTPUT × TOTAL PERIPHERAL RESISTANCE.

Mechanisms of normal maintenance of BP and the effect of age

The systolic pressure is governed by (a) cardiac action (b) the ELASTICITY and DISTENSIBILITY of the CONDUCTING ARTERIES.	Increasing AGE is normally associated with ARTERIOSCLEROSIS – loss of distensibility ⟶ ∴ Increased SYSTOLIC pressure
The diastolic pressure is maintained by the **RESISTANCE (TONE)** of arterioles (a subsidiary factor is blood viscosity)	ARTERIOLOSCLEROSIS – increased resistance ⟶ ∴ Increased DIASTOLIC pressure

Note: Diastolic pressure tends to fall after the 7th decade as cardiac output falls.

Because of the wide range in the normal population, the definition of high BP is arbitrary. The risk of complications progressively increases with BP, including within the normal range. The levels of **systolic** and **diastolic** pressure are both risk factors.

Systolic BP > 160 mmHg and Diastolic BP > 95 are generally accepted as **Hypertension**.

Modern therapy is effective in lowering BP. The decision whether or not to treat depends on the level of BP and the presence of other risk factors for cardiovascular disease.

HYPERTENSION

Aetiology

The following diagram illustrates the physiological mechanisms controlling Blood Pressure. They are presented in 2 groups but are complex and interconnected with feed-back controls.

1. **Autonomic Nervous System**

    (a) External environment
    (b) Internal environment
       e.g. baroreceptors

2. **Hormones**

    (a) Pituitary/Adrenal   (b) Renal

Note: **Nitric oxide** (NO) and **Endothelin** are both produced physiologically by endothelial cells. They have powerful and opposite effects.

    Nitric oxide ———— vasodilatation (short-acting).
    Endothelin ———— vasoconstriction (long-acting).

Their role in hypertension is not yet clear.

HYPERTENSION – ESSENTIAL AND SECONDARY

ESSENTIAL HYPERTENSION

In 95% of cases of hypertension no obvious cause is found – this is ESSENTIAL hypertension – (a diagnosis of exclusion).

A number of aetiological factors may be implicated:
1. Genetic predisposition – polygenic inheritance.
2. Racial e.g. black > white.
3. Sodium homeostasis: increased **salt intake.**
4. Lack of exercise.

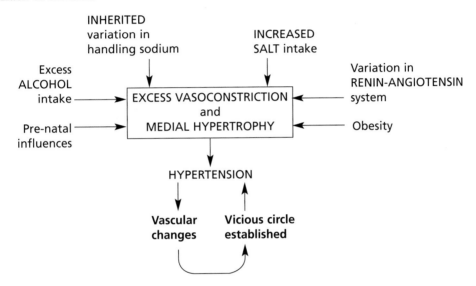

SECONDARY HYPERTENSION

5% of hypertension is a complication of other diseases. They are broadly classified as:

(a) *Kidney diseases* e.g. chronic renal failure, renal artery stenosis, polycystic kidneys. The mechanism is usually renal ischaemia with activation of the renin-angiotensin system.

(b) *Endocrine disorders* – Cushing's syndrome – corticosteroid excess;
Conn's syndrome – aldosterone excess;
Phaeochromocytoma – catecholamine excess.

(c) *Coarctation of aorta* – aortic narrowing → renal perfusion impaired
→ renin-angiotensin activation.

(d) *Eclampsia* and pre-eclampsia in pregnancy.

(e) *Drugs* e.g. steroids: oral contraceptives.

HYPERTENSION – ESSENTIAL AND SECONDARY

CLASSIFICATION – BENIGN AND MALIGNANT

In the classification of hypertension, in addition to the aetiology, two other main factors are considered.

(1) Rate of Progress	(2) Height and rapidity of rise of the BP	
Chronic – over many years	**+** Usually only mild or moderate very slow rise. (*Note:* The very old may have considerably higher BP without ill-effects)	**Benign –** during long course but eventually may have serious effects
Rapid (acute) – months or 1–2 years	**+** Usually very high and rapidly rising BP, e.g. 120 + diastolic	**Malignant –** serious damaging effects

Summary   Essential (95%)   Secondary (5%)

Benign   or   Malignant   Benign   Malignant

COMPARISON of BENIGN and MALIGNANT HYPERTENSION

	Benign	Malignant
Aetiology	Usually ESSENTIAL If secondary, commonly of endocrine type	A few cases arise out of benign essential. Majority are SECONDARY TO RENAL DISEASE
Age	Begins younger than 45 years but is prolonged into 6 and 7 decades	Young adults 25–35 years
Sex	Female > Male	Female = Male
Prevalence	VERY COMMON – at least 15% of population in Western societies	Rare
Course	VERY SLOW – many years	RAPID – months to 1–2 years
Blood pressure	Diastolic 90–120 mmHg Very slow rise	120+ Rapid rise

HYPERTENSION

COMPARISON of BENIGN and MALIGNANT HYPERTENSION *(continued)*

VASCULAR CHANGES

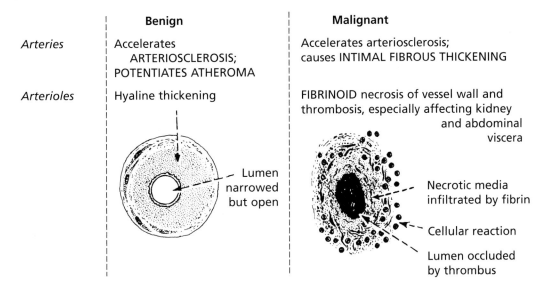

	Benign	**Malignant**
Arteries	Accelerates ARTERIOSCLEROSIS; POTENTIATES ATHEROMA	Accelerates arteriosclerosis; causes INTIMAL FIBROUS THICKENING
Arterioles	Hyaline thickening	FIBRINOID necrosis of vessel wall and thrombosis, especially affecting kidney and abdominal viscera

Benign diagram labels: Lumen narrowed but open

Malignant diagram labels: Necrotic media infiltrated by fibrin; Cellular reaction; Lumen occluded by thrombus

EFFECTS and MAIN COMPLICATIONS in VARIOUS ORGANS

Heart	Hypertrophy of left ventricle	Hypertrophy of left ventricle ± focal myocardial necrosis
Heart failure	Common	Acute heart failure
Cerebral haemorrhage	Due to rupture of damaged artery	Encephalopathy (fits and loss of consciousness) due to cerebral oedema and haemorrhage.
Kidney	Varying degrees of NEPHROSCLEROSIS but usually *not* serious.	Severe renal damage – death in uraemia
Eyes	Arterial narrowing – retinal exudation.	Papilloedema; arterial narrowing; haemorrhage and exudates.

The effects and complications are proportional to the height of the blood pressure. Therefore drug treatment which lowers the BP lowers the incidence of complications, but the diseased vessels do not return to normal and organ perfusion may be inadequate at levels of BP which would usually be considered physiological.

Note: Modern drug therapy has greatly reduced the morbidity and mortality from malignant hypertension.

ISCHAEMIC HEART DISEASE

Cardiac ischaemia is the major cause of death in affluent Western societies. It is almost always due to **atheroma** of the **coronary arteries** causing narrowing or occlusion. The effects may be of sudden or gradual onset.

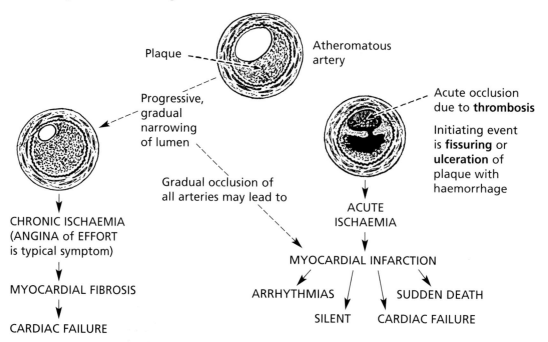

Distribution of atheromatous plaques

(1) There may be only a few plaques, but because the sites of predilection are in the proximal parts of the arteries (usually within 3 cm of the origin from the aorta), the effects of occlusion are serious.

or (2) Very numerous plaques throughout the arborisation on the surface of the heart. *Note:* The small terminal arteries penetrating the myocardium are usually not affected

(3) any combination of (1) and (2).

The site of ischaemic damage usually represents the distribution area of the diseased arterial branch.

MYOCARDIAL INFARCTION

REGIONAL INFARCTION

90% of cardiac infarcts are regional in distribution. The 3 common ones are illustrated in order of frequency.

(1) LEFT CORONARY ARTERY – ANTERIOR DESCENDING BRANCH

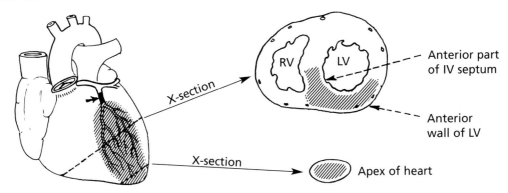

(2) RIGHT CORONARY ARTERY

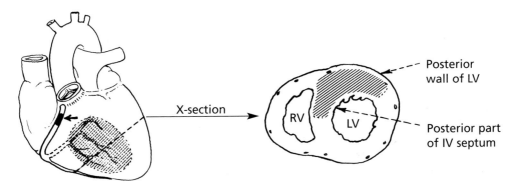

(3) LEFT CORONARY ARTERY – CIRCUMFLEX BRANCH

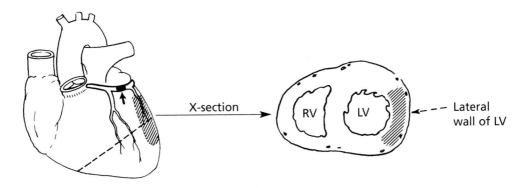

MYOCARDIAL INFARCTION

EXTENT OF DAMAGE

This depends on:

1. The inherited individual anatomical variation in distribution area, e.g. the calibres of the right coronary artery and the circumflex branch of the left coronary artery show considerable variation and are usually inversely related.

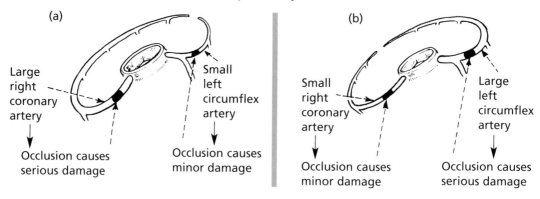

2. The efficiency of any anastomosis in the deprived distribution area. Gradual narrowing of an artery allows time for increased anastomosis to the deprived distribution area to develop, and so old age tends to be associated with improved anastomoses.

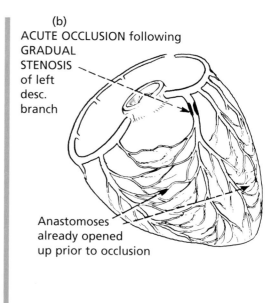

MYOCARDIAL INFARCTION

GLOBAL OR CIRCUMFERENTIAL SUBENDOCARDIAL INFARCTION

This type is not uncommon. It occurs round the circumference of the left ventricle under the endocardium in cases of severe stenosis of all the coronary arteries and is often due to hypotension. The coronaries are usually not thrombosed.

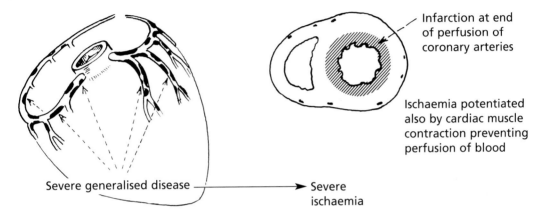

Infarction at end of perfusion of coronary arteries

Ischaemia potentiated also by cardiac muscle contraction preventing perfusion of blood

Severe generalised disease ⟶ Severe ischaemia

Global infarction is a serious condition which is not always detected by ECG.

MICROSCOPIC FOCAL INFARCTION

This is necrosis of single or small groups of muscle fibres at the margins of areas of myocardium previously damaged by ischaemia and is a component of progressive chronic ischaemia.

The **time scale** of the pathological changes following acute infarction is illustrated.

1. During the first 24 hours changes are minimal.

Time			
0–24 hrs	Minimal change	Slight blotchiness (congestion and pallor) of infarcted area	Slight separation of fibres; slight increase of leucocytes between fibres; slight disturbance of cell cytoplasm *Normal Affected fibres*

203

MYOCARDIAL INFARCTION

Time			
24 hrs –3 days	Definite changes in dead muscle	Dead muscle, paler yellow *Note:* Usually a thin layer of healthy muscle under the endocardium 	Dead muscle fibres have lost striations and nuclei; cytoplasm glassy pink (H & E staining); capillary congestion at margin; neutrophils and macrophages increasing in number
3–10 days	Healing (organisation) commencing	Margin of congestion (redness) appearing round dead muscle and resorption of muscle becoming visible at the edges 	Muscle fibres splitting up and being resorbed; granulation tissue at edges; neutrophils still present
Weeks – months	Scar tissue – healing complete	White fibrous tissue 	Scar tissue – may be occasional surviving muscle fibres embedded

These changes represent the uncomplicated continuous process of healing. However, complications are frequent, producing serious, often fatal, effects.

MYOCARDIAL INFARCTION

Time	COMPLICATIONS
Minutes, hours	**1. ARRHYTHMIAS** (a) *Ventricular fibrillation*, i.e. cardiac arrest (especially liable at onset of infarction and during first few days). (b) *Block of impulse* conduction in Bundle of His and/or its branches – usually causes slowing of ventricular rhythm or upsets the balance of ventricular contraction. **2. CARDIAC FAILURE** **3. CARDIOGENIC SHOCK** Associated with large infarcts.
Days	**4. THROMBOTIC COMPLICATIONS** **(a) MURAL THROMBOSIS** Thrombus may form on endocardium over site of infarction: potential EMBOLISM to Brain Intestine Kidney Lower limbs **(b) ATRIAL THROMBOSIS** Thrombus may form in atrial appendages – especially if atrial rhythm is disturbed **(c) LEG VEIN THROMBOSIS** Due to recumbancy and venous stasis → Pulmonary embolism may be FATAL

MYOCARDIAL INFARCTION

Time	COMPLICATIONS *(continued)*
3–14 days	5. **RUPTURE OF HEART** Potentiated by: (a) infarction of whole wall thickness (b) unusual increased neutrophil activity before organisation is established → softening of dead muscle (myomalacia cordis) **Sites affected and results** (i) *MURAL MYOCARDIUM* Infarct Blood passing through ventricular wall into pericardial sac Pericardial sac is distended with blood (tamponade); heart action impeded – DEATH (ii) *PAPILLARY MUSCLE* Infarct Rupture of muscle Sudden incompetence of mitral valve. Serious aggravation of cardiac pumping load; acute failure → often DEATH (iii) *INTERVENTRICULAR SEPTUM* Infarct Rupture with interventricular communication ⟶ Rapid combined ventricular failure DEATH

MYOCARDIAL INFARCTION

Time	COMPLICATIONS *(continued)*
3–14 days	6. **ACUTE PERICARDITIS** This may complicate the infarct.
Weeks	7. **CHRONIC HEART FAILURE** At the stage of fibrosis, chronic heart failure may supervene (+ ANGINA PECTORIS). 8. **DRESSLER'S SYNDROME** An auto-immune disorder with pericarditis and pleurisy, related to the release of antigens from damaged heart muscle.
Months	9. **CARDIAC ANEURYSM** Laminated mural thrombus may cause embolism Gradual stretching of thin fibrous scar Bulging aneurysm formed Chronic heart failure
At any time	10. **RECURRENCE OF INFARCTION** Due to further thrombotic occlusion of a coronary arterial branch.

CHRONIC ISCHAEMIC HEART DISEASE

The basic pathological process is replacement of the myocardial fibres by fibrous tissue which is laid down in two main ways depending on whether the coronary insufficiency is due to severe generalised stenosis or is the result of local infarction following thrombosis.

(1) In severe generalised coronary artery disease

(2) The coronary thrombosis, infarction, healing sequence

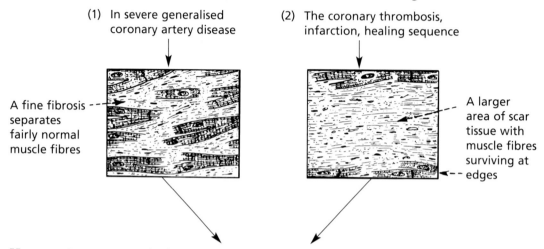

A fine fibrosis separates fairly normal muscle fibres

A larger area of scar tissue with muscle fibres surviving at edges

However, in many cases both mechanisms are present and lesions merge indistinguishably into each other.

Myocardial fibrosis tends to be progressive, reflecting the progression of the atheromatous narrowing of the arteries.

Myocardial hypertrophy from any cause is an important contributory factor in many cases.

Greater muscle mass ⟶ Greater blood supply required ⟶ Greater susceptibility to ischaemic damage

Thus hypertension, which causes left ventricular hypertrophy, is an important background factor.

ISCHAEMIC HEART DISEASE

CLINICAL, LABORATORY and ELECTROCARDIOGRAPH (ECG) EFFECTS

Cardiac Pain is caused by muscle ischaemia as follows:

It occurs in 3 main circumstances:

1. **In acute infarction** – especially in the early phases before necrosis is complete. It is usually a continuous pain – not relieved by rest.
2. **In chronic myocardial ischaemia without infarction,** e.g. ANGINA PECTORIS – episodes of cardiac pain brought on by temporary ischaemia.

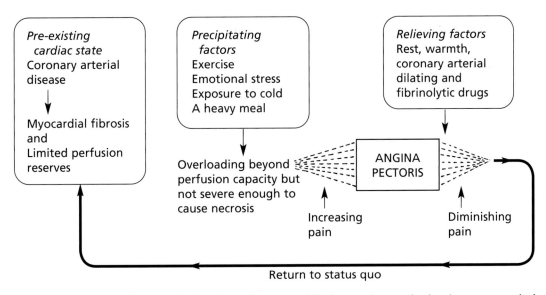

3. *Note:* The term Crescendo Angina refers to rapidly increasing anginal pain over a period of a few days without treatment, usually leading to myocardial infarction. It is due to developing thrombus or plaque rupture.

ISCHAEMIC HEART DISEASE

CLINICAL, LABORATORY and ECG EFFECTS *(continued)*

The blood in myocardial infarction

Leucocytosis

$12–15\,000/mm^3$
lasting not more
than one week

Neutrophils mobilised
from marrow by
chemotaxis of necrotic muscle

Enzyme changes

Enzymes liberated from necrotic muscle.
Two commonly used in diagnosis:

1. Troponin, within 12 hours of onset.
2. Myocardial creatine kinase (CKMB) is specific for cardiac muscle. Peak in 24 hours; falls in 72 hours.

These changes do not occur in angina pectoris since by definition necrosis has not occurred.

The Electrocardiogram (ECG)

The ventricular changes in ischaemia are reflected in the portion of ECG representing ventricular activity, i.e. the QRST complex. During excitation, contraction and restitution, the electrical potentials across the membranes of necrotic muscle fibres are strikingly different from healthy muscle. The ECG changes may be subtle but three common patterns are illustrated.

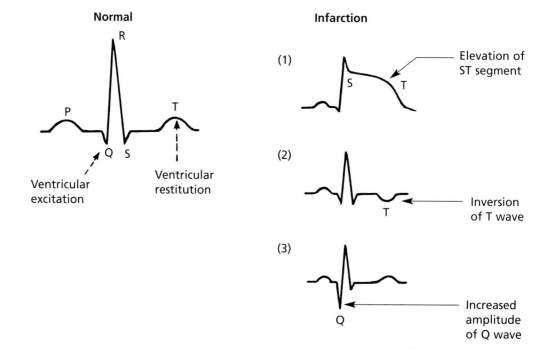

Normal

R

P   T

Q S

Ventricular
excitation

Ventricular
restitution

Infarction

(1) Elevation of ST segment

S   T

(2) Inversion of T wave

T

(3) Increased amplitude of Q wave

Q

MISCELLANEOUS AFFECTIONS OF THE MYOCARDIUM

MYOCARDITIS

Inflammation of the myocardium is rare but may be caused by a variety of agents. The process is usually acute and may be generalised, regional or focal; most patients have chest pain but recover well: less commonly heart failure develops. Some patients die suddenly. Others go on to develop cardiomyopathy years later.

Agents	Special features	Basic pathology
Viruses e.g. Coxsackie B group and influenza virus	Usually generalised: interstitial inflammation the main feature	Muscle fibre damage – necrosis and lysis of individual or small groups
Bacteria e.g. Lyme disease – *Borrelia burgdorferi*		
Toxins (incl. chemicals) Classic example – diphtheria toxin circulating in blood. Also in other severe infections e.g. typhoid, pneumonia	Usually generalised: muscle damage the main feature	
Immunological E.g. rheumatic fever – myocarditis is an important component of the disease (see p.213 for details of special pathology).		

Interstitial oedema and inflammatory cellular infiltrate

CARDIOMYOPATHY

This term refers to diseases of cardiac muscle when ischaemia, hypertension, valvular disease and inflammation have been excluded. Genetic influences are important.

3 main forms are recognised:

1. Dilated (congestive) Cardiomyopathy

All the chambers of the heart are dilated - - - - - - - - - →
and
hypertrophied - - - - - - - - - →

This is an uncommon condition which is familial in a minority of cases often due to mutations affecting cytoskeletal proteins. Patients present clinically with unexplained heart failure usually between the ages of 30 and 60 years.

MISCELLANEOUS AFFECTIONS OF THE MYOCARDIUM

CARDIOMYOPATHY *(continued)*

2a. **Hypertrophic Cardiomyopathy**

This can occur at any age, but young adults are often affected. There is often a family history presenting usually as an autosomal dominant pattern. Several genes encoding contractile protein may be involved, e.g. β-myosin heavy chain.

The effects include: sudden death, often following exercise, arrhythmias and cardiac failure.

Muscle hypertrophy is often of a particular anatomical component of the heart: histologically the enlarged muscle fibres show a striking irregularity of orientation.

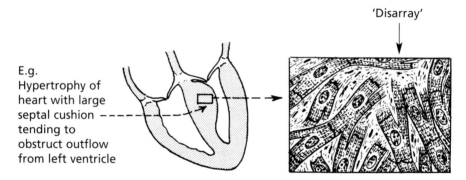

E.g.
Hypertrophy of heart with large septal cushion tending to obstruct outflow from left ventricle

'Disarray'

2b. **Restrictive Cardiomyopathy**

In this form the myocardium does not relax properly in diastole; this restricts ventricular filling and **cardiac output is reduced.**

A similar problem is seen in **Endomyocardial Fibrosis** – a disease of childhood seen mainly in Africa.

Other myocardial disorders include:

    (i) Amyloidosis (p.24).
    (ii) Haemochromatosis (p.350).
    (iii) Drugs e.g. alcohol, adriamycin, cocaine.

RHEUMATIC FEVER

In rheumatic fever (acute rheumatism), a disease of children and young adults, inflammation affects the connective tissues at many sites, of which the **heart** is the most important. The incidence in Western countries has fallen dramatically, but it is common in parts of Africa and Asia.

Aetiology
There is a strong association with streptococcal sore throat. The streptococcus is important because it shares antigens with human tissues, particularly heart muscle.

Mechanism

Throat infection due to β-haemolytic streptococcus (Group A) → IMMUNE RESPONSE → Cell mediated and ANTIBODIES to STREPTOCOCCAL ANTIGENS → CROSS-REACTION with CARDIAC and connective tissues of SUSCEPTIBLE individuals

In addition to the cardiac damage, the disease is manifest in the following ways:

1. **General manifestations** include:
   Fever with sweating and malaise: raised ESR and C-reactive protein: neutrophil leucocytosis.
2. **Indications of inflammation at local sites**
   (a) *Joints and adjacent musculofascial tissues* – causing ARTHRITIS with effusion, muscle pains and weakness.
   (b) *Serous membranes* – pericardial and sometimes pleural effusion.
   (c) *Skin* (i) a rash (erythema marginatum).
         (ii) small subcutaneous palpable nodules over bony prominences subject to pressure.
   (d) *Central nervous system* – chorea (involuntary spasmodic muscular movements).

CARDIAC MANIFESTATIONS

The inflammation is widespread throughout the heart, i.e. there is PANCARDITIS. It is convenient to consider the effects on the three anatomical cardiac layers separately – pericardial, myocardial and endocardial.

1. **Pericarditis** occurs during the acute phase of the illness and is an important cause of pericardial effusion.
2. **Myocarditis** is common during the acute phase and is usually mild: it is rarely severe enough to cause cardiac failure. The histological picture is striking and the presence of the Aschoff body is characteristic.

Oedema and lymphocyte infiltration between muscle fibres

Perivascular cellular infiltration

The Aschoff body

Central granular or hyaline debris with large mononuclear cells, some with multiple nuclei.

213

RHEUMATIC FEVER

CARDIAC MANIFESTATIONS *(continued)*

3. **Endocarditis.** Although there is a widespread histological inflammation, gross changes are seen usually on the endocardial sites subject to the greatest pressures and traumas, i.e. in the left side of the heart at the points of valve closure and at any sites of jet effect in the blood flow. The basic inflammation is complicated by ulceration of the valve surface followed by platelet and fibrin thrombosis in the form of small 'vegetations'.

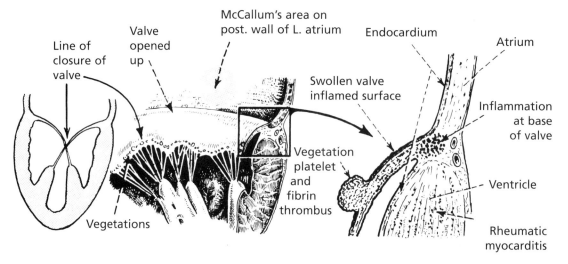

Progression of the disease

In most cases the acute phase passes off and is followed by healing with various degrees of scarring. In a significant number of cases, no florid acute phase is noticed, and in a small number, a low grade chronic inflammation is present for long periods. Repeated episodes lead to chronic valvular heart disease in about 50% of patients.

VALVULAR HEART DISEASE

The main causes are RHEUMATIC ENDOCARDITIS, degenerative changes including DYSTROPHIC CALCIFICATION and congenital heart disease. Inherited deficiencies of the ground substance of the valve are rare causes. Nowadays, with the advent of powerful antibiotics, the late effects of healed infective endocarditis are assuming greater importance.

The MITRAL and AORTIC valves, subjected to much greater pressures, are more susceptible to damage than the tricuspid and pulmonary valves. *Rheumatic mitral disease* has been very common in the past and is still seen in middle aged or older patients, but with the decline in rheumatic fever and the increasing age of the population, *calcific aortic disease* is now commoner.

MITRAL DISEASE

Stenosis is the most common result of rheumatic fever. It is the result of several components of the healing or scarring process occurring either separately or, more usually, together in varying combinations.

Normal valve
Note thin delicate curtains and chordae tendinae

Stenosis
Simple adherence of curtains: a diaphragm formed (balloon valvuloplasty or valvotomy may be possible)

OR

Adherence and distortion, thickening, shortening, calcification of valve curtains and chordae resulting in 'funnel' stenosis

(Whole valve replacement required.)

215

MITRAL VALVE DISEASE

Mitral disease *(continued)*

Incompetence may follow from the rheumatic process by a similar slow mechanism. In addition it may develop acutely due to other quite different causes:

1. In cases of left ventricular failure when severe dilatation occurs.

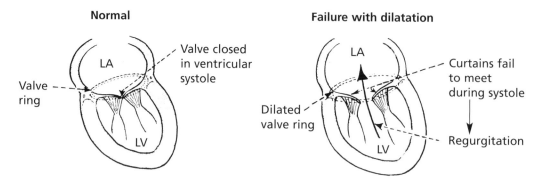

2. Necrosis with rupture of papillary muscle in acute myocardial infarction.

3. It may result from myxoid degeneration of the valve – the 'floppy valve syndrome'. More cases of this condition are now being recognised using modern non-invasive techniques to study cardiac valve function in life.

4. Infective endocarditis (see p.223).

The mechanical effects of mitral disease

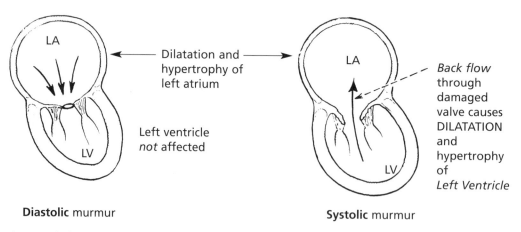

In rheumatic heart disease, pure stenosis is not uncommon; combined stenosis and incompetence is often seen.

MITRAL VALVE DISEASE

Mitral disease *(continued)*

In mitral disease, the back pressure in the left atrium is transmitted to the pulmonary veins and by raising pulmonary arterial pressure causes effects on the right side of the heart.

(a) **Compensated phase**

(1) Left atrial dilatation

↓

(2) Pulmonary congestion

↓

(3) Right ventricular hypertrophy

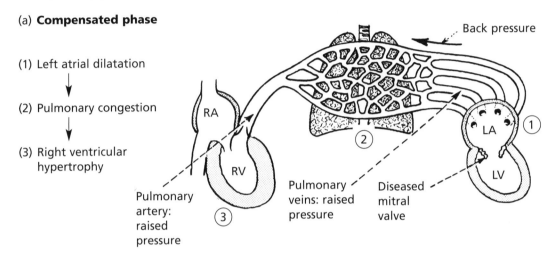

(b) **Congestive cardiac failure**

(3) Right Ventricular Hypertrophy → (4) Dilated RV → (5) Dilated RA

In the acute types of mitral incompetence, the sudden change in the intracardiac haemodynamics very seriously aggravates the heart failure already present due to the primary disease.

Complications of chronic mitral disease

1. Atrial fibrillation is common.
   Fibrillation → Thrombosis in atrial appendage → Systemic embolism
2. Infective endocarditis.

AORTIC VALVE DISEASE

STENOSIS

The main causes are RHEUMATIC SCARRING and CALCIFICATION occurring in a CONGENITALLY ABNORMAL VALVE (usually bicuspid) or one previously damaged by rheumatism or endocarditis (bacterial), but in elderly people there may be no obvious pre-existing disease.

Changes in the valve

Normal valve during ventricular systole — Delicate cusps pressed against aorta virtually no valve resistance

Aorta — Free flow of blood past valve

Scarring of cusps — Cusps adherent, thickened and distorted — Flow of blood impeded

Calcification — Anatomy of cusps obscured by hard irregular masses of calcium salts — Free flow of blood impaired

Effects

The main effect is pure HYPERTROPHY of the left ventricle to overcome the valve resistance,
e.g. 600 g
(normal – 300 g)

Ejection systolic murmur

Low pulse pressure may reduce coronary supply, rendering the hypertrophied muscle susceptible to ischaemic damage.

The heart often remains in this 'compensated' state for years but eventually failure develops with dilatation.

However SUDDEN DEATH (without pre-existing signs of failure) is a definite risk at any time, but particularly during exercise in cases of aortic stenosis.

In adults, severe aortic stenosis usually requires valve replacement.

AORTIC VALVE DISEASE

INCOMPETENCE

The main causes are scarring of the cusps due to rheumatic or infective endocarditis: less commonly dilatation of the valve ring due to disease (e.g. in ankylosing spondylitis: Marfan's syndrome) or degeneration in very old age.

Changes in the valve

Normal valve in ventricular diastole — Complete closure prevents reflux into ventricle

Aorta

Scarred valve — Failure to close allows reflux

Dilatation of valve ring

Disease of aortic wall

Cusps healthy but too small for enlarged aperture → reflux

Gradual distension and distortion of ring

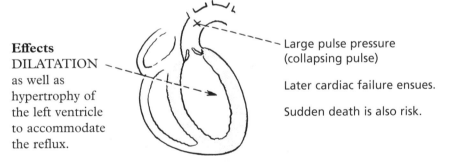

Effects
DILATATION as well as hypertrophy of the left ventricle to accommodate the reflux.

Large pulse pressure (collapsing pulse)

Later cardiac failure ensues.

Sudden death is also risk.

Diastolic murmur: 'water-hammer' pulse.

Aortic stenosis and incompetence often exist together and the effects are compounded.

TRICUSPID AND PULMONARY VALVES

Diseases of these valves on the right side of the heart are not common. However functional tricuspid incompetence due to severe cardiac dilatation is an important end stage in progressive cardiac failure.

Progressive failure → Dilatation → TRICUSPID INCOMPETENCE → Right atrial failure → Severe systemic venous congestion (congestive cardiac failure)

INFECTIVE ENDOCARDITIS

This is a disease of the heart valves particularly: the mural endocardium is only occasionally affected by late spread from the valves.

In the classical situation, bacteria settle on previously diseased valves. In drug abusers using the intravenous route, normal valves may be affected.

There is a spectrum between 2 extremes classically called acute and subacute and the disease evolves in one of 2 main patterns depending on the type of bacteria.

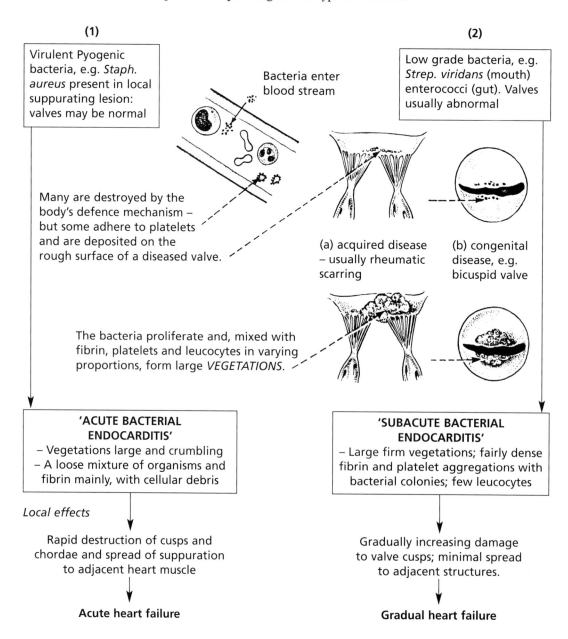

(1)

Virulent Pyogenic bacteria, e.g. *Staph. aureus* present in local suppurating lesion: valves may be normal

Bacteria enter blood stream

(2)

Low grade bacteria, e.g. *Strep. viridans* (mouth) enterococci (gut). Valves usually abnormal

Many are destroyed by the body's defence mechanism – but some adhere to platelets and are deposited on the rough surface of a diseased valve.

(a) acquired disease – usually rheumatic scarring

(b) congenital disease, e.g. bicuspid valve

The bacteria proliferate and, mixed with fibrin, platelets and leucocytes in varying proportions, form large *VEGETATIONS*.

'ACUTE BACTERIAL ENDOCARDITIS'
– Vegetations large and crumbling
– A loose mixture of organisms and fibrin mainly, with cellular debris

Local effects

Rapid destruction of cusps and chordae and spread of suppuration to adjacent heart muscle

Acute heart failure

'SUBACUTE BACTERIAL ENDOCARDITIS'
– Large firm vegetations; fairly dense fibrin and platelet aggregations with bacterial colonies; few leucocytes

Gradually increasing damage to valve cusps; minimal spread to adjacent structures.

Gradual heart failure

INFECTIVE ENDOCARDITIS

In addition to the local effects, the course of the disease is influenced by other important complications.

So-called

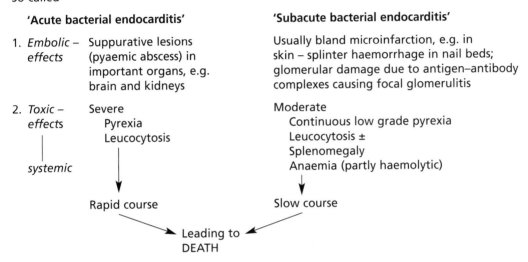

'Acute bacterial endocarditis'	**'Subacute bacterial endocarditis'**
1. *Embolic –* Suppurative lesions *effects* (pyaemic abscess) in important organs, e.g. brain and kidneys	Usually bland microinfarction, e.g. in skin – splinter haemorrhage in nail beds; glomerular damage due to antigen–antibody complexes causing focal glomerulitis
2. *Toxic –* Severe *effects* Pyrexia Leucocytosis	Moderate Continuous low grade pyrexia Leucocytosis ± Splenomegaly Anaemia (partly haemolytic)

systemic

Rapid course   Slow course

Leading to
DEATH

This classical situation is nowadays modified by immunosuppressive drugs, antibiotics and intracardiac prostheses including catheter lines from peripheral veins.

Immunosuppression
This allows opportunistic infection by a much wider range of organisms, e.g. bacteria not usually pathogenic, and fungi.

Antibiotics
1. Their effects blur the distinction between the two types and allow healing but often with serious scarring of the valve.
2. The structure of the vegetation is important; in some cases the bacterial colonies are protected from the antibiotic.

Antibiotic in blood stream

Colonies embedded in firm fibrin, platelets and collagen

∴ Large prolonged dosage of antibiotic required

Cardiac prostheses and catheter lines act as a focus for bacterial growth and infective endocarditis is a serious complication.

CARDIAC ARRHYTHMIAS

CARDIAC ARRHYTHMIAS and DISEASES of the CONDUCTING SYSTEM

Of the wide variety of cardiac arrhythmias which have now been studied in detail using the electrocardiograph, the majority are due to (A) functional disturbances of the intrinsic excitability of the cardiac muscle at various sites or of the cardiac neurohumoral controls; only a minority are due to (B) organic disease of the conducting system itself. Organic heart disease particularly of ischaemic type is a common concomitant.

(A) **Important disorders of cardiac muscle excitability**

1. **Atrial fibrillation**
    In this common disorder, continuous incoordinate movement of the atrial muscle completely negates its role as a priming pump and the atria become functionally inert. There is no specific pathological change in the atrial wall, but atrial dilatation associated with cardiac disease is usually a precondition.

    Predisposing conditions

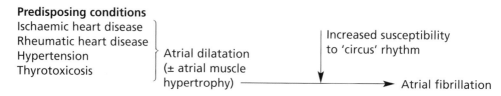

    Ischaemic heart disease ⎫
    Rheumatic heart disease ⎬ Atrial dilatation (± atrial muscle hypertrophy) ——→
    Hypertension
    Thyrotoxicosis ⎭

    Increased susceptibility to 'circus' rhythm ↓ ——→ Atrial fibrillation

    There are two main effects:

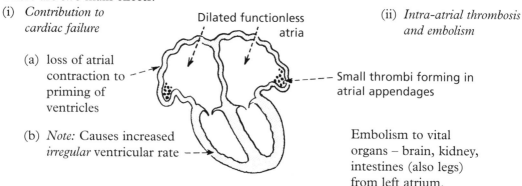

    (i) *Contribution to cardiac failure*

    Dilated functionless atria

    (ii) *Intra-atrial thrombosis and embolism*

    (a) loss of atrial contraction to priming of ventricles

    Small thrombi forming in atrial appendages

    (b) *Note:* Causes increased *irregular* ventricular rate

    Embolism to vital organs – brain, kidney, intestines (also legs) from left atrium.

2. **Ventricular paroxysmal tachycardia and fibrillation**
    These very serious conditions are usually superimposed upon and aggravate pre-existing severe myocardial disease – usually ischaemic in type. In fibrillation, a form of cardiac 'arrest', cardiac function ceases.

CARDIAC ARRHYTHMIAS

Cardiac arrhythmias *(continued)*

(B) Diseases of the conducting system

The usual disorder is slowing of the impulse and it is most often associated with organic disease in the adjacent cardiac tissue.

Associated conditions

Cardiac ischaemia — Acute infarction ⎫ —— are the most common
— Fibrosis ⎬ and important

Others are – myocarditis, calcification around the valve rings and drugs, e.g. digitalis, propranolol.

Sites of disorder   **Effects**

- - SA node – Sinus bradycardia
Paroxysmal supraventricular tachycardia

- - AV node   *Heart block*
and   1st degree: only mild delay in conduction
Bundle of   ∴ no effect on ventricular rate
His   2nd degree: moderate delay, missed
   ventricular beats
   3rd degree: complete block, idioventricular
   rhythm established, 25–50 per min

Left and   *Bundle branch block*
right —— Causes loss of efficiency of
bundles   ventricular contraction

The 3 important components of arrhythmias are:
Tachycardia, bradycardia and irregularity.
The effect of any arrhythmia on cardiac function depends essentially on its effect on ventricular output.

Tachycardia
pulse rate over 160/min ——→ Diastolic time too short to ——→ Low cardiac
allow adequate ventricular   output
↓ filling; also impairment of
coronary flow
Seriously aggravated
by **Irregularity**

↑

Bradycardia
– pulse rate less than 60/min ——————————————

Failure

CONGENITAL HEART DISEASE

Developmental abnormalities of the heart are relatively common; clinically significant defects occur in 7–11 per 1000 live births and the rate is significantly higher in stillbirths. The severity varies from minor aberrations to complex distortions incompatible with life. Many patients now live normal lives after cardiac surgery.

Aetiology

This is often obscure. Hereditary factors are of limited importance, Down syndrome often causes septal defects. Possible environmental factors are complex and numerous.

Examples include: virus infection, e.g. rubella; teratogen, e.g. thalidomide (historically); altitude at birth (patent ductus arteriosus is commoner at high altitudes).

The initial damage which is sustained during the early formative stages in the 2nd and 3rd months of pregnancy is modified by later fetal and postnatal growth and development.

Single anatomical abnormalities occur, but often there are multiple defects which are associated in groups of which the more common are given specific names.

Abnormal development occurs:

(1) At the emergence of the great vessels

↓

Stenoses cause impedence to blood flow

(2) During formation of the septa between right and left sides and following failure of closure, e.g. ductus and foramen ovale.

↓

Abnormal apertures allow shunting of blood

This is a huge subject:

Fallot's tetralogy illustrates these main points:

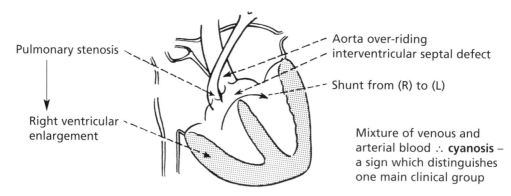

Pulmonary stenosis

↓

Right ventricular enlargement

Aorta over-riding
interventricular septal defect

Shunt from (R) to (L)

Mixture of venous and arterial blood ∴ **cyanosis** – a sign which distinguishes one main clinical group

Often complications – pulmonary hypertension, increased blood volume, polycythaemia, and infective endocarditis – increase the disability.

Surgical repair is the ideal treatment.

DISEASES OF THE PERICARDIUM

PERICARDITIS

Pericarditis is commonly a complication of diseases of the heart or adjacent structures or of generalised disorders. In some cases no cause can be found.

In **acute pericarditis**, fibrin exudation is common: sometimes exudation of serous fluid is the main feature. Haemorrhagic effusion is usually due to infiltration by tumour. Purulent pericarditis complicating bacterial infections is rare.

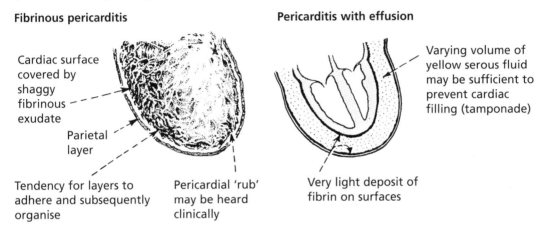

Fibrinous pericarditis

Cardiac surface covered by shaggy fibrinous exudate

Parietal layer

Tendency for layers to adhere and subsequently organise

Pericardial 'rub' may be heard clinically

Pericarditis with effusion

Varying volume of yellow serous fluid may be sufficient to prevent cardiac filling (tamponade)

Very light deposit of fibrin on surfaces

Diseases which may lead to pericarditis

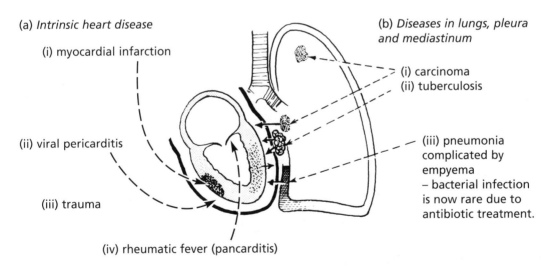

(a) *Intrinsic heart disease*

  (i) myocardial infarction

(ii) viral pericarditis

(iii) trauma

(iv) rheumatic fever (pancarditis)

(b) *Diseases in lungs, pleura and mediastinum*

(i) carcinoma
(ii) tuberculosis

(iii) pneumonia complicated by empyema
– bacterial infection is now rare due to antibiotic treatment.

(c) *Generalised disorders*

  (i) uraemia
  (ii) connective tissue diseases e.g. SLE, rheumatoid disease

DISEASES OF THE PERICARDIUM

CHRONIC PERICARDITIS may be due to tuberculosis, viral infection or rheumatoid arthritis; sometimes the cause cannot be determined. The basic changes are organisation and calcification. In extreme cases, cardiac function is impaired.

Dense fibrous calcified tissues – causing close adherence of the pericardial layers; preventing proper cardiac filling;
– this extreme condition is called **constrictive pericarditis.**

Venous ostia

PERICARDIAL HAEMORRHAGE occurs most commonly as a result of **cardiac rupture** complicating acute infarction. The other main cause is rupture of dissecting **aortic**

aneurysm back into the pericardium. The pericardial sac becomes distended with blood (tamponade) and death follows rapidly due to compression of the heart.

Compression of heart

Cardiac rupture into pericardium

CARDIAC TUMOURS

Primary tumours in the heart are very rare. Secondary tumours, especially from the lungs, affecting the pericardium by direct spread and the heart by blood spread are fairly common in advanced malignant disease.

Atrial 'myxoma' is a rare tumour affecting usually the left atrium in which a smooth, pale, soft, rounded mass is attached by a pedicle to the endocardium. It can cause serious effects by occluding the mitral valve opening or by embolisation. Mesothelioma may present primarily in the pericardium.

Rhabdomyomas are occasionally seen in childhood associated with tuberous sclerosis.

DISEASES OF ARTERIES

ARTERITIS

The term 'arteritis' refers to a group of conditions with inflammation of the vessel wall, usually due to immune mechanisms. Large, medium or small arteries may be affected.

Polyarteritis nodosa (PAN)

This is a disease affecting the medium and small arteries and arterioles. In the acute phase, there are signs of generalised illness with fever, etc., but the disease often becomes chronic and relapsing.

The typical lesion is a focal necrosis of the arterial wall.

In microscopic polyarteritis, a form of glomerulonephritis is associated with affection of afferent arterioles.

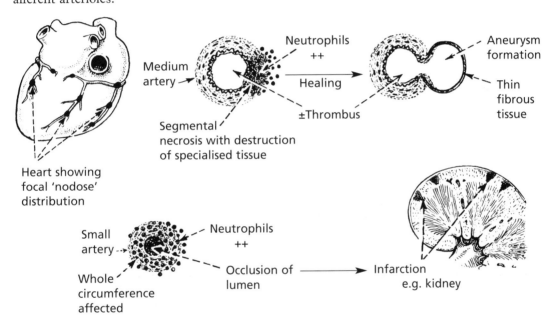

Any artery may be affected, but damage to the HEART, KIDNEYS, BRAIN and GUT is particularly important. When the arteries supplying peripheral nerves are affected symptoms of 'neuritis' may be striking.

Other forms of arteritis include e.g. *Wegener's granulomatosis* in which destructive lesions of the nasal mucosa, the lungs and the kidneys result.

Aetiology PAN appears to be due to antigen: antibody complexes. Hepatitis B infection is the source of antigen in some cases. Anti-neutrophil cytoplasmic antibodies (ANCA) occur in various forms of vasculitis – p-ANCA in microscopic polyarteritis and c-ANCA in Wegener's granulomatosis.

Arteritis may also complicate other conditions (usually the *connective tissue diseases*, see p.625), e.g. rheumatoid arthritis, systemic lupus erythematosus (SLE).

227

DISEASES OF ARTERIES

BUERGER'S DISEASE (thromboangiitis obliterans)

In this very painful condition, the inflammation involves the small peripheral arteries of the legs and often the arms. Typically the victim is a young Jewish male (20–40 years) **heavy cigarette smoker.**

Cross-section of neurovascular bundle

Artery thrombosed

Veins thrombosed

Nerves affected causing pain

Acute inflammation with neutrophils affecting veins and perivascular tissues as well as the arterial wall

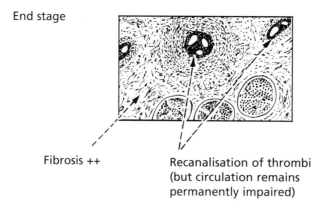

End stage

Fibrosis ++

Recanalisation of thrombi (but circulation remains permanently impaired)

GANGRENE of the toes may follow as more vessels become involved.

DISEASES OF ARTERIES

Temporal arteritis (Giant-cell arteritis/cranial arteritis)

This disease of unknown aetiology affects elderly people (over 65 years). It may cause severe facial pain and headache and may be associated with ocular symptoms and cause blindness. In a significant number of old people, there are no symptoms.

Some cases occur along with polymyalgia rheumatica – a disease in which there are generalised muscle pains and systemic malaise. Commonly, branches of the external carotid arteries are affected, but sometimes other caudal arteries and even the aortic arch may also be involved.

There is inflammation of the vessel wall complicated by thrombosis.

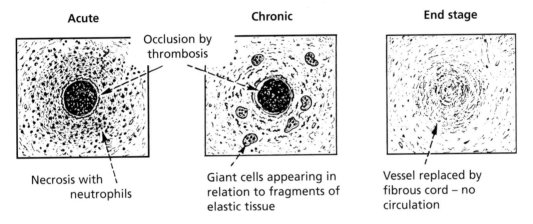

Acute	Chronic	End stage

Occlusion by thrombosis

Necrosis with neutrophils

Giant cells appearing in relation to fragments of elastic tissue

Vessel replaced by fibrous cord – no circulation

Takayashu's disease

In this rare disease, the typical victim is a young female (20–30 years). The patchy arteritis is more severe and affects the aorta and its primary branches, leading to ischaemia of BRAIN (cerebral arteries), EYES (ophthalmic arteries), FACE (carotid arteries), ARMS ('pulseless' disease), HEART (coronary orifices), KIDNEYS (causing HYPERTENSION) in varying combinations.

The important vascular changes in diabetes mellitus are described on page 646.

ANEURYSMS

A local enlargement of an artery is called an **aneurysm**. Although localised, it often reflects the presence of more widespread arterial disease.

MECHANISM of FORMATION

The two main forces concerned in maintenance of the integrity of the shape of an artery are:

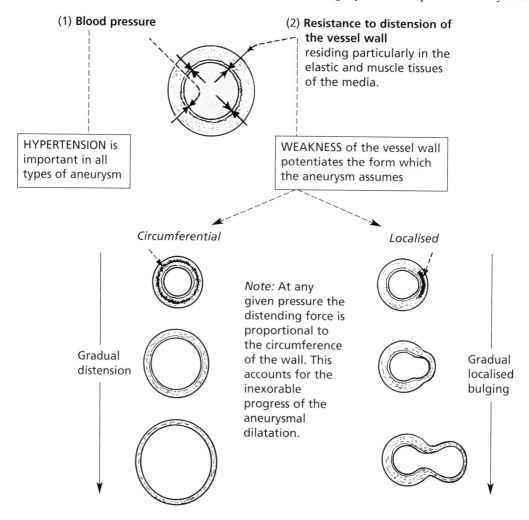

(1) **Blood pressure**

(2) **Resistance to distension of the vessel wall** residing particularly in the elastic and muscle tissues of the media.

HYPERTENSION is important in all types of aneurysm

WEAKNESS of the vessel wall potentiates the form which the aneurysm assumes

Circumferential

Localised

Gradual distension

Note: At any given pressure the distending force is proportional to the circumference of the wall. This accounts for the inexorable progress of the aneurysmal dilatation.

Gradual localised bulging

Causes

Aneurysms may be due to: acquired diseases of vessel wall (atheroma, arteritis, syphilis (now rare)); congenital weakness (berry aneurysms, p.232, 543); hypertension; trauma.

ANEURYSMS

TYPES of ANEURYSM

There are two main varieties:

(1) **Fusiform**

(2) **Saccular**

These are well illustrated in the aorta.

Fusiform aneurysm of abdominal aorta – usually due to atheroma; often below renal arteries and may also affect iliac arteries.

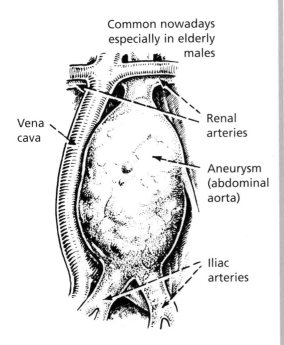

Common nowadays especially in elderly males

Vena cava

Renal arteries

Aneurysm (abdominal aorta)

Iliac arteries

Complications
1. Local pressure effects – usually not serious.
2. Thrombosis with embolism to legs.
3. Fatal retroperitoneal or intraperitoneal haemorrhage.

Saccular aneurysm of aortic arch – now usually due to atheroma: in the past, syphilis.

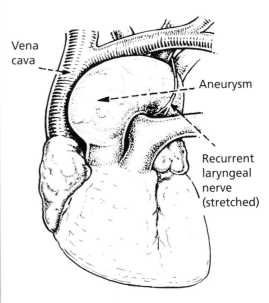

Vena cava

Aneurysm

Recurrent laryngeal nerve (stretched)

Complications
1. Pressure effects
    (a) on nerves, e.g. recurrent laryngeal nerve paralysis
    (b) on bones e.g. vertebral, sternal or rib erosion
    (c) on neighbouring viscera, e.g. oesophagus, heart, lungs.
2. Fatal haemorrhage.

ANEURYSMS

OTHER VARIETIES of ANEURYSM

1. **Dissecting aneurysm**
   Classically begins in the arch of aorta.
   Predisposing causes: (a) HYPERTENSION (common)
                       (b) Atheroma
                       (c) Medial degeneration (rare) seen in Marfan's syndrome due to mutation of the fibrillin gene.

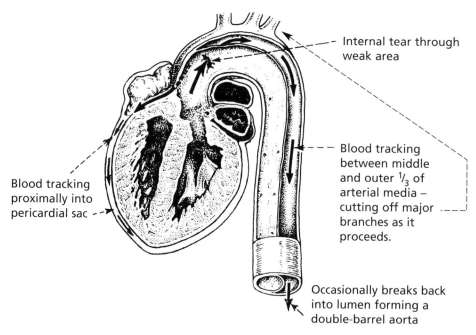

Internal tear through weak area

Blood tracking between middle and outer $\frac{1}{3}$ of arterial media – cutting off major branches as it proceeds.

Blood tracking proximally into pericardial sac

Occasionally breaks back into lumen forming a double-barrel aorta

2. **'Berry' aneurysm** occurs in medium-sized vessels at the base of the brain, e.g. on Circle of Willis. Associated with congenital deficiency of arterial media. Rupture causes subarachnoid haemorrhage.

Circle of Willis

3. **Microaneurysm** – associated with hypertension and affects smaller arteries and arterioles, especially in the brain.

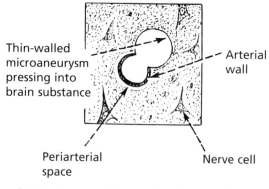

Thin-walled microaneurysm pressing into brain substance

Arterial wall

Periarterial space

Nerve cell

Rupture causes intra-cerebral haemorrhage.

ARTERIAL DISEASES – MISCELLANEOUS

RAYNAUD'S PHENOMENON
This is essentially spasmodic attacks of pallor of the fingers (the toes, ears and nose may also be affected) due to intense constriction of the small arteries and arterioles in response to cold. The cause is not known.

The condition affects 5–10% of young women in temperate climates.

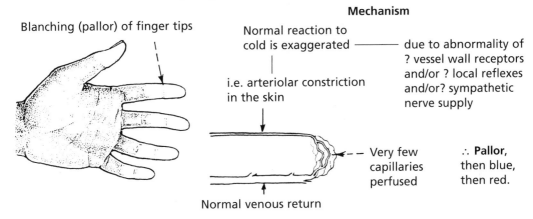

Blanching (pallor) of finger tips

Mechanism

Normal reaction to cold is exaggerated —— due to abnormality of ? vessel wall receptors and/or ? local reflexes and/or? sympathetic nerve supply

i.e. arteriolar constriction in the skin

Very few capillaries perfused

∴ **Pallor,** then blue, then red.

Normal venous return

This condition may continue for many years and NO PERMANENT DAMAGE RESULTS.

A **Secondary form** of Raynaud's Phenomenon may occur as a symptom in other conditions. Examples include the 'connective tissue diseases', systemic sclerosis (see p.625) and systemic lupus erythematosus (SLE); cold agglutinins causing vascular blockage due to agglutination of red cells; the use of heavy pneumatic drills disturbing neurovascular controls in the hands.

In these circumstances the disease is serious and disabling, the trophic changes adding significantly to the damage caused by the primary diseases elsewhere in the body.

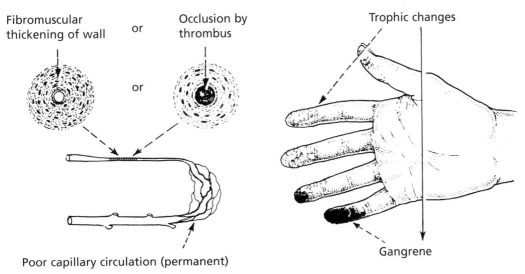

Fibromuscular thickening of wall   or   Occlusion by thrombus

or

Trophic changes

Poor capillary circulation (permanent)

Gangrene

DISEASES OF VEINS

Diseases of the veins are important because they can be associated with:

(1) *Acute* severe, sometimes fatal, complications

(2) *Chronic* disability

Embolism to pulmonary arteries

Thrombosis of veins (phlebothrombosis)

Rupture with **haemorrhage** from oesophageal varices

Ulcer →

Haemorrhoids (piles)

Aching pains due to varicose veins

↓

Ulcers

ACUTE PHLEBOTHROMBOSIS AND THROMBOPHLEBITIS

The veins of the lower limbs are very common sites of acute thrombosis, especially after surgical operations and during illnesses with enforced recumbency.

In the majority of cases the thrombosis is the primary event and mild inflammation follows as a reaction. Phlebothrombosis is the preferred name.

Thrombophlebitis is reserved for cases in which the thrombosis is secondary to inflammation in or adjacent to the vein.

ACUTE PHLEBITIS
Suppurative (pyogenic)

Secondary to bacterial infection
e.g. a very rare complication of appendicitis

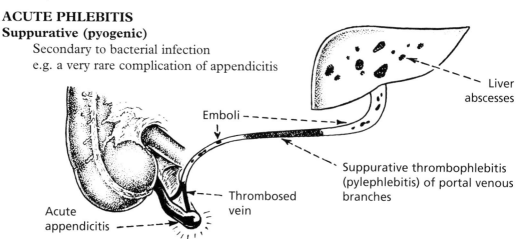

Emboli - - -

Liver abscesses

Suppurative thrombophlebitis (pylephlebitis) of portal venous branches

Thrombosed vein

Acute appendicitis - - -

DISEASES OF VEINS

VEINS in MALIGNANT DISEASE

(a) Venules are easily invaded and infiltrated by carcinoma and are an important route in the metastatic spread of the tumour.

(b) Large veins, particularly in the mediastinum and pelvis, may be compressed from outside by the tumour – the resulting obstruction causing serious effects.

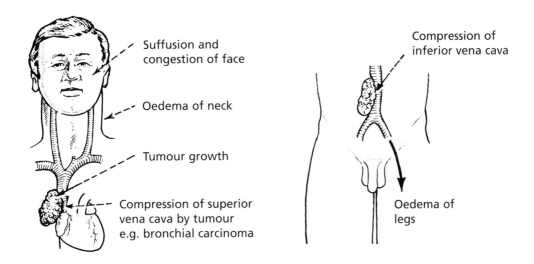

Suffusion and congestion of face

Oedema of neck

Tumour growth

Compression of superior vena cava by tumour e.g. bronchial carcinoma

Compression of inferior vena cava

Oedema of legs

Migratory (thrombophlebitis migrans)

In this rare condition the thrombosis is not confined to the lower limb veins and can affect veins anywhere in the body. A striking feature is the appearance and disappearance of thrombosis apparently at random sites.

The mechanism is not fully understood but usually a **malignant tumour** is in the background – sometimes the phlebitis is the first clinical sign of an occult tumour but more often it complicates the terminal stages of tumour growth.

VARICOSE VEINS

This is a very common condition, the incidence increasing with **age**, and particularly high in **females** – often a sequel of pregnancy. The veins become prominent and tortuous and bulge outwards under the skin; the legs are particularly affected.

A **varix** is a localised bulge in a vein analogous to a saccular aneurysm in an artery. It is almost always associated with more generalised varicosity of the vein.

Aetiology

A vein wall, thin and composed of musculoelastic tissues, is designed to conduct blood at low pressures: the physiological movement of the blood is influenced mostly by pressure gradients derived from outside the vein wall.

Varicose veins arise when the vein wall is subjected to an increased expanding pressure (tension) over long periods.

Mechanism

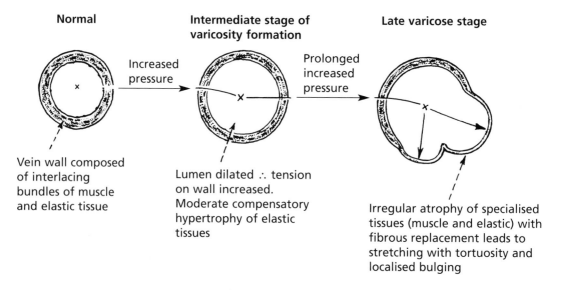

Normal

Vein wall composed of interlacing bundles of muscle and elastic tissue

Increased pressure

Intermediate stage of varicosity formation

Lumen dilated ∴ tension on wall increased. Moderate compensatory hypertrophy of elastic tissues

Prolonged increased pressure

Late varicose stage

Irregular atrophy of specialised tissues (muscle and elastic) with fibrous replacement leads to stretching with tortuosity and localised bulging

VARICOSE VEINS

FACTORS WHICH INFLUENCE THE BASIC MECHANISM

(a) Acting on the vein wall

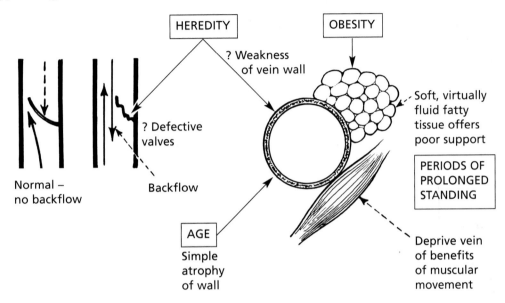

HEREDITY

OBESITY

? Weakness of vein wall

? Defective valves

Soft, virtually fluid fatty tissue offers poor support

PERIODS OF PROLONGED STANDING

Normal – no backflow

Backflow

AGE

Simple atrophy of wall

Deprive vein of benefits of muscular movement

(b) Increasing the intraluminal pressure

1. Obstruction to venous flow – usually in the pelvis – by:
   Pregnancy
   Tumour
   Constipation with
     loaded colon
   Thrombosis in veins
     (also may destroy valves)
   Constrictions on limbs.

2. Special anatomical considerations.

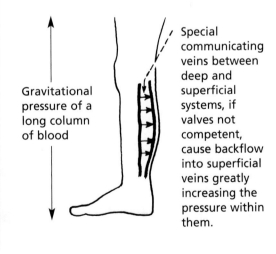

Gravitational pressure of a long column of blood

Special communicating veins between deep and superficial systems, if valves not competent, cause backflow into superficial veins greatly increasing the pressure within them.

237

VARICOSE VEINS

Effects

1. Symptoms of leg fatigue and aching pains.
2. Trophic changes – varicose eczema with pigmentation due to haemosiderin deposition – may proceed to ULCERATION: very slow to heal.
3. Haemorrhage is a rare complication.
4. Thrombosis is a frequent complication.
   Note: Superficial venous thrombosis is not usually associated with embolism; deep venous thrombosis is the dangerous condition.

VARICOSE VEINS IN SPECIAL SITES

Oesophageal varices

Haemorrhage

Usually due to portal venous obstruction when portal-systemic venous anastomoses open up.

Complicated by serious haemorrhage which may be fatal

Varicocele

Affects the pampiniform plexus: feels like a 'bag of worms'. It may cause dull aching and, because the increased vascularity raises the scrotal temperature, the condition has been incriminated in some cases of infertility.

Haemorrhoids

Varices of the anorectal veins; usually associated with constipation.

Complications are: 1. rectal bleeding

3. Prolapse.

2. acute pain due to local haematoma (not a true haemorrhoid).

DISEASES OF LYMPHATICS

The lymphatic vessels participate in disease processes in two main ways:

1. They afford a natural route by which diseases can spread.
2. They may become obstructed, with serious results.

1. LYMPHATICS as a mechanism by which DISEASE SPREADS

Small lymphatics are thin-walled vessels which have a simple endothelial layer and readily allow entry of tumour cells, bacteria and foreign material often within phagocytes.

The mechanism is important in the spread of (a) infection and (b) tumours.

Malignant cells

Acute lymphangitis
The lymphatics draining an area infected by pyogenic bacteria (especially streptococci) may themselves become acutely inflamed.

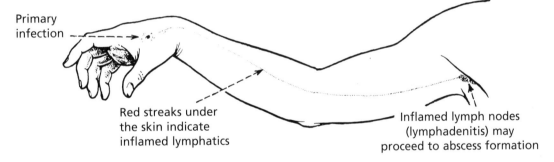

Primary infection

Red streaks under the skin indicate inflamed lymphatics

Inflamed lymph nodes (lymphadenitis) may proceed to abscess formation

Chronic infections such as tuberculosis also spread by lymphatics.

Spread of tumours
This is an important route of spread of malignant tumours, especially carcinoma.

Disposal of particulate matter
This was formerly seen in the lungs where inhaled soot could be seen clearly indicating the lymphatic system under the pleura.

Soot (carbon) is relatively inert, but other dusts may initiate serious disease.

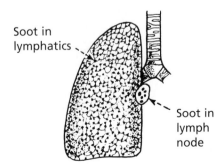

Soot in lymphatics

Soot in lymph node

LYMPHATIC OBSTRUCTION

LYMPHATIC OBSTRUCTION

This is usually due to acquired disease but rarely there is a congenital deficiency of lymphatics (Milroy's syndrome).

The main causes of acquired obstruction are:

(a) **Tumour growth**

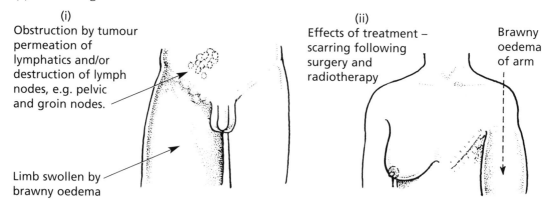

(i)
Obstruction by tumour permeation of lymphatics and/or destruction of lymph nodes, e.g. pelvic and groin nodes.

Limb swollen by brawny oedema

(ii)
Effects of treatment – scarring following surgery and radiotherapy

Brawny oedema of arm

(b) **Blocking by parasites** – e.g. adult worms of filariasis in the tropics.

Effects of chronic lymphatic obstruction:
– accumulation of fluid in the tissues causes swelling of the affected part (lymphoedema).

Special varieties of lymphoedema

Peau d'orange – where the lymphatics of the skin are blocked by tumour.

Elephantiasis – where a limb and/or the scrotum is massively enlarged due to filarial lymphatic blockage.

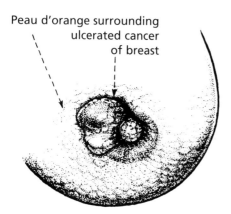

Peau d'orange surrounding ulcerated cancer of breast

VASCULAR TUMOURS

Benign tumours of endothelial cells – ANGIOMAS – illustrate the difficulty in defining the borderline between the tumours (neoplasms) and hamartomas (developmental abnormalities). These are discussed on page 132.

Other varieties include:

1. PYOGENIC GRANULOMA

This striking lesion appears on the skin at a site subject to trauma and infection, e.g. around the finger nails, the nostrils or the tongue.

It not uncommonly occurs during pregnancy.

It grows over several days to form a small red nodular excrescence up to about 1 cm in diameter and is usually ulcerated. – – – – – –

Neutrophils

Sprouting capillaries

Narrow neck

The lesion is entirely benign despite its rapid evolution and responds to simple removal.

2. TELANGIECTASIS

Small localised dilatations of small blood vessels. There are two main types: congenital and acquired.

(a) *Congenital.* In the rare hereditary haemorrhagic telangiectasia, the small lesions occur in the skin and mucous membranes and may be associated with bleeding (especially from the nose).

(b) *Acquired.* The small lesions, affecting the face and neck, are known as **spider naevi.**

The mechanism of their development is probably related to oestrogen excess, since they occur in pregnancy and in serious liver disease (oestrogen catabolism diminished) where they are an important diagnostic sign.

Telangiectasia may be seen in skin damaged by radiotherapy.

Dilated vessels radiating from central vessel

VASCULAR TUMOURS

3. LYMPHANGIOMA

Lymphangiomas are much rarer than haemangiomas and are usually without serious pathological significance.

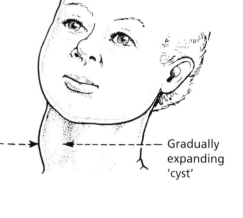

Sometimes the abnormal lymphatic vessels become enormously distended and form fluctuant swellings with local pressure effects, e.g. 'cystic hygroma' of neck of babies and children.

Gradually expanding 'cyst'

4. GLOMANGIOMA (glomus tumour) –

arises from a specialised type of arteriolovenous junction which includes a rich neural component. A common site is the finger tip, perhaps under the nail; a very small but often excruciatingly *painful tumour.*

Microscopically it consists of a complex of blood vessels lined by endothelium but cuffed by round clear cells with contractile properties (myoid cells). It is rich in nerve fibres.

ANGIOSARCOMAS

These are uncommon malignant tumours of endothelial cells. They may affect the skin.

Lesions of the scalp occur in the elderly. They appear as spreading 'bruise-like' areas often with a central nodule. Chronic sun exposure is thought to be important.

Lesions often arise in the limbs in areas of lymphoedema e.g. in the past following irradiation and lymph node clearance for carcinoma of breast.

Angiosarcoma – multiple nodules

Angiosarcoma of the liver is associated with exposure to vinyl chloride monomer.

KAPOSI'S SARCOMA

This tumour has greatly increased in incidence in the wake of the spread of AIDS and HIV infection.

It is a tumour of endothelial cells due to infection by Herpes virus type 8 often occurring in immunocompromised patients.

It occurs in 3 main groups of patients.

(a) In IMMUNOSUPPRESSION – especially in AIDS but also in transplant patients.
(b) **Sporadic** (classic) – affecting elderly males (especially Askanazy Jews) living in the Mediterranean littoral.
(c) **Endemic** – mainly in central Africa, typically affecting young adults.

The disease presents as dark coloured (due to high blood content) **subcutaneous nodules** or plaques resembling bruises.

(a) The nodules may be **multiple** and fairly randomly distributed – this is seen particularly in AIDS cases.

(b) In 'classic' Kaposi, the tumour begins as a **solitary** nodule particularly on the limbs.

(c) In the African endemic Kaposi, lymph nodes are commonly affected.

The histological appearances are of malignant spindle cells lining a network of sieve-like spaces containing extravasated red cells.

243

RESPIRATORY SYSTEM

UPPER RESPIRATORY TRACT

ACUTE INFLAMMATION
Infections of the nose, nasal sinuses, pharynx and larynx are common. They are usually mild and self-limiting. Most cases are due to viral infection, but this is often followed by bacterial superinfection.

1. Viral infection
This phase is characterised by features of acute inflammation but without the exudation of neutrophils.

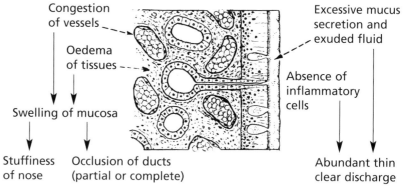

Congestion of vessels

Oedema of tissues

Swelling of mucosa

Stuffiness of nose

Occlusion of ducts (partial or complete)

Excessive mucus secretion and exuded fluid

Absence of inflammatory cells

Abundant thin clear discharge

Viruses involved
A wide variety, of which the major types are:

(i) **rhinoviruses**
(ii) **coronaviruses** — responsible for more than half of cases of the common cold;
(iii) **myxoviruses** (e.g. influenza), **paramyxoviruses** (e.g. respiratory syncytial virus) can also invade the lower respiratory tract.

The viruses adhere to cell surface proteins e.g. on cilia; ⟶ enter the cells and replicate ⟶ and kill them

Bacteria can readily invade the damaged tissue

2. Bacterial phase
Many bacteria are commensal in the respiratory tract (e.g. *Streptococcus mutans, Haemophilus influenzae*) and can superinfect the damaged tissue, which then exhibits the typical features of acute inflammation including exudation of neutrophils.

Congested vessels with margination of neutrophils

Mucoid secretion

Fluid exudate

Loss of surface epithelium

Neutrophil exudate

Mucopurulent discharge

The wide variety of different viruses involved prevents protective immunity.

RHINITIS

COMMON COLD (Acute coryza)

This common respiratory inflammation usually involves the nose and adjacent structures.

The 2 phases, *viral* and *bacterial,* are typically seen in this disease.

The drainage from the sinuses, especially the maxillary, is often blocked by swelling of the mucosa — giving rise to sinusitis.

The infection is acquired by droplet spread of viruses by sneezing.

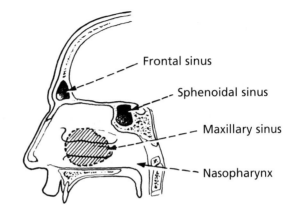

ALLERGIC RHINITIS 'Hay fever'

An allergic (immediate type hyper-sensitivity) type of inflammation (p.103) is often seen. Patients develop immediate symptoms of sneezing, itching and watery rhinorrhoea.

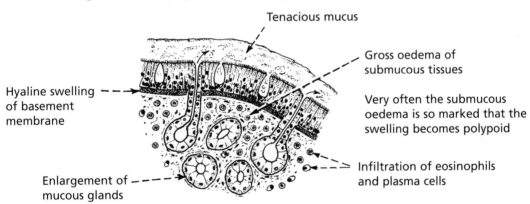

The repeated attacks frequently lead to chronic changes in the mucosa with polyp formation.

RHINITIS

NASAL POLYPS

These form particularly on the middle turbinate bones and within the maxillary sinuses.

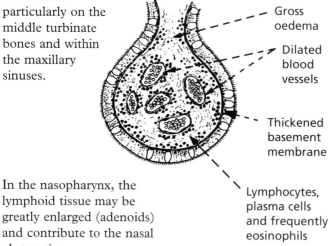

Gross oedema

Dilated blood vessels

Thickened basement membrane

Lymphocytes, plasma cells and frequently eosinophils

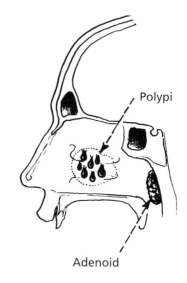

Polypi

Adenoid

In the nasopharynx, the lymphoid tissue may be greatly enlarged (adenoids) and contribute to the nasal obstruction.

ALLERGIES

Seasonal allergy
This is due to pollens liberated from trees and grass.

Non-seasonal allergy
The main cause is the house dust mite, *Dermatophagoides pteronyssinus*. Allergy to pets is common e.g. cats – the allergens are usually salivary proteins from cat fur.

Feather pillow – invisible infestation

VASOMOTOR RHINITIS

This is a clinical diagnosis. The pathological changes are, to some extent, similar to those of allergic rhinitis, but the condition is more continuous, less spasmodic. Although the cause is unknown, viral infections in a polluted atmosphere (usually an urban setting) are thought to initiate the 'sensitivity' and non-specific stimuli such as bright light and smells precipitate an attack.

ACUTE PHARYNGITIS, TRACHEITIS AND LARYNGITIS

ACUTE PHARYNGITIS and TRACHEITIS

Most sore throats are caused by **viruses** – including adenovirus and Epstein–Barr virus.

Bacteria include *Streptococcus pyogenes, Haemophilus parainfluenzae* and *Corynbacterium diphtheriae.*

Tonsillitis is a common acute inflammation, historically due to streptococcal infection but, with the introduction of antibiotics, viruses are the initiating infective agents in most cases.
Acute phase ⟶ may progress to (a) acute suppuration (quinsy)
 or (b) CHRONIC TONSILLITIS

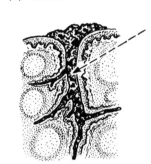

Swollen, red tonsils with purulent exudate at mouths of crypts.

Dilated crypts containing inspissated exudate – harbouring bacteria and fungi.

Liability to relapse to acute inflammation.

Diphtheria, now uncommon in countries where vaccination is widespread, is a serious infection.

The formation of a pseudomembrane is striking.

Normal

Basement membrane

Membrane consisting of fibrin, necrotic epithelium, neutrophils and numerous bacteria

Congested vessels

This pseudomembrane may spread to block the larynx, causing respiratory obstruction.

The EXOTOXIN of diphtheria is encoded by a bacteriophage (a virus which infects the bacterium). It can cause myocarditis (p.211) and neuropathy (p.573).

In **Acute epiglottitis**, typically due to *Haemophilus influenzae*, there is severe inflammation and oedema. In young children, the larynx becomes obstructed necessitating tracheostomy and administration of antibiotics.

Acute laryngitis is often due to parainfluenza viruses. Acute *oedema of the glottis* is seen in some cases of anaphylaxis (p.102) and angioneurotic oedema.

OTHER DISORDERS OF THE LARYNX

CHRONIC LARYNGITIS

Cigarette smoking, repeated attacks of infection and atmospheric pollution may lead to chronic inflammation of the larynx.

Two main features are (a) changes in the lining epithelium and (b) increase in mucus secretion.

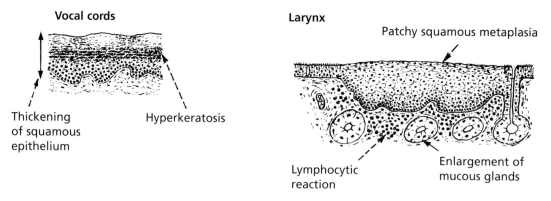

Vocal cords

Thickening of squamous epithelium

Hyperkeratosis

Larynx

Patchy squamous metaplasia

Lymphocytic reaction

Enlargement of mucous glands

The following sequence of events tends to take place:

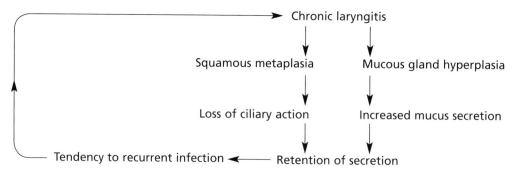

Chronic laryngitis

Squamous metaplasia

Mucous gland hyperplasia

Loss of ciliary action

Increased mucus secretion

Tendency to recurrent infection

Retention of secretion

Tuberculosis – this can cause severe ulceration of the larynx and is usually secondary to pulmonary tuberculosis.

Vocal cord nodule (singer's node)
This is found in singers and those who abuse their voice. Small smooth nodules may be seen on one or both vocal cords where the cords impact during phonation.

They consist of squamous epithelium overlying fibrin-rich and myxoid stroma.

TUMOURS OF THE UPPER RESPIRATORY TRACT

BENIGN TUMOURS

(a) Epithelial

Papillomas may be single but are often multiple and due to infection by papilloma virus. The epithelium may be one of two types:

Squamous cell

Transitional cell

In transitional papillomas, the abnormal epithelium grows down the glandular ducts and the name 'inverted papilloma' is applied. Such tumours often recur after incomplete removal.

(b) Connective tissue

Haemangiomas, especially of the nasal septum, can cause persistent nose bleeds. A special form, angiofibroma, affects male children and grows throughout childhood but typically regresses.

MALIGNANT TUMOURS

These are mainly squamous carcinomas and are commonly seen in the larynx. Intraepithelial neoplasia (carcinoma-in-situ) is a frequent precursor.

Smoking and alcohol consumption are aetiologically important. The rate of growth and spread is influenced by the site within the larynx.

Tumours of the true cord tend to stay localised and have a better prognosis than supraglottic (X) and subglottic (Y) tumours – the looser surrounding tissues allow early local and cervical node spread.

Nasopharyngeal carcinoma is common in Eastern countries and is associated with Epstein–Barr virus infection.

Adenocarcinoma of the nose is a rare tumour, sometimes seen in woodworkers.

LUNGS – ANATOMY

ACINUS

This is the functional unit of the lung, where gas transfer takes place. It consists of the respiratory bronchiole and associated alveolar ducts and sacs supplied by one terminal bronchiole.

LOBULE

This is served by one preterminal bronchiole and is the smallest anatomic compartment of lung that is grossly apparent. It contains 3 to 30 acini and is bound by connective tissue septa. These connective tissue septa may be accentuated in smokers.

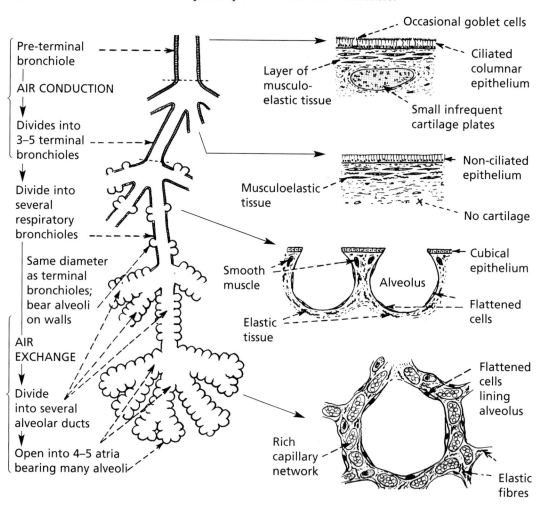

The total area for air exchange is very large (equivalent to a tennis court) allowing considerable reserve capacity.

LUNGS – ANATOMY

HISTOLOGY of the ALVEOLUS

Two types of cell (pneumocytes) line the alveoli:

Type 1 –
     are flattened cells which cover >90% of the surface.

Type 2 –
     These rounded granular cells secrete surfactant and undergo hyperplasia when Type 1 cells are injured.

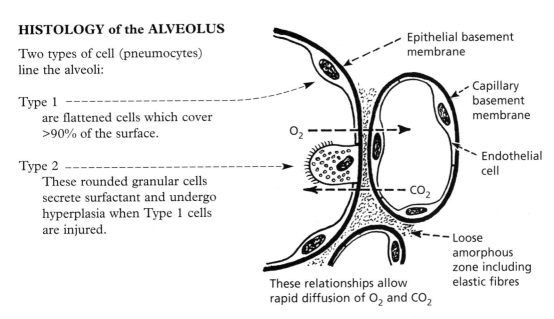

Epithelial basement membrane

Capillary basement membrane

Endothelial cell

O_2

CO_2

Loose amorphous zone including elastic fibres

These relationships allow rapid diffusion of O_2 and CO_2

Macrophages and mast cells are also present in the alveoli.

PULMONARY VASCULATURE

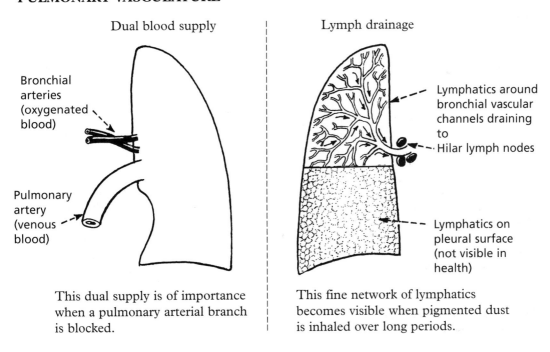

Dual blood supply

Bronchial arteries (oxygenated blood)

Pulmonary artery (venous blood)

Lymph drainage

Lymphatics around bronchial vascular channels draining to

Hilar lymph nodes

Lymphatics on pleural surface (not visible in health)

This dual supply is of importance when a pulmonary arterial branch is blocked.

This fine network of lymphatics becomes visible when pigmented dust is inhaled over long periods.

RESPIRATION

The normal intake of air is around 7 litres per minute; of this, after allowing for non-functioning dead space (trachea, bronchi, etc.), approximately 5 litres per minute are available for alveolar ventilation. A definite flow of air is maintained as far as the terminal bronchiole. Beyond this point the actual flow ceases and gas exchange is effected by diffusion.

A single terminal bronchiole (TB) gives rise to

3–5 respiratory bronchioles (RB)
Diameter of each RB = diameter of TB. Air flow stops.

Each RB gives rise to several alveolar ducts (AD) of similar diameter to respiratory bronchiole ◄——— From this point on, disparity of air pressure falls to zero and movement of respiratory gases is by diffusion.

Three factors are involved in the maintenance of adequate respiration:

1. Adequate intake of air –
2. Rapid diffusion along alveolar ducts and through alveolar walls – – – – – – – – – – – – – – – – – – –
3. Adequate perfusion of pulmonary circulation

Interference with any of these factors will result in respiratory embarrassment (dyspnoea) and even respiratory failure.

Inadequate air supply to alveoli (hypoventilation)

This may be due to lesions and diseases which interfere with the mechanics of respiration, such as central nervous lesions affecting the respiratory centre, paralysis of muscles of respiration as in poliomyelitis, injuries and deformities of the thoracic skeleton (e.g. fracture of ribs, kyphosis) and pleural disease preventing lung expansion as in pleural effusion or pneumothorax.

The most common cause of hypoventilation is bronchial obstruction. This may be reversible due to bronchial spasm as in asthma or irreversible in chronic obstructive pulmonary disease (p.258).

RESPIRATION

Impaired diffusion of gases

Three mechanisms may interfere with diffusion:

1. Reduction in the total alveolar surface available for diffusion, e.g. consolidated airless lobe in pneumonia, fibrosis of lung, tumour growth, advanced tuberculosis.
2. Increase in distance over which diffusion takes place as in emphysema.

3. Increase in the thickness of the alveolar capillary membrane. Diffusion of gas across the membrane is so rapid this can be of little practical importance. CO_2 is more soluble than O_2 and diffusion through the alveolar wall is 20 times as rapid as O_2, therefore while blood O_2 progressively falls there is usually no retention of CO_2.

Altered pulmonary perfusion

Interference with the pulmonary circulation may occur in 4 main ways:

1. Occlusion of larger vessels by multiple emboli.
2. Slowing of the pulmonary circulation as in venous congestion due to left heart lesions or congenital left-right shunts.
3. Reduction in the pulmonary capillary bed by diffuse lung disease such as fibrosis, emphysema or extensive tuberculosis.
4. Pulmonary vascular spasm due to hypoxia. Permanent changes can occur in the vessels if the hypoxia is unrelieved.

Note: In addition to hypoxaemia, inadequate perfusion tends to cause retention of carbon dioxide.
In chronic lung disease, ventilation, diffusion and perfusion disorders are present in varying degrees.

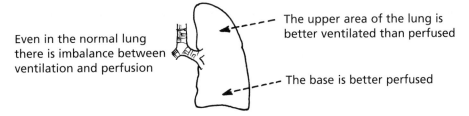

In many lung diseases this imbalance is increased. Admixture of well and poorly oxygenated blood results in hypoxaemia.

ACUTE BRONCHITIS

This is an inflammation of the large and medium bronchi. The condition may be serious if associated with pre-existing respiratory disease. Mucous and serous glands in the walls of the bronchi provide abundant mucoid secretion during the inflammation. Ciliated epithelia lining the bronchi aid passage of the exudate upward and help prevent spread down to the bronchioles.

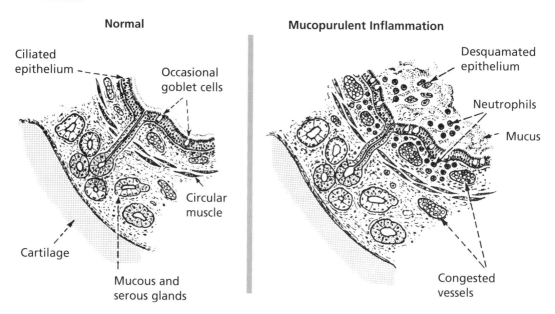

In most cases, the process is initiated by a viral or mycoplasmal infection. It is a common complication of influenza and measles. This initial phase is followed by bacterial invasion. *Streptococcus pneumoniae* and *Haemophilus influenzae* are commonest, but *Staphylococcus aureus* and *Streptococcus pyogenes* may be found, especially in infants.

The condition is usually mild, and spread to the bronchioles is unusual in healthy adults due to the effective ciliary action of the bronchial epithelium. Spread may occur however in debilitated people. Bronchiolitis and bronchopneumonia result and can prove fatal. Equally important is the serious effect of repeated attacks of acute infection in patients with CHRONIC BRONCHITIS (p.258).

In **children:**

1. Whooping cough (due to *Bordetella pertussis*) may cause permanent damage due to the severity of the infection and the stress on the airways during the coughing and whooping attacks.
2. **Bronchiolitis** in the very young (<2 years), in the majority of cases, is due to *Respiratory Syncytial Virus* and the risk of progression to **bronchopneumonia** is high.

BRONCHIAL ASTHMA

In asthma, there are spasmodic attacks of reversible bronchial obstruction with wheezing and dyspnoea and often a dry cough. The prevalence has markedly increased in recent years, possibly in part due to air pollution. There are 2 main patterns:

1. **Atopic asthma** (p.103)
   - typically starts in childhood.
   - often a strong family history of asthma or atopic conditions (e.g. eczema).
   - attacks provoked by IgE type I hypersensitivity reaction to inhaled allergens, e.g. pollen, cats, house mite dust.

2. **Non-atopic asthma**
   - usually in middle age.
   - usually no history of atopy: family history uncommon.
   - no particular antigens incriminated.

Other varieties include occupational asthma and aspirin-induced asthma.
The basic mechanism is as follows:

Activation of T-helper 2 lymphocytes

IL-4 and IL-6 → Recruitment of mast cells

IL-5 and GM-CSF → Maturation and priming of eosinophils

Release of mediators including histamine, leukotrienes and prostaglandins

Smooth muscle contraction
Bronchial oedema
Mucus plugging

ACUTE ASTHMA
Recurrent episodes of inflammation lead to irreversible damage

The **histological changes** are a combination of allergic reaction and muscular hypertrophy, the result of prolonged spasm.

Congested vessels

Oedematous submucosa

Eosinophils

Mucus secreting glands

Viscid secretion composed of:
Eosinophils
Desquamated epithelium
Thick mucus

Basal layer of cells

Thickened and hyalinised basement membrane

Hypertrophy of muscle

Sputum
In some cases the following may be seen:

1. *Curschmann's spirals* – appear as small white granules in sputum.

Charcot–Leyden crystals – in association with eosinophils.

257

CHRONIC OBSTRUCTIVE PULMONARY DISEASE (COPD)

This term describes three entities that show considerable clinical overlap:
1. Chronic bronchitis
2. Emphysema
3. Small airways disease

COPD is common accounting for approximately 5% of male deaths in the U.K.

Aetiology The main factors are:
1. SMOKING – by far the major risk factor and dose related.
2. α_1-antitrypsin deficiency. Reduced levels of this protease inhibitor correlate with lung damage, especially in smokers.
3. OCCUPATION, especially exposure to dusts, e.g. coal mining.

CHRONIC BRONCHITIS

The clinical definition is based on the presence of a productive cough lasting at least 3 months and occurring annually for at least 2 years.

Pathologically the following changes are seen:

The increase in thickness of the mucous gland layer is striking: at post-mortem the Reid index is measured – i.e. the ratio of the submucous layer (X) to the whole thickness (Y): a value greater than 1:2 is significant.

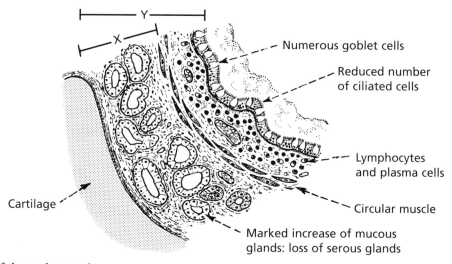

- Numerous goblet cells
- Reduced number of ciliated cells
- Lymphocytes and plasma cells
- Circular muscle
- Marked increase of mucous glands: loss of serous glands
- Cartilage

The effect of these changes is:

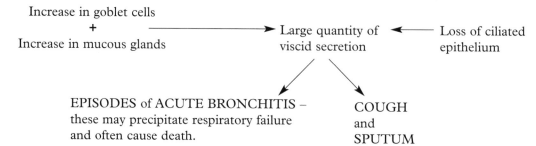

Increase in goblet cells
+
Increase in mucous glands → Large quantity of viscid secretion ← Loss of ciliated epithelium

EPISODES of ACUTE BRONCHITIS – these may precipitate respiratory failure and often cause death.

COUGH and SPUTUM

EMPHYSEMA

This is defined as a permanent dilatation of air spaces distal to the terminal bronchiole due to destruction of their walls without fibrosis. It is an important component of COPD (p. 258) and has the same aetiological factors.

Changes seen on clinical examination

Anatomical changes due to increased use of accessory muscles of respiration and increased lung volume.

Normal

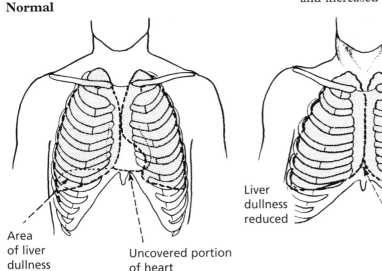

Area of liver dullness

Uncovered portion of heart

Prominent sternoclavicular muscles

Shoulders held high

Chest 'barrel shaped'

Ribs almost horizontal

Liver dullness reduced

Heart covered by lungs

Pathological changes At post-mortem the lungs are over-inflated

When removed the lung tends to collapse unless it is inflated with fixative and cut later.

External appearance

Cut surface

Dilated bullae usually towards the periphery of the upper parts

Rupture of a bulla can cause pneumothorax

Edges of lung are rounded

On the sectioned lung 2 main patterns are seen.
1. **Panacinar emphysema** and 2. **Centriacinar (centrilobular) emphysema.**

EMPHYSEMA

PANACINAR EMPHYSEMA

The enlarged air spaces are distributed across the entire acinus.

Histological section

Naked eye cut surface   Normal lung   Panacinar emphysema

Distension of alveolar ducts

Alveolar walls thin, ruptured with retracted ends.

Special stains show loss of elastic tissue. The capillaries are stretched and thinned. The reduction in blood supply is probably a factor in leading to rupture of alveoli.

There is little evidence of bronchiolitis. The voluminous lungs produce characteristic radiological changes. The distension eventually spreads to involve the respiratory bronchiole, i.e. the whole acinus is affected – panacinar emphysema.

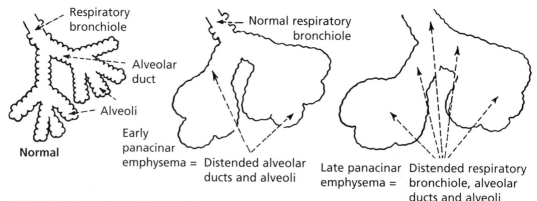

Respiratory bronchiole

Normal respiratory bronchiole

Alveolar duct

Alveoli

Normal

Early panacinar emphysema = Distended alveolar ducts and alveoli

Late panacinar emphysema = Distended respiratory bronchiole, alveolar ducts and alveoli

CENTRILOBULAR EMPHYSEMA

In this form the dilated air spaces immediately surround and involve the respiratory bronchioles.

Naked eye appearance   Histological section

Normal alveoli

Dilated spaces around respiratory bronchioles

Narrowed terminal bronchiole showing chronic inflammation

Distended respiratory bronchioles

Chronic inflammation of the respiratory bronchioles is an important feature: eventually, in many cases, the distension extends to produce panacinar emphysema.

EMPHYSEMA

Aetiology

The essential cause is thought to be an imbalance between protease and anti-protease activity. The enzyme elastase is also important.

The imbalance may be due to:

(a) Reduced inhibitor e.g. α_1-antitrypsin (α_1AT) deficiency inherited as an autosomal dominant characteristic.

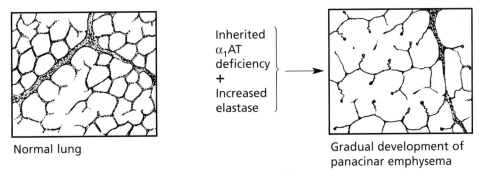

Normal lung

Inherited
α_1AT
deficiency
+
Increased
elastase

Gradual development of panacinar emphysema

(b) Excess enzyme production e.g. due to SMOKING

SMOKING → inflammation of bronchioles → ↑ proteases → centrilobular emphysema

Emphysema is an important component of lung damage due to dust inhalation (*pneumoconiosis*) (see p.272).

Functional effects of Chronic Obstructive Pulmonary Disease (COPD)

Patients with COPD tend to fall into 2 groups depending on whether or not they tolerate hypoxia.

(a) PINK PUFFERS	(b) BLUE BLOATERS
Do NOT tolerate hypoxia.	Tolerate hypoxia.
Severe breathlessness.	Severe hypoxaemia and hypercapnia.
Hyperventilation.	Right ventricular hypertrophy.
Relatively normal blood gases.	Cor Pulmonale with peripheral oedema.
	Secondary polycythaemia.

Eventually many patients develop severe chronic respiratory failure and may die during an acute episode of bronchitis.

BRONCHIECTASIS

Bronchiectasis means a permanent dilatation of one or more bronchi. There are 2 main subdivisions

1. **Obstructive** due to tumour, foreign body or enlarged lymph nodes
2. **Post-infective** due to repeated respiratory infection e.g. Cystic Fibrosis or immunodeficiency syndromes.

Pathogenesis

Recurrent inflammation

BACTERIAL GROWTH

DESTRUCTION of TISSUE

Squamous metaplasia of epithelium (loss of cilia)

RETENTION of SECRETION

Effects

1) Large quantities of secretion are retained in the bronchi and putrefactive bacteria produce a foul smell

2) Pyaemia giving rise to brain abscess or meningitis may result from involvement of a pulmonary vein branch by the suppurative process

3) Suppuration is common in the cavities and local complications arise e.g.
    lung abscess
    bronchopleural fistula
    empyema

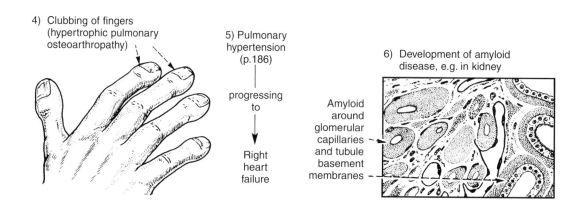

4) Clubbing of fingers (hypertrophic pulmonary osteoarthropathy)

5) Pulmonary hypertension (p.186)

progressing to

Right heart failure

6) Development of amyloid disease, e.g. in kidney

Amyloid around glomerular capillaries and tubule basement membranes

PNEUMONIA – BRONCHOPNEUMONIA

Pneumonia is an inflammatory process involving the alveolar tissue of the lungs. It is discussed under 3 main headings:

1. Bronchopneumonia
2. Lobar pneumonia
3. Miscellaneous pneumonias

Bronchopneumonia – patchy consolidation

Lobar pneumonia – whole lobe affected

1. BRONCHOPNEUMONIA

Bronchopneumonia caused by a variety of bacteria is the commonest form. It may affect all ages, but it is particularly frequent in 4 circumstances:

(a) as a terminal event in a chronic debilitating disease
(b) in infancy
(c) in old age
(d) as a manifestation of secondary infection in viral conditions e.g. influenza, measles.

Bronchopneumonia is primarily an inflammation spreading from terminal bronchioles to their related alveoli.
The lesions are initially focal, involving one or more lobules.
First red, then grey, they show a central bronchiole containing pus.

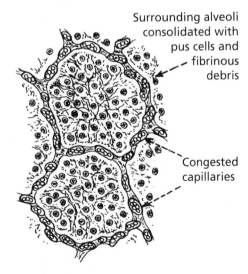

Ciliated epithelium destroyed

Congested vessels and emigration of neutrophils

Inflamed bronchiole filled with pus

Surrounding alveoli consolidated with pus cells and fibrinous debris

Congested capillaries

Possible sequels

1. Resolution – complete or partial (antibiotic and physiotherapy are important).
2. Patchy scarring.
3. Rarely, continuing sepsis with lung abscess formation.

LOBAR PNEUMONIA

2. LOBAR PNEUMONIA

As the name suggests, a complete lobe or even two lobes of a lung are affected, the most striking changes occurring in the alveoli. The disease is now rare in Western countries. It is seen typically in adults aged 20–50 years with males predominating and is caused by *Streptococcus pneumoniae*. Occasionally *Klebsiella pneumoniae* is the agent in the debilitated elderly, diabetics and alcoholics.

 The whole affected lobe progresses uniformly through 4 distinct phases illustrating the classic progression of an acute inflammation: this has been so radically altered by antibiotic treatment that the following description is to some extent historical.

Clinically, the onset is acute with fever and often rigors. There is a dry cough and rusty sputum; dyspnoea and often chest pain due to pleurisy.

The **Pathology** is described in 4 phases merging sequentially: all the alveoli in the lobe are uniformly affected.

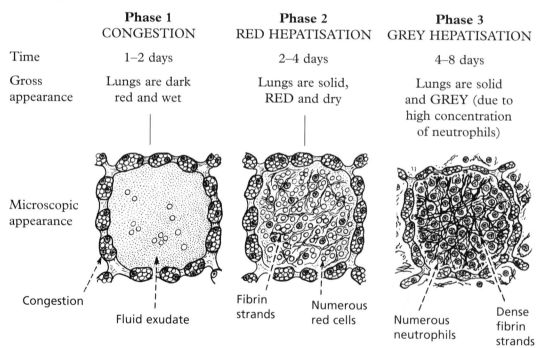

	Phase 1 CONGESTION	**Phase 2** RED HEPATISATION	**Phase 3** GREY HEPATISATION
Time	1–2 days	2–4 days	4–8 days
Gross appearance	Lungs are dark red and wet	Lungs are solid, RED and dry	Lungs are solid and GREY (due to high concentration of neutrophils)
Microscopic appearance			

Congestion

Fluid exudate

Fibrin strands

Numerous red cells

Numerous neutrophils

Dense fibrin strands

Phase 4 – RESOLUTION begins dramatically on day 8–10 and restoration to normal is rapid.

LEGIONNAIRE'S DISEASE

Previously confused with pneumococcal pneumonia, Legionnaire's disease occurs in small epidemics, is more common in males and is due to a tiny Gram-negative bacillus – *Legionella pneumophila*. The death rate can be high – up to 20%. Infection is associated with inhalation of aerosol from contaminated water storage systems.

Clinical features

Two phases are recognised:

Prodromal phase – vague flu-like illness lasting about 5 days.

Active phase

A dry cough develops. Vomiting and diarrhoea may be severe.
Patient becomes somnolent, confused and signs of consolidation appear.

Laboratory findings

Hyponatraemia. Lymphopenia. Neutrophils normal.
Signs of disseminated intravascular coagulation may develop. Serology may show an increase in antibody titre after 10–15 days.

Pathology

Both lungs are consolidated, dark red, heavy and oedematous. Fibrinous pleurisy or pleural effusion may be found.

Histology

Two stages are evident:

First stage

– – Dilated, congested alveolar capillaries

– – Fibrinous exudate containing red cells
and a moderate number of neutrophils

Second stage

Neutrophils disappear – replaced by
scanty lymphocytes and macrophages

Alveolar walls
inconspicuous
and avascular

Small abscesses may destroy bronchioles;
and lung parenchyma may show necrosis

The exudate may organise, causing an increasing interstitial fibrosis with permanent loss of lung function.

VIRAL PNEUMONIAS

INFLUENZA

In most cases, influenzal infection is confined to the upper respiratory tract, but in debilitated persons and during epidemics, the whole respiratory tract is affected.

Trachea and bronchi

Intense inflammation with haemorrhage develops.

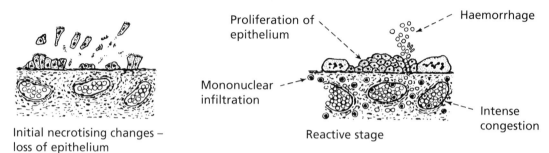

Initial necrotising changes – loss of epithelium

Proliferation of epithelium

Mononuclear infiltration

Haemorrhage

Intense congestion

Reactive stage

Pneumonia changes

The lungs are bulky, purple red and exude blood-stained froth when cut. The microscopic changes vary from one part to another.

Hyaline membrane formation

Intense interstitial mononuclear reaction

Fibrin

Swelling of basement membrane and loss of epithelium

Oedema fluid and large numbers of red cells

Mononuclear cells

Hyaline membrane

Infective agents

Of the three main types A, B and C, type A is the most virulent, and mutants of this type are responsible for most epidemics and the fatalities which occur.

Secondary infection is common, the bacteria most frequently involved being *Staphylococcus aureus*, *Haemophilus influenzae* and *Streptococcus pneumoniae*.

SARS

Severe acute respiratory syndrome is a recently recognised infectious atypical pneumonia caused by a novel corona virus, the SARS-associated corona virus. The disease was first recognised in Asia in February 2003 and caused a pandemic over the ensuing months.

ATYPICAL PNEUMONIAS

There are a number of pneumonic conditions due to *viruses* and *bacteria* in which a common pattern of pathological change is observed.

1. Necrotising bronchiolitis

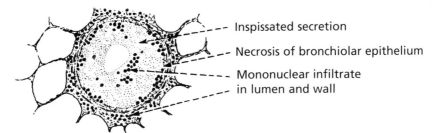

- - - Inspissated secretion

- - - Necrosis of bronchiolar epithelium

- - - Mononuclear infiltrate
in lumen and wall

2. Interstitial pneumonia

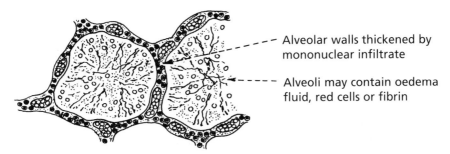

- - - Alveolar walls thickened by
mononuclear infiltrate

- - - Alveoli may contain oedema
fluid, red cells or fibrin

3. Reactive changes

The lining epithelial cells of bronchioles and alveoli are stimulated by the presence of the virus.

Cuboidal cells - - - →

Multinucleated - - -
cells

Occasionally found:

Intranuclear
inclusion body - - -

Cytoplasmic
inclusion body - - - →

Variations in the basic pattern occur in different infections. Confluent consolidation is often found in psittacosis and ornithosis (excreted by infected birds) and in measles giant cell pneumonia. Interstitial pneumonia is produced by cytomegalovirus and in rickettsial infections such as Q fever and 'scrub typhus'. In mycoplasma pneumonia, inflammation spreads from the bronchioles into the lung parenchyma and may become chronic with fibrosis.

PNEUMONIA – SPECIAL TYPES

ASPIRATION PNEUMONIA

This is due to inhalation of food or infected material from the mouth or pharynx. It may occur during anaesthesia or coma or may complicate conditions associated with frequent regurgitation e.g. oesophageal obstruction, pyloric stenosis.

In adult cases the inhalation of acid gastric contents may cause an initial shock reaction: in other cases the onset is insidious.

Possible progression is as follows:

Inhalation of ⟶ Secondary ⟶ Bronchopneumonia
foreign material   infection   lung abscess

Histologically 'foreign material', usually vegetable matter, may be seen evoking — — — a foreign body giant cell reaction.

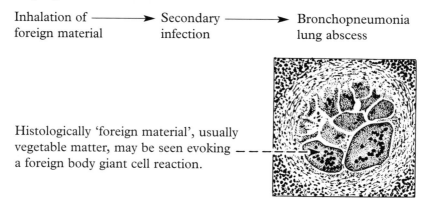

Lipid pneumonia

– The exogenous form is due to long-continued inhalation of small quantities of oily material usually derived from nasal medicaments: it is often clinically silent.

– The endogenous form is derived from tissue lipid debris distal to local bronchial obstruction.

Miscellaneous pneumonias

Opportunistic infections are seen in therapeutically immunosuppressed patients and in AIDS cases.

The causative agents include:

Viruses e.g. *Cytomegalovirus*
Bacteria e.g. *Mycobacterium avium intracellulare*
Fungi e.g. *Pneumocystis carinii, Cryptococcus neoformans, Aspergillus fumigatus, Candida albicans.*

LUNG ABSCESS

This is now an uncommon condition due to prompt treatment of preceding infection. The usual causes are:

1. Inhalation of infected material from the larynx or pharynx.

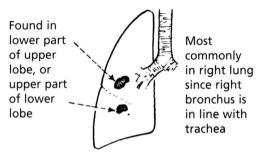

Found in lower part of upper lobe, or upper part of lower lobe

Most commonly in right lung since right bronchus is in line with trachea

2. Obstruction of a bronchus by tumour growth or foreign body. Site depends on size of bronchus affected.

Near hilum if large bronchus

At periphery if small bronchus

3. Infection of pre-existing cavities, e.g. in tuberculosis or bronchiectasis.
4. Pneumonia. Abscess is most likely to occur in debilitated persons with bronchopneumonia.

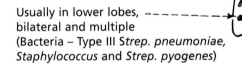

Apical abscess may occur in klebsiella infection

Usually in lower lobes, bilateral and multiple
(Bacteria – Type III *Strep. pneumoniae,* *Staphylococcus* and *Strep. pyogenes*)

Rarer causes of abscess are: pyaemia, trauma to lung, extension from suppuration in mediastinum, spinal column or subphrenic region, and infection with *Entamoeba histolytica*.

Sequelae of lung abscess

1. Small abscesses may heal.
2. Subpleural abscesses may extend to cause empyema.
3. Bronchopleural fistula resulting in pyopneumothorax is a further complication following on (2).
4. If a large pulmonary vessel is eroded, fatal haemorrhage can occur.
5. Rarely, blood spread leads to meningitis or cerebral abscess.

TUBERCULOSIS (TB)

The lungs are more commonly affected by TB than any other organ. The incidence of TB in developed countries is rising, partly due to AIDS. Drug resistant strains of Mycobacteria are an increasing problem.

There are 2 patterns of pulmonary tuberculosis — primary and secondary.

PRIMARY INFECTION

This occurs in patients, usually children, who have not been previously exposed to TB or vaccinated against it.

Infection is by inhalation.

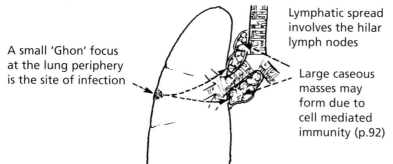

A small 'Ghon' focus at the lung periphery is the site of infection

Lymphatic spread involves the hilar lymph nodes

Large caseous masses may form due to cell mediated immunity (p.92)

The COMBINATION of Ghon focus + hilar nodes is termed the primary complex.

In most patients, the lesions undergo fibrosis or calcification and heal. Spread can, however, occur.

SECONDARY INFECTION

This is a recurrence of TB in later life — either reactivation or reinfection. The patients have immunity to TB and develop a cell mediated response leading to CASEATION.

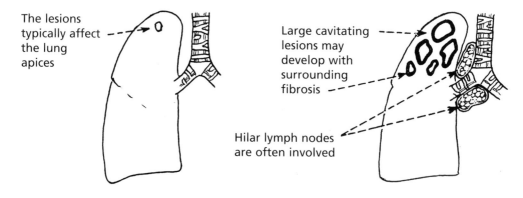

The lesions typically affect the lung apices

Large cavitating lesions may develop with surrounding fibrosis

Hilar lymph nodes are often involved

SPREAD OF TUBERCULOSIS

SPREAD OF TUBERCULOSIS

This is typically seen in secondary TB, but may also complicate primary infection.

The infection can spread by several pathways.

(a) **Direct spread** e.g. to pleura and pericardium.

(b) **By the bronchi.**

Tubercle bacilli may spread to the larynx or by the bronchi to give tuberculous bronchopneumonia ('Galloping consumption').

Consolidation is seen throughout large areas of lung parenchyma.

This occurs particularly in the immunosuppressed.

(c) **By the pulmonary veins.**

This may lead to isolated blood borne infection e.g. tuberculous meningitis (p.553), renal TB and bone TB e.g. Pott's disease of the spine: or to miliary spread throughout the body.

Kidney   Spine

(d) **By the pulmonary arteries** (probably by lymphatics draining into the inferior vena cava).

In this, miliary spread occurs throughout the lung fields alone.

The clinical course of tuberculosis is variable and depends on the immune status of the individual, the response of the bacteria to drugs, and intercurrent disease.

The **histological** features are as described on page 72.

Miliary tubercles, approximately 1–2 mm, are seen throughout the lung fields.

PNEUMOCONIOSES (DUST DISEASES)

The reaction to inhaled dust varies very considerably. Some dusts, e.g. pure carbon, are inert: others, e.g. silicates, cause severe lung disease.

Basic Pathology

1. *Inorganic dust* particles reaching the lungs are ingested by alveolar macrophages.

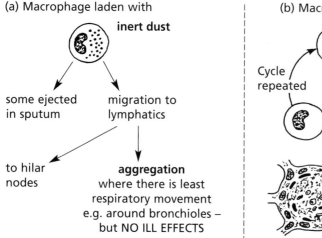

(a) Macrophage laden with **inert dust**

some ejected in sputum → migration to lymphatics

to hilar nodes

aggregation where there is least respiratory movement e.g. around bronchioles – but NO ILL EFFECTS

(b) Macrophage laden with **damaging dust**

Cycle repeated

→ **death of cell**

liberation of silica

recruitment of new macrophage

accumulation of silica in alveoli and local lymphatics

↓ progressive FIBROSIS

2. *Organic dust* particles which cause lung disease by a different mechanism include FUNGI encountered in many occupations, e.g. farmers, malt workers, bird fanciers.

The basic pathology is an immunological sensitivity reaction and the term hypersensitivity pneumonitis is used.

Inhalation of antigen → Antigen-antibody complex → Inflammation

Removal of antigen → Resolution

Repeated exposure → Chronic inflammation and fibrosis

ANTHRACOSIS

Pure carbon is biologically inert and is deposited as in (a) above with no ill effects. Damage to the lung seen in coal-miners and in populations exposed to carbon polluted atmosphere is potentiated by the content of silicates and other pollutants.

Coal-miner's Pneumoconiosis

1. Simple aggregation of coal dust particles may progress with the formation of small dust nodules and mild centrilobular emphysema (p.260) with MINIMAL FUNCTION LOSS.
2. In a few cases, Progressive Massive Fibrosis supervenes with SEVERE DISABILITY.

The cause is unknown, theories include silicates in dust; concomitant tuberculosis; sensitivity reaction.

Irregular masses of black fibrous tissue in the upper lobes with cavities filled with black fluid

Simple anthracotic changes

PNEUMOCONIOSES (DUST DISEASES)

The severe diseases caused by inorganic dust inhalation, usually occupationally, are described.

1. **Silicosis** – stone workers, sandblasters, miners.
2. **Asbestosis** – shipbuilding, insulation, electrical work.

The damage caused depends on:

(a) The type of dust
e.g. soluble/insoluble.

(b) The shape of the particle e.g.

Fibres align in the long axis of the airways helping them to reach the lung.

(c) The size of the particle — particles longer than 5 µm are likely to be trapped in the nose and large airways.

(d) The amount of exposure — large amounts overwhelm the defence mechanisms (especially lung macrophages).

SILICOSIS

The lung lesions are slowly progressive over many years. Silicates are particularly damaging to lung macrophages.

Chronic exposure ⟶ Death of macrophages ⟶ Release of cytokines ⟶ Fibrosis

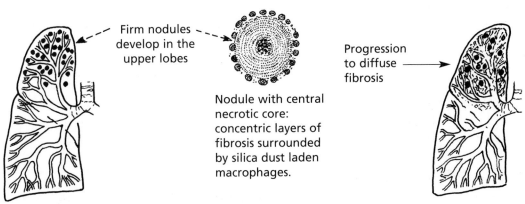

Firm nodules develop in the upper lobes

Nodule with central necrotic core: concentric layers of fibrosis surrounded by silica dust laden macrophages.

Progression to diffuse fibrosis

Patients develop increasing breathlessness and may die of respiratory failure and cor pulmonale.

The silicotic lung is particularly susceptible to **tuberculosis** and, historically, this was an important cause of death.

ASBESTOSIS

Asbestos is the generic name for a group of fibrous silicates widely used in heavy industry for insulation (particularly in shipbuilding).

There are two distinct forms of asbestos – serpentine (curly and flexible) and amphibole (straight and stiff). Amphibole fibres (crocidolite and amosite) are more pathogenic than serpentine fibres (principally chrysotile).

Asbestosis results from chronic exposure.

Diffuse fibrosis is most marked in lower lobes

↓

often progressing to honeycombing

Some asbestos fibres become encrusted with iron and protein

~20μm

The ASBESTOS BODIES are markers of asbestos exposure and can be identified in SPUTUM or lung tissue.

Other important complications are:

1. Lung cancer

Asbestos workers have an increased risk of lung cancer, especially if they also smoke. Risk of cancer = risk due to smoking × risk due to asbestos.

2. Pleural pathology

(a) Pleural plaques

These are dense areas of hyaline fibrosis on the parietal pleura.

They cause no morbidity but are markers of exposure.

Rarely there is diffuse pleural fibrosis

(b) Mesothelioma (Malignant tumour of the pleura)

This can occur up to 40 years after a brief exposure to asbestos (particularly crocidolite).

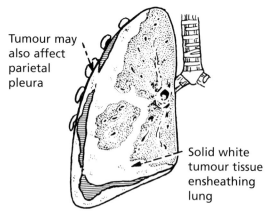

Tumour may also affect parietal pleura

Solid white tumour tissue ensheathing lung

Note: Mesothelioma may also affect the pericardium and peritoneum.

INTERSTITIAL PULMONARY FIBROSIS

Interstitial Pneumonia

This encompasses a group of conditions in which the lung is altered by a combination of interstitial inflammation and fibrosis. These may present as an acute or chronic illness.

Several histological patterns are recognised:

1. **Diffuse Alveolar Damage (DAD, Hamman–Rich Syndrome) and Usual Interstitial Pneumonia (UIP)**

   Initiation of inflammation at alveolar (and bronchiolar) level (probably basically an auto-immune reaction).

Hyaline membrane

Loss of type I pneumocytes; increase in type II.

Progression to FIBROSIS

Loss of specialised structure and alveolar space

Macrophages and lymphocytes

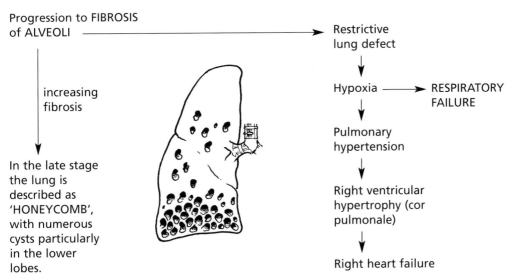

Progression to FIBROSIS of ALVEOLI

increasing fibrosis

In the late stage the lung is described as 'HONEYCOMB', with numerous cysts particularly in the lower lobes.

Restrictive lung defect

↓

Hypoxia ——→ RESPIRATORY FAILURE

↓

Pulmonary hypertension

↓

Right ventricular hypertrophy (cor pulmonale)

↓

Right heart failure

Infection is a common terminal event, and there is an increased risk of lung cancer.

INTERSTITIAL PULMONARY FIBROSIS

2. Desquamative interstitial pneumonia (DIP)

3. Organising pneumonia

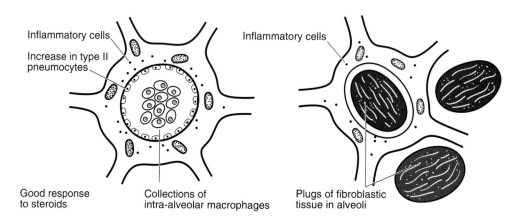

In many cases there is no recognisable cause. However similar pathological pictures may be seen in:

1. Pneumoconiosis
2. Sarcoidosis
3. Collagen vascular disease, e.g. rheumatoid arthritis, SLE
4. Drugs, e.g. bleomycin, amiodarone
5. Poisons, e.g. paraquat
6. Infections, e.g. atypical pneumonias.

LUNG CANCER

Lung cancer (carcinoma of the bronchus) is the commonest form of cancer and one which is largely preventable. Approximately 35 000 patients die of lung cancer in the United Kingdom each year.

Gross Pathology

The tumour arises from the main bronchi or their large branches (central) or at the periphery of the lung (peripheral)

Most patients present with cough, haemoptysis or chest pain, but metastases may be the first sign.

The lung distal to the tumour may collapse or become consolidated
(Retention pneumonia).

Central tumours arise from the bronchial mucosa and form a friable mass which often partly obstructs the bronchial lumen.

Tumour spread

(a) LOCAL SPREAD

(ii) Pleural involvement often results in a haemorrhagic effusion.

(iii) Hilar lymph nodes are often involved – with extension into mediastinal nodes.

(i) The tumour directly invades adjacent lung tissue. Invasion of a large blood vessel may lead to severe haemorrhage (Haemoptysis).

(iv) Direct spread to the pericardium may cause pericardial effusion with subsequent involvement of the myocardium.

LUNG CANCER

LOCAL SPREAD (continued)

(v) Apical tumours (**Pancoast tumour**) can involve structures in the neck.

Involvement of the brachial plexus can give sensory and motor symptoms

Involvement of cervical sympathetic chain causes Horner's syndrome:
Ptosis – drooping eyelid.
Enophthalmos – sunken eye.
Miosis – small pupil.
Anhydrosis – loss of sweating.

(iv) Spread to the mediastinum

(a) The superior vena cava can be obstructed – venous congestion in head and neck.

(b) Nerves may be involved –
Recurrent laryngeal ⟶ vocal cord paralysis.
Phrenic ⟶ paralysis of diaphragm.

(b) DISTANT SPREAD

Haematogenous spread is common, usually due to invasion of pulmonary veins. The common sites are: LIVER, BONE, BRAIN, ADRENAL (the last is usually asymptomatic but is found frequently at autopsy).

Lymphatic spread to cervical nodes and retrograde spread to the abdomen occurs.

NON-METASTATIC EFFECTS
These include:

1. ACTH secretion ⟶ Adrenal hyperplasia ⟶ Raised blood cortisol ⟶ Cushing's syndrome.

2. ADH secretion ⟶ Retention of water ⟶ Dilutional hyponatraemia

3. Parathyroid hormone related peptide (PTHrP) secretion ⟶ Hypercalcaemia (p.25).

Other syndromes include: encephalopathy, cerebellar degeneration, neuropathy, myopathy, Eaton Lambert myasthenia-like syndrome, etc.

LUNG CANCER

HISTOLOGICAL TYPES

Four main types are recognised

1. Small cell	20%.	The
2. Squamous carcinoma	30%.	proportions
3. Adenocarcinoma	40%.	vary between
4. Large cell carcinoma	10%.	series.

The separation of small cell carcinoma from non-small cell variants is extremely important as the former tumour is treated by chemotherapy.

SMALL CELL LUNG CARCINOMA

This is the most aggressive form of lung cancer and metastasises early and widely. It does respond well, at least initially, to chemotherapy – some patients survive for up to 2 years.

Almost no cytoplasm

Spindle-shaped dark nuclei; may appear to be rounded or oval. May be arranged in sheets, cords or small round aggregates.

Clusters of hyperchromatic cells with nuclear moulding may be seen on sputum cytology

The tumour arises from neuro-endocrine cells and expresses markers such as NCAM-1. It is the form which most commonly has endocrine and other non-metastatic humoral effects.

SQUAMOUS CARCINOMA

These tend to arise centrally from major bronchi, within dysplastic squamous epithelium following squamous metaplasia.

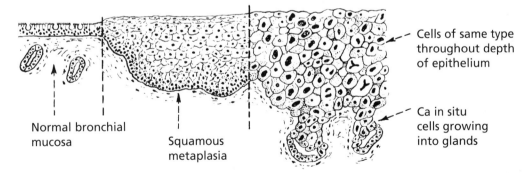

Cells of same type throughout depth of epithelium

Ca in situ cells growing into glands

Normal bronchial mucosa

Squamous metaplasia

Although squamous carcinoma is often slow growing, there is often extensive destruction of local tissues. The affected bronchi are often blocked, leading to retention pneumonia or collapse.

279

LUNG CANCER

HISTOLOGICAL TYPES *(continued)*

ADENOCARCINOMA

This tumour is a common tumour in women and is seen in non-smokers, but is also associated with smoking. At least two-thirds arise in the periphery of the lung, sometimes in relation to scarring.

Two main patterns are seen:

(a) A well defined mass of malignant cells arranged in acini with a fibrous stroma.

(b) Growth of tumour cells along the alveolar walls (so-called 'bronchioalveolar carcinoma')

Normal alveoli

Tumour cells spreading along alveolar walls

LARGE CELL CARCINOMA

As the name suggests, this tumour consists of large malignant cells without any specific differentiation. This is therefore a diagnosis of exclusion. The tumour usually arises centrally.

AETIOLOGY OF LUNG CANCER

The main factors are:

1. *Cigarette smoking* – This is by far the major cause, established by epidemiological and animal studies. Cigarette smoke contains carcinogens such as 3,4 benzpyrene and nitrosamines. Passive smoking is also significant.

2. *Industrial and atmospheric pollution* — There is a large number of pollutant industrial processes e.g. asbestos workers, miners exposed to irradiation (e.g. radon, uranium) and metal smelters (e.g. chromium and nickel).

Lung cancer is more common in urban than in rural areas.

SECONDARY LUNG TUMOURS

It must always be remembered that many other cancers spread to the lungs both by blood and lymphatic routes.

OTHER TUMOURS OF THE BRONCHI AND LUNGS

Benign tumours of the bronchi and lung are unusual. There are 2 main types.

1. SQUAMOUS PAPILLOMA

Polypoid tumours, usually multiple, at mouths of large bronchi

Papillomas are similar to the papillary tumours of the larynx. They occur in young people and on occasion may cause stridor due to partial bronchial obstruction. They are due to papilloma virus infection (types 6 and 11). Malignant change is exceptional.

2. CHONDROID HAMARTOMA

These are uncommon lesions of the lung which consist of lobules of cartilage and cleft-like spaces lined by bronchial epithelium. Their importance is that they appear as 'coin lesions' on chest X-ray and may simulate primary or secondary tumours. Current evidence suggests they are benign neoplasms rather than hamartomas.

CARCINOID TUMOURS

These tumours account for 1–2% of primary lung neoplasms. They often appear around the age of 50 years. Usually the tumour is situated in a primary bronchus or at the lung periphery. The tumour is a smooth surfaced yellow nodule.

Histologically these resemble carcinoid tumours of the appendix (see p.334). A small proportion of these tumours metastasise to regional lymph nodes – all are potentially malignant.

Central tumours tend to block the bronchus in which they arise.

Atypical carcinoid tumours: This sub-group of tumours shows nuclear pleomorphism, mitotic activity and necrosis. Over half eventually metastasise.

Tumours of bronchial glands
Both benign and low grade malignant tumours of the bronchial glands are occasionally seen. These present as obstructing lesions.

COLLAPSE OF LUNG

There are 2 basic causes of collapse of the lung.

(1) **Pressure** on the visceral pleura by fluid or air – this is discussed in more detail on pages 283 and 284.

(2) **Bronchial obstruction** causing absorption collapse. The illustration shows collapse of a lung segment.

Absorption of air from alveoli

↓

COLLAPSED segment dark red in colour (haemoglobin not oxygenated).

The commonest causes are bronchial tumour and inhaled foreign body.

Sequel – if the obstruction is not relieved, infection ± fibrosis follows.

ATELECTASIS AND HYALINE MEMBRANES

Respiratory difficulties arising shortly after the birth of a baby are associated with pathological changes in the lungs.

Aetiology — there are 2 main factors

(1) *Premature birth* — (a) immaturity of lungs — deficiency of SURFACTANT (surfactant facilitates alveolar expansion and forms a protective layer between air and alveolar lining cells).

(b) immaturity of respiratory centre.

(2) *Cerebral damage* — respiration depressed.

Atelectasis means failure of the lungs to expand at birth.

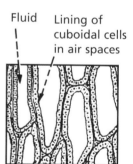

If respiration is not fully established, difficulties continue with the formation of HYALINE MEMBRANES due to the precipitation of protein along respiratory bronchioles and alveolar ducts.

ADULT RESPIRATORY DISTRESS SYNDROME (ARDS)

The adult lung may show similar changes with hyaline membranes secondary to a wide variety of disorders: severe shock, inhalation of irritant gases and pure oxygen, paraquat ingestion and uraemia are examples.

The mechanism is illustrated under Shock Lung (p.173).

DISEASES OF THE PLEURA

INFLAMMATION (PLEURISY)

There are several causes.

(a) *Infection* – usually due to spread from pneumonia or tuberculosis.
      – following penetrating injury e.g. stab wound.
(b) *Autoimmunity* – e.g. rheumatoid arthritis, systemic lupus erythematosus.
(c) *Overlying a pulmonary infarct (p.162).*

FIBRINOUS PLEURISY

Fibrinous exudate on parietal and visceral layers ⟶ Pleural friction rub, pleuritic chest pain due to movement on respiration

The exudate is absorbed but organisation may lead to pleural adhesions.

If fluid accumulates in excess, there is a pleural effusion – pain and friction rub disappear as the inflamed layers are separated.

If infection of the pleura proceeds, an empyema (a collection of pus in the pleura) may form. This is now unusual.

PLEURAL EFFUSION

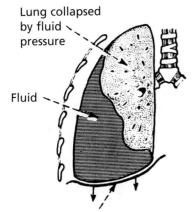

Lung collapsed by fluid pressure

Fluid

Diaphragm depressed

The accumulation of fluid within the pleura can be explained as a form of local oedema.

The composition of the fluid is related to the underlying cause.

TRANSUDATE	EXUDATE
e.g. in heart failure	e.g. in fibrinous pleurisy
– low protein content;	– high protein content;
– few inflammatory cells.	– numerous inflammatory cells.

Examination of the pleural fluid may show mesothelial cells, lymphocytes, macrophages, neutrophils and sometimes tumour cells.

DISEASES OF THE PLEURA

PNEUMOTHORAX

This is the accumulation of air in the pleural space. It may follow blunt trauma or penetrating wound e.g. stabbing. Older patients with emphysema may develop spontaneous pneumothorax. In young people this is usually due to rupture of small bullae.

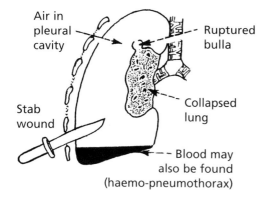

Air in pleural cavity

Ruptured bulla

Collapsed lung

Stab wound

Blood may also be found (haemo-pneumothorax)

In a TENSION PNEUMOTHORAX there is a valve effect – air continues to enter the pleura during inspiration but cannot exit during expiration.

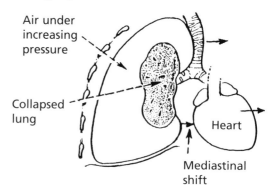

Air under increasing pressure

Collapsed lung

Heart

Mediastinal shift

Patients complain of chest pain and breathlessness.

PLEURAL MALIGNANCY

Metastatic tumours affect the pleura in 2 ways.

(a) By LYMPHATIC spread – with numerous small nodules e.g. breast carcinoma.

(b) By DIRECT spread e.g. lung cancer.

There is usually a pleural effusion in which tumour cells can be found.

Malignant Mesothelioma

This primary pleural malignancy is usually due to asbestos exposure — often many years before.

The tumour may encase the entire lung and
        grow into the interlobar fissures

The tumour can metastasise to other sites, but most patients die due to the local respiratory effects.

Histologically, the tumour shows a mixture of epithelial and sarcomatous tissues.

There is often a malignant pleural effusion.

GASTROINTESTINAL TRACT

THE MOUTH

INFLAMMATION

A wide variety of inflammatory conditions is seen.

VIRAL INFECTIONS

Herpes simplex virus (usually type I) infects the mouth in young children – numerous vesicles and ulcers are seen. The virus can become latent in the trigeminal ganglion and repeated 'cold sores' occur on the lip in later life.

Coxsackie viruses can cause oral blistering (e.g. herpangina; hand, foot and mouth disease). Koplik's spots are a feature of measles.

FUNGAL INFECTION

Candida albicans is an oral commensal in 20–40% of the population. Infection is seen in infants, in patients on broad spectrum antibiotics, steroid or cytotoxic therapy and also in the immunosuppressed and diabetics. Extensive oral candida is common in patients with AIDS.

BACTERIAL INFECTIONS

Acute ulcerative gingivitis and oropharyngitis (Vincent's angina) is due to coinfection with *Fusibacterium fusiformis* and *Borrelia vincenti*.

Syphilis, now uncommon in the West, can involve the mouth as a primary chancre, irregular lines of ulceration – snail track ulcers of the secondary stage, and as small gummas (tertiary).

Oral tuberculosis, usually due to coughed up bacilli from pulmonary TB, is now uncommon. Ulcers may occur on the tongue.

Aphthous ulcers

Around 30% of the population are troubled by these painful, usually small, ulcers on the cheek, tongue and gums. The aetiology is unknown; in some individuals they are provoked by stress or local trauma.

Dermatoses e.g. lichen planus – can affect the oral mucosa.

Blisters and inflammation

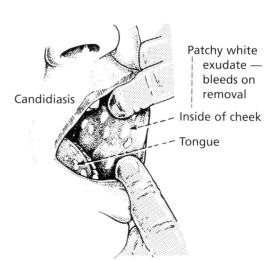

Candidiasis

Patchy white exudate — bleeds on removal

Inside of cheek

Tongue

ORAL CANCER

Oral cancer accounts for 2% of cancers in the United Kingdom. There is wide geographical variation – commoner in S. East Asia. Males are at least twice as commonly affected as women – it is a disease of the elderly.

Aetiology

The major causes are:

1. Tobacco – especially pipe and cigar smoking. Chewing tobacco, sometimes mixed with betel nuts (in Eastern countries) is also implicated.
2. Alcohol, especially spirits.
3. Exposure to ultra-violet light (cancer of the lip).
4. Human papilloma virus (type 16) may be involved.

Pathology

Almost all cases are **squamous cell carcinomas**. The lip, tongue, floor of mouth, tonsil and fauces are affected in that order of frequency.

Ulcerated nodule often on the lower lip with raised edges.

Histologically it is a well-differentiated keratinising growth.

Growth is relatively slow but eventually dissemination to the submandibular nodes takes place and thence to the deeper cervical nodes

Tongue/Floor of mouth

Carcinoma of the tongue and other sites within the mouth is a more aggressive growth than tumours of the lips. Starting as a nodule in the buccal sulcus adjacent to the tongue, it quickly breaks down to form an irregular ulcer with ragged edges.

Local infiltration leads to fixation of the tongue. Spread may be extensive to floor of mouth, fauces, pharynx, and into the medullary cavity of the mandible via occlusal ridge gaps particularly in the edentulous patient.

Lymph node involvement occurs early, usually to the deeper cervical nodes.

287

MOUTH

ERYTHROPLAKIA and LEUKOPLAKIA

Many oral cancers arise from dysplastic squamous epithelium.

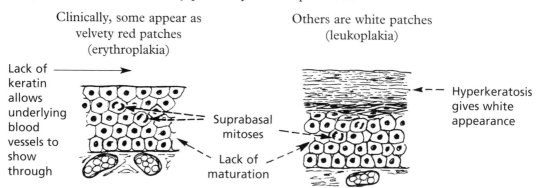

Clinically, some appear as velvety red patches (erythroplakia)

Others are white patches (leukoplakia)

Lack of keratin allows underlying blood vessels to show through

Suprabasal mitoses

Lack of maturation

Hyperkeratosis gives white appearance

Not all examples of leukoplakia are premalignant; this is simply a descriptive term for a white patch.

It may also be due to: – chronic irritation (e.g. dentures)
– pipe smoking
– Candida.

A distinctive form – 'hairy leukoplakia' – occurs on the lateral border of the tongue in patients with HIV/AIDS. It appears to be due to Epstein–Barr virus infection, often with superimposed candida.

Pigmentations

Dark pigmentations of the gums are seen in chronic poisoning with heavy metals; lead (blue), bismuth (grey), mercury (purplish). Melanotic pigmentation of the mouth is seen in Addison's disease and the Peutz–Jeghers syndrome.

Benign Tumours

A variety of benign tumours are seen e.g. squamous papillomas. Haemangiomas (often on the lips or tongue) can interfere with swallowing and may bleed after biopsy.

Granular cell tumour

This is a rare tumour and its importance lies in the fact that it may be mistaken for carcinoma of the tongue.

Overlying epithelium shows very irregular downgrowths – but it is not neoplastic (so-called pseudoepitheliomatous hyperplasia)

Large granular cells (thought to arise from Schwann cells) between and around muscle cells of tongue

Note: Epulis is a clinical term applied to swellings at the gum margin. Most of them are granulomas associated with chronic gingivitis. A few are true neoplasms.

DENTAL CARIES AND PERIODONTAL DISEASE

These two very common processes are primarily of importance to dentists but an understanding is also valuable for doctors.

DENTAL CARIES

This is the commonest disease of teeth.

Poor oral hygiene + high sugar intake lead to formation of plaque.

Plaque includes masses of bacteria e.g. *Streptococcus mutans* + sugar

} Lactic acid and proteolytic enzymes

remove calcified parts of tooth (CARIES)

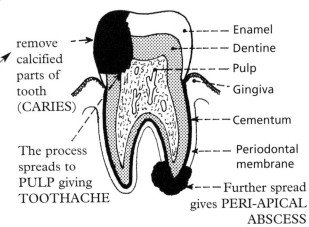

— Enamel
— Dentine
— Pulp
— Gingiva
— Cementum
— Periodontal membrane
— Further spread gives PERI-APICAL ABSCESS

The process spreads to PULP giving TOOTHACHE

PERIODONTAL DISEASE

This is the major cause of tooth loss in middle age. It is essentially due to gingivitis.

A pouch is formed between the gingiva and the neck of the tooth.

Bacteria e.g. bacteroides, fusobacterium, cause inflammatory reaction.

Inflammation spreads to the periodontal membrane.

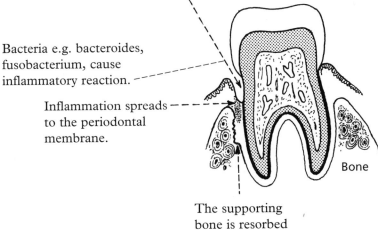

Bone

The supporting bone is resorbed

Loosening of tooth

DISEASES OF THE SALIVARY GLANDS

INFLAMMATION

Simple bacterial infection of these glands is uncommon. It may occur during a prolonged illness, particularly if a calculus has formed in a duct.

More commonly acute inflammation is due to the virus of mumps, which produces acute swelling, particularly of the parotid glands, with oedema and mononuclear infiltration of the interstitial tissue.

The testes and pancreas may also be inflamed and atrophy may follow.

Chronic inflammation is rare. It may occur as a manifestation of sarcoidosis. The parotid gland becomes swollen and there may be an accompanying irido-cyclitis. This has given rise to the term 'uveo-parotid fever'. The parotid gland shows a chronic inflammatory reaction with granulomas typical of sarcoidosis.

Parotid

Pancreas

Testes

Sjögren's syndrome

In this auto-immune condition there is a destruction of the gland tissue of the salivary, lacrimal and conjunctival glands by an infiltrate of lymphocytes (so-called lympho-epithelial lesions) and plasma cells. The duct epithelia often undergo reactive hyperplasia. It results in dryness of the mouth, caries due to lack of saliva, and ulceration of the conjunctiva caused by lack of secretion from the lacrimal and conjunctival glands. Polyarthritis is often present and the serum contains autoantibodies and rheumatoid factor.

Occasionally a B-cell lymphoma arises from the lymphoid proliferation.

Calculus formation

This can affect the submandibular or, less often, the parotid duct. Blockage of the duct leads to episodes of swelling after food and eventually to atrophy of the gland. Occasionally acute inflammation may be superimposed.

SALIVARY GLAND TUMOURS

The majority (80%) of tumours arise in the parotid gland and most in this site are benign.

The remaining 20% occur in the submandibular and minor salivary glands – in these sites 30–40% are malignant.

SALIVARY GLANDS – TUMOURS

PLEOMORPHIC SALIVARY ADENOMA (P.S.A.)

This is the commonest tumour of the salivary glands and most often occurs in the parotid. The term 'pleomorphic' applies not to the nuclei of the cells but to the different types of tissue found. These are derived from the epithelial and myoepithelial cells.

To the naked eye, the tumour appears rounded or lobulated and encapsulated. Microscopically the cellular pleomorphism assumes several forms.

The **epithelial** elements form duct-like structures often with 2 cell layers - - - ▶

or

trabeculae - - - - - - - ▶

(Squamous differentiation may be seen)

The **myoepithelial** elements are seen as - - - ▶ cellular clumps

or

may be separated by a myxoid ground substance - - - ▶

Cartilagenous metaplasia may - - - ▶ also occur.

Although the tumour appears encapsulated, there are frequently small lobules which extend - - - - ▶ into the adjacent tissue.

If the tumour is 'shelled out' these lobules are left behind and cause local recurrence. For this reason superficial parotidectomy is usually performed, ensuring complete removal of the tumour.

— Main tumour mass

MALIGNANT CHANGE

Under 5% of these tumour become malignant, often after many years. Most of these are adenocarcinomas. CARCINOMA-IN-P.S.A. has a poor prognosis.

WARTHIN'S TUMOUR

This is a benign lesion, mainly in the parotid of elderly men. It consists of tall epithelial cells with eosinophilic cytoplasm (oncocytes) and a striking reactive lymphoid infiltrate.

SALIVARY GLANDS – CARCINOMAS

Adenocarcinomas of the salivary glands may arise de novo or from pre-existing P.S.A. They may affect major or minor glands. The prognosis is variable.

Three unusual subtypes are worth noting.

1. **Acinic cell carcinoma**
   Approximately 1/4 of all malignant parotid tumours are of this type. It grows slowly, recurs after removal and sometimes there is late extension to the regional lymph nodes and distant organs.

Closely aggregated cells containing secretory granules and sometimes glycogen.

2. **Adenoid cystic carcinoma**
   This usually occurs in minor salivary glands and accounts for 7% of salivary gland tumours. It extends by direct spread, but metastases can occur to lymph nodes, lungs and bones. There is a special tendency to spread along nerve sheaths.

Cribriform pattern. Solid masses of epithelium enclosing small cystic spaces containing mucin. The cells resemble basal cells.

3. **Muco-epidermoid carcinoma**
   The behaviour of this type varies, but all tend to recur and infiltrate locally. More aggressive tumours metastasise to the lymph nodes and may invade the blood stream. They are generally found in the major salivary glands and form 3 or 4% of all tumours of these glands.

Squamoid cells

Mucus-secreting cells

OESOPHAGUS

The oesophagus is a muscular tube 25 cm long; it is lined by stratified squamous epithelium which is resistant to damage by heat, cold and mechanical trauma.

INFLAMMATION

Reflux oesophagitis

This is the commonest form of inflammation due to reflux of gastric acid through a relaxed lower oesophageal sphincter, into the lower oesophagus. It is a common concomitant of hiatus hernia.

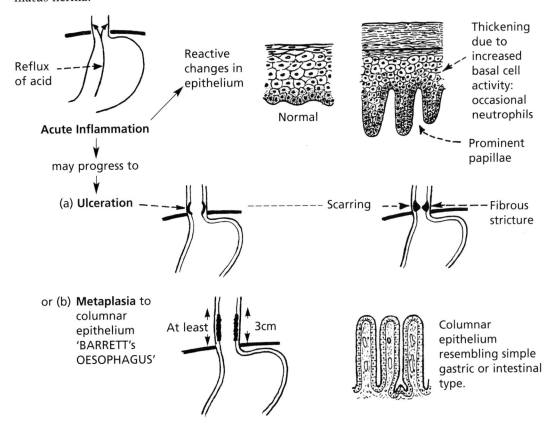

Note: This is an important premalignant lesion: the increased risk of CANCER developing is 30–40 fold.

METAPLASIA ⟶ DYSPLASIA (detected ⟶ ADENOCARCINOMA by endoscopy and biopsy)

Other forms of oesophagitis

(1) Infection by *Herpes simplex virus*, cytomegalovirus and *Candida albicans* occurs particularly in the immunosuppressed and AIDS.

(2) Ingestion of drugs, e.g. tetracycline and non-steroidal anti-inflammatory drugs, may cause ulceration of the distal oesophagus.

OESOPHAGUS

HIATUS HERNIA

In hiatus hernia part of the stomach herniates into the thorax. This is common, particularly in the elderly, though often asymptomatic. Two forms are seen:

1. **Sliding hernia**

   – the distal oesophagus and proximal stomach slide proximally so the latter lies in the thorax. Most cases are of this type.

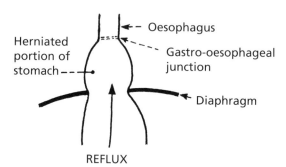

2. **Rolling hernia**

   – a loop of stomach rolls upwards and passes through the diaphragm alongside the oesophagogastric junction. Since the junction is preserved reflux is unusual.

DIVERTICULA

These are relatively rare and are of 2 varieties.

1. Pulsion type

Involves pharynx (pharyngeal pouch). Sac is distended during swallowing of food. By pushing down behind oesophagus, it may compress this structure. Abnormal function of the upper oesophageal sphincter is an aetiological factor.

2. Traction type

This is due to traction of fibrous tissue produced by mediastinal inflammation, e.g, tuberculosis of lymph nodes.

Rarely, there may be a congenital diverticulum at the level of the bifurcation of the trachea.

OESOPHAGUS

Obstruction usually leads to dysphagia – difficulty in swallowing. The causes form 2 main groups:

1. **Strictures** of the oesophageal wall due to:
   – inflammation caused by acid reflux or caustic ingestion.
   – carcinoma.
   – historically mucosal webs at the upper end were a feature of the Plummer–Vinson syndrome in chronic untreated iron deficiency anaemia.

2. **Functional** obstruction

Achalasia of the oesophagus develops in young adults and may cause severe obstruction.

Above the obstruction the oesophagus is dilated, the muscle is hypertrophied and the mucosa may be ulcerated. Narrowing occurs at the lower end.

It is due to a conduction failure in the peristaltic mechanism preventing opening of the cardiac sphincter. Reduced numbers of ganglion cells are found in the myenteric plexus.

(In South American trypanosomiasis the myenteric plexus may be destroyed and long-standing diabetic autonomic neuropathy may cause a similar problem.)

In **Systemic sclerosis**, replacement of muscle by fibrous tissue may seriously disturb oesophageal peristalsis.

OESOPHAGEAL VARICES

These are important lesions which occur secondarily to portal hypertension caused by cirrhosis of the liver (see p.350).

Fibrosis in the liver obstructs the flow of blood from the gastrointestinal tract in the portal system. Anastomotic channels connecting the portal and systemic venous systems open up and become distended. The most important are the oesophageal tributaries of the azygos vein which connect through the diaphragm with the portal system. They become varicose, and are easily traumatised by the passage of food, leading to haemorrhage which can be fatal.

Spontaneous rupture of the oesophagus is a rare condition of uncertain aetiology. Tears without rupture but causing haemorrhage and haematemesis may also occur (Mallory–Weiss syndrome).

Congenital abnormalities include stenosis and atresia with fistula formation.

OESOPHAGUS

TUMOURS

Benign tumours of the oesophagus are very rare. They are almost always of connective tissue origin (usually leiomyomas) and form polyps within the lumen, causing obstruction.

Carcinoma

Carcinoma of the oesophagus occurs at three levels: ⟶ (1) At level of bifurcation of trachea. This is the commonest site

(2) Upper end of oesophagus at level of cricoid cartilage

(3) Lower end of oesophagus

At the upper and middle third, SQUAMOUS CARCINOMA.
At the lower end, ADENOCARCINOMA (associated with Barrett's oesophagus).
The disease is more common in men by at least 2 to 1.
Two forms of growth are seen.

(1) Scirrhous encircling the tube and causing constriction

(2) Soft polypoidal growth filling lumen

In both instances the growth tends to extend in a longitudinal manner in the submucosal lymphatics. This means that the surgeon has to remove the tumour with wide margins.

Spread

At the common site, near the tracheal bifurcation, spread may involve the trachea or a bronchus, ulcerating the wall and resulting in aspiration pneumonia. Tumours at other levels may involve the trachea or other mediastinal structures. Lymph node involvement is common. Death usually results from the oesophageal obstruction, but the patient may survive long enough for metastases to appear in other organs, e.g. liver.

Aetiological factors

The incidence shows a geographical variation, being common in China and Africa. Smoking and dietary factors including alcohol consumption are important in the aetiology of squamous carcinoma. Post-cricoid carcinoma in women is a rare late complication of the dysphagia complicating iron deficiency anaemia. The incidence of adenocarcinoma is rising and is attributable to Barrett's oesophagus and reflux.

STOMACH

The stomach is divided into five anatomical regions:

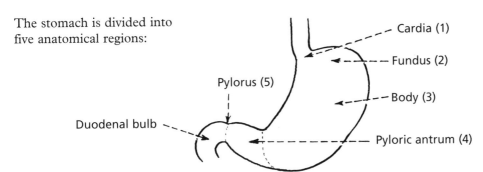

- Cardia (1)
- Fundus (2)
- Body (3)
- Pyloric antrum (4)
- Pylorus (5)
- Duodenal bulb

It has three secretory areas:

1. Cardiac

Pits

Mucous glands

2. Body and Fundus

This is the main specialised secreting area.

Pit

Parietal oxyntic cells secreting HCl and intrinsic factor

Chief or pepsin secreting cells

3 types of cell

- Mucous
- Parietal
- Chief

3. Antrum and Pylorus

Prominent pits

Mucus secreting glands including endocrine cells

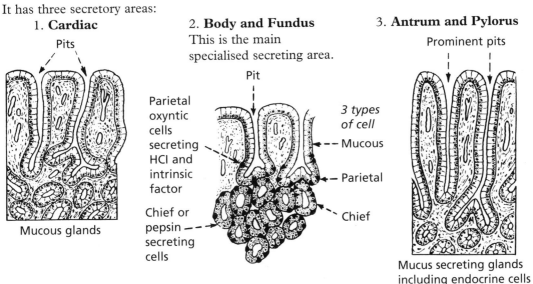

Note: (i) Mucus is secreted throughout the gastric mucosa: the specialised secretory cells are confined to the body and fundus.

(ii) There is a rapid turnover of the epithelial cells.

Vascular supply

Along the lesser curvature, run the right and left gastric arteries, which anastomose directly.

The greater curvature shows 3 arterial supplies:

- Branches from the splenic artery
- Right and left gastroepiploic arteries

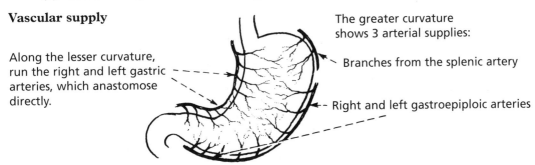

The arteries anastomose freely in the muscular, submucous and mucous coats, except along the lesser curvature of the pyloric antrum and the first part of duodenum. In this area, there is little anastomosis between the terminal branches in the mucosa.

297

GASTRITIS

ACUTE INFLAMMATION

Mild acute gastritis is an acute inflammation with neutrophil reaction in the superficial layers of the mucosa. Pain and sickness have a multitude of causes varying from hot fluids, alcohol and aspirin which act as direct irritants, to infections such as childhood fevers, viral infections and bacterial food poisoning.

A more acute form, known as acute haemorrhagic or erosive gastritis, is associated with ingestion of irritant drugs, particularly aspirin and non-steroidal anti-inflammatory drugs (NSAIDs) and is also a complication of shock states.

Haemorrhagic erosions

These are tiny ulcers, a few millimetres in diameter, which are formed by the digestion of the mucous membrane overlying small haemorrhages. They are usually multiple and affect all parts of the stomach. They occur mostly on the apex of mucosal folds and involve only the mucosa.

Note that the changes are superficial so that restoration to normal can very quickly occur.

Naked eye appearance

Erosion of mucosa with bleeding and loss of gland duct epithelium

Neutrophil infiltration

Stress ulcers

Occasionally, particularly in severe shock, there is deeper acute ulceration with considerable haemorrhage and even perforation.

Parietal cells

Muscle layer

Oedema resulting in swelling of mucosa and separation of glands

CHRONIC GASTRITIS

Although chronic gastritis is a common disorder it very rarely arises from the types of acute inflammation described above.

Our understanding of the aetiology and mechanisms of GASTRITIS and GASTRODUODENAL ULCERATION was radically altered by the discovery of a specific infective agent, *Helicobacter pylori*, with a high world wide prevalence.

GASTRITIS

CHRONIC GASTRITIS *(continued)*

The SYDNEY SYSTEM is a classification incorporating two separate divisions: (1) HISTOLOGICAL and (2) ENDOSCOPIC.
The histological classification has 3 main elements:

(a) AETIOLOGY	(b) TOPOGRAPHY i.e. site affected: antrum, body or both.	(c) MORPHOLOGY including information on activity and intestinal metaplasia – graded as mild, moderate or severe.

The two main types of chronic gastritis are examples of this classification in use:

(a) Auto-immune associated chronic pangastritis.
(b) *H. pylori* associated chronic gastritis of the antrum.

The endoscopic classification uses the same topography and categorises the gastritis in terms of the endoscopic appearances.

AUTO-IMMUNE ASSOCIATED GASTRITIS

Prevalence: 5% of chronic gastritis cases are of this type.
Aetiology: Evidence for auto-immune mechanisms:
    (1) Presence of antibodies to parietal cells and intrinsic factor.
    (2) Associated with other auto-immune disorders, e.g. thyroiditis.
Sites affected: The fundus and body predominantly.
Morphological changes are progressive over several years with gradual thinning of the mucosa.

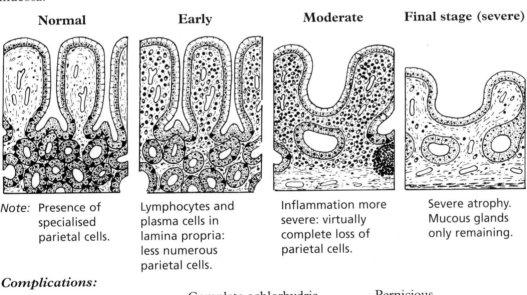

Normal	**Early**	**Moderate**	**Final stage (severe)**
Note: Presence of specialised parietal cells.	Lymphocytes and plasma cells in lamina propria: less numerous parietal cells.	Inflammation more severe: virtually complete loss of parietal cells.	Severe atrophy. Mucous glands only remaining.

Complications:

(1) Loss of parietal cells ⟶ Complete achlorhydria / Absence of intrinsic factor ⟶ Pernicious anaemia (see p.389)

(2) There is a definite association with the development of GASTRIC CARCINOMA often preceded by INTESTINAL METAPLASIA.

299

GASTRITIS

CHRONIC GASTRITIS *(continued)*

Helicobacter pylori ASSOCIATED CHRONIC GASTRITIS

Prevalence: 80% of chronic gastritis cases are of this type. The organism has a world wide distribution. In Western countries the prevalence of *Helicobacter* is over 30% by 30 years of age. In developing countries it is even higher.

Aetiology: *Helicobacter pylori* is a Gram-negative spiral bacterium ($\smallsmile$, $\frown$) which is specifically adapted to colonise the gastric mucosa: this continues indefinitely.

Site affected: The antrum and pyloric canal particularly.

Morphological changes are essentially superficial with inflammation involving the upper half of the mucosa.

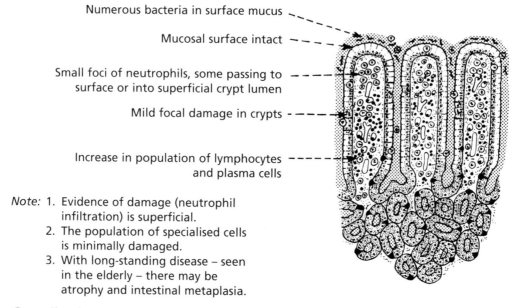

Numerous bacteria in surface mucus

Mucosal surface intact

Small foci of neutrophils, some passing to surface or into superficial crypt lumen

Mild focal damage in crypts

Increase in population of lymphocytes and plasma cells

Note: 1. Evidence of damage (neutrophil infiltration) is superficial.
2. The population of specialised cells is minimally damaged.
3. With long-standing disease – seen in the elderly – there may be atrophy and intestinal metaplasia.

Complications:

(1) GASTRIC and DUODENAL ulcer (see p.303).
(2) Progression to CARCINOMA, often preceded by INTESTINAL METAPLASIA.
(3) Association with LYMPHOMAS.

OTHER FORMS of CHRONIC GASTRITIS

These include eosinophilic gastritis often associated with food allergy, and reflux gastritis due to reflux of duodenal contents.

In some cases, continuing damage by the agents causing acute gastritis (e.g. drugs) progresses to a chronic form.

PEPTIC ULCERATION

Peptic ulcers occur when acid-containing gastric juices breach the mucosa of the gut.

Chronic peptic ulcers are found in 3 main sites.

2. Gastric ulcers usually affect the antrum on the lesser curve.

3. Reflux of acid may lead to oesophageal ulcers.

1. The first part of the duodenum. The incidence has fallen in recent years.

Occasionally a peptic ulcer arises at a site of heterotopic gastric mucosa e.g. Meckel's diverticulum.

Ulcer

Small intestine

Peptic ulcers are usually solitary, but in 10% a second ulcer is found, e.g. on the opposite side of the duodenum (kissing ulcer).

A **typical chronic peptic ulcer** is a punched out oval ulcer 2–3 cm in diameter.

The ulcer bed consists of fibrin and debris.

The surrounding mucosa often shows stellate folds due to scarring.

Mucosa

Granulation tissue grows into the debris

Blood vessels in the base show endarteritis

Muscle

In long standing lesions fibrous tissue replaces muscle.

Acute gastric ulcers (often called stress ulcers) may be seen in patients with severe burns, after major trauma or with raised intracranial pressure. These may cause bleeding, but usually heal completely. Acute ulcers may also be due to treatment with non-steroidal anti-inflammatory drugs (NSAIDs).

PEPTIC ULCERATION

SEQUELS and COMPLICATIONS

1. **Healing** is common, particularly when treated.

2. **Scarring** may lead to stricture formation.

Lesions of the lesser curvature produce an 'hour glass' stomach.

Stomach dilated. Vomiting leads to metabolic alkalosis.

Lesions of duodenum or pylorus lead to gastric outlet obstruction.

3. **Perforation** of an ulcer causes **acute peritonitis**. This may be

Generalised   or   **Localised**

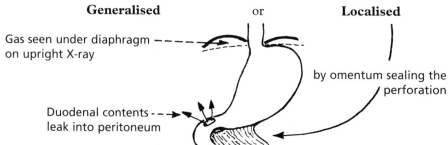

Gas seen under diaphragm on upright X-ray

by omentum sealing the perforation

Duodenal contents leak into peritoneum

Note: Loculation of pus may occur e.g. subphrenic abscess.

4. Haemorrhage

Minor haemorrhage is common but may not be apparent clinically.

Major haemorrhage can lead to haematemesis, to 'coffee ground' vomit or to melaena (tarry black stools).

It is no longer believed that there is a significant risk of malignant transformation of peptic ulcers.

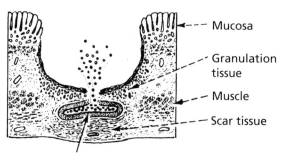

Eroded artery in ulcer base

PEPTIC ULCER – AETIOLOGY

Normally gastric mucosal damage is prevented by a balance between the damaging agents and the mucosal defences.

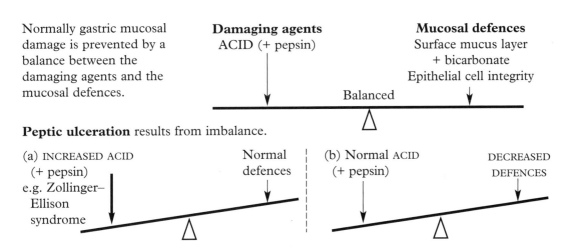

Damaging agents
ACID (+ pepsin)

Mucosal defences
Surface mucus layer
+ bicarbonate
Epithelial cell integrity

Balanced

Peptic ulceration results from imbalance.

(a) INCREASED ACID (+ pepsin) e.g. Zollinger–Ellison syndrome

Normal defences

(b) Normal ACID (+ pepsin)

DECREASED DEFENCES

Although the mechanisms in gastric and duodenal ulcers differ, in both *HELICOBACTER PYLORI* infection is important.

Gastric ulcer

Colonisation of antrum by *H. pylori* (70%).

High magnification

NSAIDS → REDUCED MUCOSAL DEFENCES

DUODENO-GASTRIC REFLUX (including bile; aggravated by smoking)

ACID (usually low or normal)

Helicobacter in surface mucus

Focal epithelial cell damage

Focal neutrophil infiltration

Duodenal ulcer (DU)

The main factors are **hyperacidity** and *H. pylori* infection (>90% of cases).

H. pylori ⟶ Gastric infection

Increased gastrin

Hyperacidity (genetic factors also important)

H. pylori infection of duodenum + other factors, e.g. stress, smoking

ACID

METAPLASIA

Focal metaplasia of tips of duodenal villi

Gastric type mucus and *Helicobacter pylori*

Cell damage

↓

Neutrophils

↓

Duodenitis

DUODENITIS → ULCER

Note: DU is cured when *H. pylori* is eliminated and acid reduced.

GASTRIC CARCINOMA

This very important tumour has an especially high incidence in Japan, Chile and Italy. Its incidence has fallen in the United Kingdom and the U.S.A. since the 1930s.

Tumours are divided evenly between the proximal and distal stomach.

Morphologically, there are several types.

1. EXOPHYTIC

These exophytic tumours are commonly seen in the fundus.

Eventually the tumour spreads through the stomach wall
to the serosa
and is often
ulcerated on
the surface.

2. ULCERATIVE

These tumours, often in the antrum, produce large irregular ulcers with a rolled edge.

The rolled edge rather than the ulcer base should be biopsied.

3. DIFFUSE PATTERN

In this form of tumour the entire gastric wall is thickened. Ulceration is usually minimal, but the mucosal folds are prominent.

This is sometimes knows as 'leather-bottle stomach' (linitis plastica).

Histologically, gastric cancers tend to fall into one of two types (Lauren classification),

(a) Intestinal

Malignant cells arranged in **acini** invade through the muscle of the stomach wall.

(b) Diffuse

Typically seen in linitis plastica. These tumours consist of **signet ring cells.**

Extracellular mucin may also be present.

Globules of mucin push the nucleus to one side.

GASTRIC CARCINOMA

Gastric carcinomas are aggressive tumours with both local and distant spread.

LOCAL spread

DISTANT spread

1. By lymphatics e.g. to supraclavicular node (Troisier's sign).

2. To lungs but usually late.

To oesophagus

1.* Mucosal and **submucosal** lymphatic spread

to duodenum*

3. **Haematogenous to liver** (via portal vein)

2. To draining lymph nodes

3. To adjacent viscera including liver

4. Transcoelomic to ovaries (Krukenberg tumours)

* *Note:* The duodenal mucosa is resistant to direct mucosal spread.

Staging is by the T.N.M. system (Tumour: nodes: metastases).

EARLY GASTRIC CANCER

Early gastric cancers are common in populations where there is screening e.g. Japan. The prognosis is far better than for deeply penetrating 'advanced' tumours.

By definition, the tumour is confined to the mucosa or mucosa and submucosa.

There is often extensive lateral spread within the mucosa.

The muscular layers are not involved

GASTRIC CARCINOMA

Aetiology

It has long been recognised that gastric cancer occurs in achlorhydric states, especially with chronic atrophic gastritis.

It is now clear that *Helicobacter pylori* is a major carcinogenic factor for these tumours arising in the distal stomach. Acid reflux is responsible for those in the proximal stomach.

OTHER GASTRIC TUMOURS

Benign gastric polyps are often seen at endoscopy.

Gastrointestinal stromal tumours (GISTs) arise from within the stomach wall and may cause haemorrhage. All are potentially malignant.

GASTRIC LYMPHOMAS account for 5% of gastric malignancy. They are usually 'B' cell lymphomas of MALT type (p.436). They are strongly associated with *Helicobacter pylori* infection and some lymphomas respond to eradication of *H. pylori*.

SMALL INTESTINE – MALABSORPTION

The main function of the small intestine is digestion and absorption of food.
Malabsorption may be due to disorders of the small bowel, pancreas and biliary tract.

COELIAC DISEASE

This important cause of malabsorption is due to sensitivity to gliadin, a component of the wheat protein **gluten**. The clinical features depend on the age at presentation.

Infancy   – Failure to thrive, diarrhoea (steatorrhoea)

Childhood – Growth retardation, nutritional deficiencies e.g. anaemia.

Adults   – Anaemia, altered bowel habit, weight loss.

In coeliac disease there is partial or complete villous atrophy.

These changes are seen in biopsies of the jejunum (Crosbie capsule) and distal duodenum (by endoscope). The changes revert to normal if gluten is removed from the diet. Serological tests are available with anti-endomysial antibodies (directed against tissue transglutaminase).

The basic mechanism is as follows:

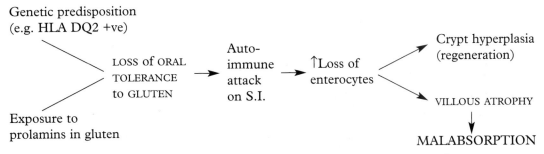

Patients with coeliac disease also have increased prevalence of autoimmune diseases e.g. diabetes, autoimmune thyroiditis and of lymphocytic colitis, a cause of unexplained diarrhoea.

They are at increased risk of developing small bowel **lymphoma**.

MALABSORPTION

Other causes of malabsorption in the small bowel include:

1. TROPICAL SPRUE

This is a disease of unknown aetiology occurring in the tropics but largely excluding Africa. Villous atrophy is seen and patients develop steatorrhoea, weight loss and deficiency of B12 and Folate, leading to megaloblastic anaemia. Treatment with folic acid and antibiotics cause the disease to remit.

2. GIARDIASIS

An infection with the protozoan *Giardia lamblia*, giardiasis is associated with diarrhoea and malabsorption. Patients with hypogammaglobulinaemia are especially at risk.

3. WHIPPLE'S DISEASE

In this rare condition, mainly of middle aged men, malabsorption, arthritis, lymphadenopathy and skin pigmentation are seen.

Large macrophages fill the lamina propria. They contain mucopolysaccharides (are periodic acid Schiff (PAS) positive). Electron microscopy shows numerous intracellular bacteria – now thought to be a gram-positive organism *Tropheryma whippelii*. Antibiotics are curative.

4. CROHN's DISEASE (p.309)

5. After SMALL BOWEL RESECTION

6. BIOCHEMICAL DISORDERS e.g. disaccharidase deficiency, abetalipoproteinaemia

7. BACTERIAL COLONISATION of the small bowel e.g. Blind Loop Syndrome.

Pancreatic diseases e.g. cystic fibrosis (p.375) and obstructive jaundice (p.341) also cause malabsorption.

CROHN'S DISEASE

Crohn's disease and ulcerative colitis are two forms of **non-infective inflammatory bowel disease.** They have similarities and striking contrasts (p. 311).

CROHN'S DISEASE

Patients, usually young adults, present with diarrhoea, abdominal pain and weight loss. Although the disease can affect any part of the G.I. tract from the mouth to the anus, the great majority of lesions are seen in the distal *small bowel* and *colon*.

The disease is discontinuous, with 'skip' lesions and normal intervening bowel.

Peri-anal lesions are common.

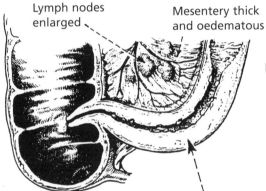

Lymph nodes enlarged

Mesentery thick and oedematous

Mucosal 'cobblestone' appearance.

Linear 'fissured' ulcers

Surviving mucosa forming 'cobbles'

In its classic form, 'regional ileitis', the terminal ileum is thickened and the lumen narrowed and ulcerated.

Transmural inflammation extending to serosa

Mucosa inflamed but architecture preserved

Deep fissuring ulcers

Granulomas associated with lymphatics are present in 2/3 of cases.

LOCAL COMPLICATIONS

Transmural inflammation ⟶ adhesions between viscera; fistulae to bowel, bladder, vagina.

Lumenal narrowing ⟶ intestinal obstruction.

Ileal involvement ⟶ malabsorption, especially of Vit B12.

Cancer ⟶ increased risk of colonic and **small intestinal** cancer, but not so great as the risk of colonic cancer in ulcerative colitis.

ULCERATIVE COLITIS

Clinical features

Patients, usually young adults, present with diarrhoea, often bloody. The disease has a remitting/relapsing course. In severe cases weight loss and anaemia are common. The disease begins in the rectum and shows continuous spread proximally.

Ileal inflammation can occur – 'backwash ileitis'

Continuous spread of varying length.

Rectum always involved

Anal lesions are uncommon.

The whole colon is affected in 20% of cases

In the established disease the **gross appearances** are striking.

Microscopy shows the evolution.

The ulcers are linear and may lie over the taenia coli

Swollen surviving islands of mucosa forming pseudo-polyps.

Early phase

Mucosa acutely congested especially over the tips of mucosal folds

Neutrophils in the crypts form 'crypt abscesses'

Muscularis mucosae

Established phase

Epithelium lost with ulceration

The inflammation is usually **confined to the mucosa**

Periods of remission occur when many of the ulcerated areas heal.

The crypts of Lieberkühn do not reform completely.

Granulation tissue

Ultimately the surface may be covered by a simple layer of mucus-secreting epithelium without glands.

LOCAL COMPLICATIONS

Toxic megacolon: In a small number of patients inflammation is very severe and the colon becomes greatly dilated and thinned. There is a high risk of perforation with peritonitis.

Dysplasia and Colonic cancer: Patients with (a) early onset, (b) total colonic involvement and (c) long-lasting (10–20 years) disease have a greatly increased risk. These patients require colonoscopic surveillence with biopsy to look for dysplasia and cancer.

CROHN'S DISEASE AND ULCERATIVE COLITIS

The aetiology of these two conditions is uncertain. Both have mild familial tendency (approximately 10%). Infection by organisms unknown has been suggested for each. Granulomas in Crohn's disease suggest mycobacterial infection (*M. pseudotuberculosis* is a possible candidate). Food allergy and stress may be involved in ulcerative colitis. Ex-smokers and non-smokers have a higher risk of ulcerative colitis; the converse is true for Crohn's disease.

EXTRA-GASTROINTESTINAL COMPLICATIONS – both diseases.

1. Eye disorders – conjunctivitis and uveitis in <5%.
2. Joints – seronegative arthritis with spinal and peripheral joint involvement approximately 15% (p.621).
3. Liver – sclerosing cholangitis and cholangiocarcinoma may be seen in ulcerative colitis, but very rarely in Crohn's disease.
4. Erythema nodosum and pyoderma gangrenosum may be found in both.

Macroscopic differences in the pathology of U.C and C.D

	Ulcerative colitis	Crohn's disease
1.	Lesions continuous – mucosal	Skip lesions – transmural
2.	Rectum always involved	Rectum normal in 50%
3.	Terminal ileum involved in <10% (backwash ileitis – mild)	Terminal ileum involved in 30%
4.	Granular, ulcerated mucosa; no fissuring	Discretely ulcerated mucosa; cobblestone appearance; fissuring
5.	Often intensely vascular	Vascularity seldom pronounced
6.	Normal serosa	Serositis common
7.	Muscular shortening of colon	Fibrous shortening; strictures common
8.	Fistulae rare	Enterocutaneous or intestinal fistulae in 10%
9.	Malignant change – well recognised	Malignant change – less common
10.	Anal lesions uncommon	Anal lesions in 75%; anal fistulae; ulceration or chronic fissure.

Rarely it may be impossible to distinguish between ulcerative colitis and Crohn's disease.

MICROSCOPIC COLITIS

This term describes two forms of colitis which are often overlooked because the colon appears normal on colonoscopy. Both tend to occur in middle aged women who present with chronic watery diarrhoea. The diagnoses depend on identification of characteristic histological findings.

COLLAGENOUS COLITIS

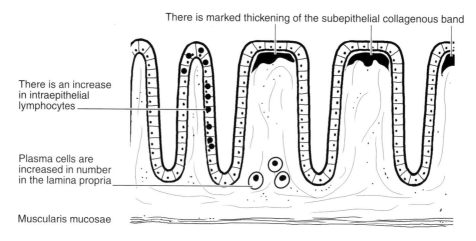

There is marked thickening of the subepithelial collagenous band

There is an increase in intraepithelial lymphocytes

Plasma cells are increased in number in the lamina propria

Muscularis mucosae

Patients often have concomitant diseases, typically autoimmune, such as rheumatoid arthritis, coeliac disease and diabetes.

LYMPHOCYTIC COLITIS

There is a marked increase in intraepithelial lymphocytes akin to those seen in coeliac disease

It is likely that collagenous and lymphocytic colitis are part of the spectrum of the same disease. A relapsing and remitting course is often seen.

INTESTINAL INFECTIONS

Viruses, bacteria, protozoa and worms can all infect the gastrointestinal tract. There are 3 main patterns of infection:

1. Organisms remain within the lumen of the gut and release toxins which damage the surface epithelium e.g. cholera.
2. Organisms invade the wall of the gut, but remain localised to the gut wall e.g. bacillary dysentery.
3. Organisms invade the gut wall and spread systemically through the blood stream e.g. typhoid.

Acute diarrhoeal diseases

In these disorders, infection, mainly of the small bowel, produces little mucosal inflammation, but there is often profuse watery diarrhoea. In adults this may be mild but, especially in infants, dehydration can lead to death.

Responsible organisms include: *E. coli, Vibrio cholerae,* rotaviruses, *Cryptosporidium parvum.*

Cholera is the classic example of the effects of toxin production.

Note: There is minimal epithelial cell damage.

INTESTINAL INFECTIONS

INTESTINAL INFECTIONS *(continued)*

E. coli 0157 is a strain which produces exotoxin causing haemorrhagic colitis often complicated by renal failure in the elderly or the haemolytic uraemic syndrome in children. The contamination is on meat or meat products and outbreaks and sporadic cases occur worldwide.

Toxic enteritis (Food poisoning)

Many bacteria can elaborate enterotoxins in food before it is consumed: although cooking kills the bacteria the preformed toxin may be heat resistant. *Staphylococcus aureus* and *Bacillus cereus* (in rice particularly) are good examples.

In **ROTAVIRUS infection**, seen especially in children under 5 years, the mechanism is different.

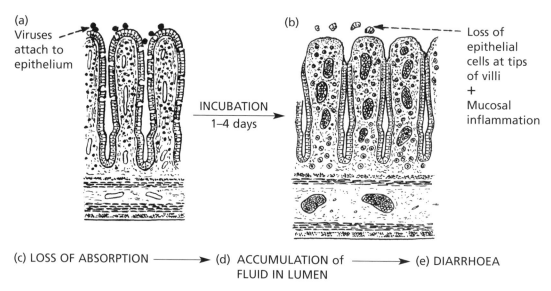

(a) Viruses attach to epithelium

INCUBATION 1–4 days

(b) Loss of epithelial cells at tips of villi
+
Mucosal inflammation

(c) LOSS OF ABSORPTION ⟶ (d) ACCUMULATION of FLUID IN LUMEN ⟶ (e) DIARRHOEA

Note: Recovery is usually rapid and complete, providing dehydration is treated.

TYPHOID

Salmonella infections

Salmonella infections vary from food poisoning, usually a mild inflammation with diarrhoea, to typhoid fever which if untreated is often fatal.

TYPHOID FEVER

Following ingestion of *S. typhi*, the disease process falls into three distinct phases.

Ingestion of *S. typhi*
(contaminated water
or food)

Phase I
Invasion of intestinal
lymphoid tissue and
proliferation of bacteria.
This phase lasts for 2
weeks.

ASYMPTOMATIC

Phase II
Invasion of blood stream
causing bacteraemia.

FEVER: TOXAEMIA
'Rose spots' in skin,
Splenomegaly,
Toxic cardiopathy,
POSITIVE BLOOD CULTURE,
Appearance of antibodies to
   S. typhi – WIDAL TEST.

Phase III
Localisation of bacteria in
intestinal lymphoid tissue,
mesenteric nodes, GALL-
BLADDER, liver, and
sometimes the bones.

INTESTINAL LESIONS
Endocarditis,
Meningitis,
Arthritis,
FAECAL and URINE CULTURE
   POSITIVE,
WIDAL TEST – RISING TITRES.

Blood
vessels

Spleen

Liver

Gall-
bladder

Intestine

TYPHOID

TYPHOID FEVER *(continued)*

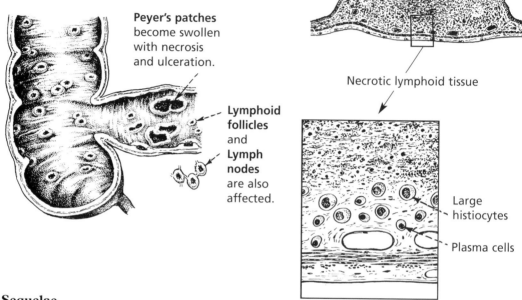

Peyer's patches become swollen with necrosis and ulceration.

Lymphoid follicles and **Lymph nodes** are also affected.

Necrotic lymphoid tissue

Large histiocytes

Plasma cells

Sequelae

1. Healing is the usual outcome.

2. Deep intestinal ulceration
   - haemorrhage.
   - perforation and peritonitis (usually fatal).

3. Persistent infection (1–3%) – usually GALLBLADDER or urinary tract.

   These carriers appear healthy but are an important source of outbreaks.

PARATYPHOID FEVER

This disease is clinically indistinguishable from typhoid fever but is usually much less severe.

The pathological changes resemble those of typhoid fever but are commonly limited to a small portion of the bowel. Frequently there is an absence of ulceration.

Two serological types of the paratyphoid organism are recognised, A and B. Type B is a common cause of enteric fever in Europe. As in typhoid, patients often become 'carriers'.

Note: TAB vaccination, using antigens derived from *S. typhi* and *paratyphi A and B*, produces a very effective active immunity.

BACILLARY DYSENTERY

This is an acute inflammation of the large intestine, varying in severity according to the infecting agent.

The bacteria adhere to and *invade* the mucosa. They remain localised to the gut.

Excess mucus secretion

Acute congestion

Neutrophil exudate

Crypt abscess

Shigella sonnei
Mild acute inflammation of colon.
Commonest form in the United Kingdom.

Small haemorrhages

Loss of epithelium and superficial destruction

Acute inflammation

Abscess

Shigella flexneri
Severe acute inflammation.

Pseudomembrane of fibrin, mucus and necrotic cells

Necrosis of surface tissues, later spreading to deeper layers

Oedema and inflammation in submucosa

Shigella dysenteriae
Most severe type, occurs in tropics.

Irregular spreading ulcers with thin shredded margins are formed by shedding of necrotic material.

Clinical manifestations

There is acute diarrhoea with abdominal pain, tenesmus and the passage of blood-stained mucus. *S. dysenteriae* infections are often associated with severe toxaemia and sometimes a shock-like condition. Blood, mucus and neutrophils are found in the faeces, and in the early stages the bacilli can be isolated.

Healing by resolution with complete restoration of the mucosa is usual. Only in exceptional cases does relapse occur with consequent scarring.

AMOEBIC DYSENTERY

This is due to infection by *Entamoeba histolytica* in food and water. It is most often seen in tropical and subtropical countries.

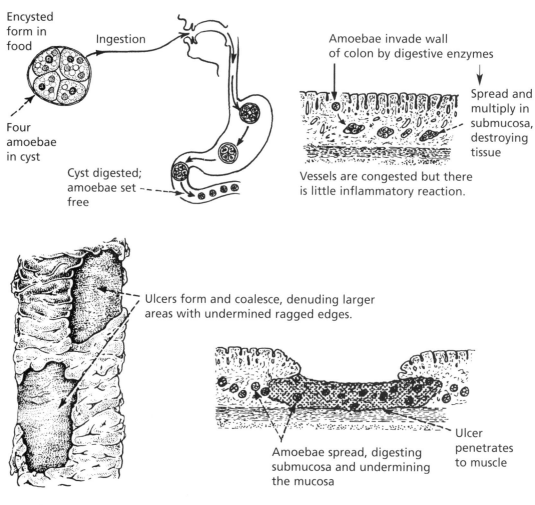

Encysted form in food

Ingestion

Four amoebae in cyst

Cyst digested; amoebae set free

Amoebae invade wall of colon by digestive enzymes

Spread and multiply in submucosa, destroying tissue

Vessels are congested but there is little inflammatory reaction.

Ulcers form and coalesce, denuding larger areas with undermined ragged edges.

Amoebae spread, digesting submucosa and undermining the mucosa

Ulcer penetrates to muscle

Healing of the ulcers with fibrosis occurs. The disease persists with overgrowth of fibrous tissue, adhesions to various structures and fistulae may occur. Occasionally the amoebae may invade portal venous tributaries and cause amoebic abscess of the liver (p.360).

Large numbers of motile amoebae can be found in the faeces during the acute phase of the disease. Later, in the chronic state, they are frequently in an encysted form. Mucus and blood are abundant.

Note: Non-pathogenic amoebae can be found in the colon of healthy individuals.

TUBERCULOUS ENTERITIS AND PSEUDOMEMBRANOUS COLITIS

1. **Primary tuberculous infection** usually follows ingestion of infected milk containing bovine tubercle bacilli and affects the small bowel. It is similar to primary tuberculosis of the lung – a small mucosal lesion and enlarged caseous lymph nodes. These usually heal with fibrosis and calcification.

2. **Secondary tuberculosis**
   This is due to swallowing tubercle bacilli from open pulmonary tuberculosis. The mucosal lesion is prominent and lymph nodes less affected. The lesions start in the Peyer's patches.

Shallow ragged ulcers

Ulcers may coalesce to form a large circumferential ulcer.

Caseating granulomas in all layers.

As in the lung, there is a good deal of fibrous granulation tissue surrounding the caseous lesions and the vessels undergo obliteration. For this reason, perforation and haemorrhage are uncommon. Adhesions to other loops of bowel are common and the caseating process may erode through the walls and cause fistula formation with short circuiting and resulting malabsorption. If the fibrous adhesions are dense, obstruction may arise.

PSEUDOMEMBRANOUS COLITIS

Varying lengths of colon show focal inflammation with the formation of surface yellow plaques (pseudomembranes). Most cases are associated with the use in elderly patients of antibiotics.

Microscopic

Foci of mucus, fibrin, epithelial debris and a few neutrophils erupt on the mucous surface

Naked eye appearance

The lesions may coalesce forming typical adherent plaques over large areas, resulting in a fatal outcome. The lesions are caused by toxins from *Clostridium difficile* – an anaerobe normally present in small numbers which proliferate due to elimination of competing bacteria by the antibiotic. The toxin can be found in the stools.

APPENDICITIS

Acute appendicitis is a common cause of abdominal pain requiring surgery, particularly in the West where there is low roughage diet.

Appendicitis usually follows obstruction of the lumen with distal infection and ulceration. The usual causes are:

(a) Viral infection → reactive hyperplasia of lymphoid follicles. (Infection by *Yersinia enterocolitica* can have similar effects.)
(b) Inspissated faeces (faecoliths).

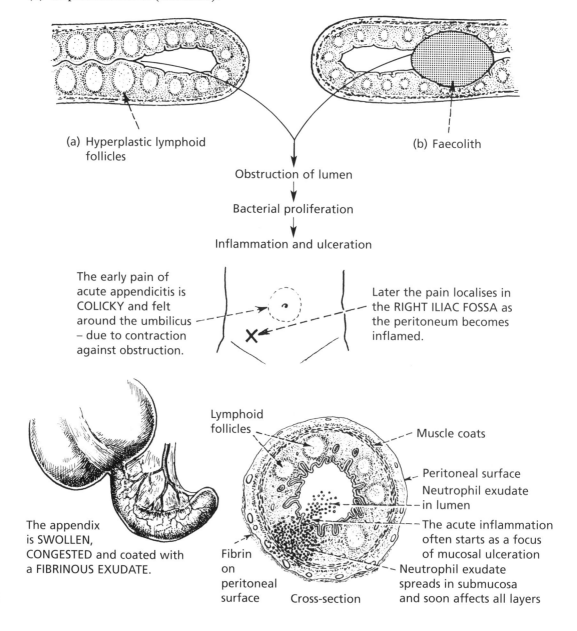

(a) Hyperplastic lymphoid follicles

(b) Faecolith

Obstruction of lumen

Bacterial proliferation

Inflammation and ulceration

The early pain of acute appendicitis is COLICKY and felt around the umbilicus – due to contraction against obstruction.

Later the pain localises in the RIGHT ILIAC FOSSA as the peritoneum becomes inflamed.

The appendix is SWOLLEN, CONGESTED and coated with a FIBRINOUS EXUDATE.

Lymphoid follicles

Muscle coats

Peritoneal surface

Neutrophil exudate in lumen

The acute inflammation often starts as a focus of mucosal ulceration

Fibrin on peritoneal surface

Neutrophil exudate spreads in submucosa and soon affects all layers

Cross-section

APPENDICITIS – SEQUELS

If untreated the appendicitis may become suppurative or gangrenous. The following complications are fortunately rare.

1. **General peritonitis** is the most important complication since it results in toxaemia and may be fatal. It is especially associated with gangrenous appendicitis but may complicate any type of acute appendicitis.

2. **Appendix abscess**
   This arises in the following way:

Abscess in appendix wall → Perforation + Fibrinous adhesions to adjacent structures (particularly the greater omentum) → Localised abscess in right iliac fossa

Further complications may arise due to spread of infection:

(a) Along the right paracolic gutter to produce a subphrenic abscess between the diaphragm and liver

(b) Into the pelvis to form abscesses around bladder and rectum. In the female the uterus and fallopian tube may be involved.

Appendix abscess

Rectum

Pelvic abscess

Bladder

3. **Adhesions**
   Intestinal obstruction may result from constricting bands, or volvulus may be induced.

4. **Liver abscesses and portal pylephlebitis**
   These are now rare. They are due to spread of infection to the mesenteric veins resulting in septic embolism. Liver abscesses usually arise from infective emboli, but occasionally there may be a spreading suppurating thrombosis culminating in hepatic sepsis.

MUCOCELE
This term describes dilatation of the appendix by accumulation of mucus, usually due to mucinous cystadenoma.

DIVERTICULAR DISEASE

Diverticula are common in the **sigmoid colon**, affecting at least 10% of adults in societies where the diet lacks fibre (low residue).

Reduced dietary fibre – low residue in distal colon $\longrightarrow$ Induces muscular hypertrophy $\longrightarrow$ Increased intraluminal pressure $\longrightarrow$ Outpouching of mucosa

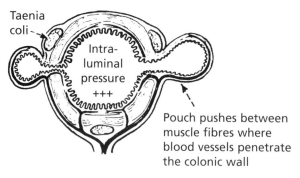

Taenia coli

Intra-luminal pressure +++

Pouch pushes between muscle fibres where blood vessels penetrate the colonic wall

Complications

Diverticulitis is common

Inflammation and ulceration $\longleftarrow$ abscess formation
fistulae (e.g.colo-vesical)
haemorrhage

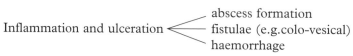

Repeated attacks

$\downarrow$

Fibro-muscular thickening

$\downarrow$

Stenosis

Note: This may simulate carcinoma

Other diverticula are also found in the caecum and small intestine: in the latter, colonisation by bacteria which utilise Vit B12 may lead to macrocytic anaemia.

Inspissated faeces

Inflammatory fibromuscular thickening

Meckel's diverticulum of the small intestine is present in 2% of the population.

It is a remnant of the **vitello-intestinal duct** about 60 cm proximal to the ileo-caecal valve.

Complications are rare:

(1) The wide communication with the bowel precludes stasis and inflammation.

(2) Rarely ectopic gastric or pancreatic tissue cause local damage (p.301).

ISCHAEMIA AND THE INTESTINES

ACUTE VASCULAR OCCLUSION

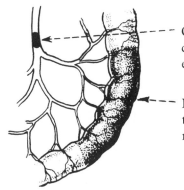

Occlusion of the superior mesenteric artery is usually due to thrombosis complicating atheroma, or embolism from the left side of the heart or aorta.

Infarction of a loop or much of the small bowel leads to abdominal pain. The infarcted bowel must be removed surgically. Many of these elderly patients die.

ISCHAEMIC COLITIS

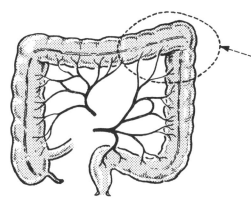

The colon is more vulnerable to chronic ischaemia than the small bowel.

Ischaemic colitis commonly affects the splenic flexure – the watershed zone. It often occurs in patients with arterial disease with hypotension e.g. due to shock or cardiac failure.

Milder ischaemia ⟶ mucosal ulceration

                     ↓

                  healing with stricture

Severe ischaemia ⟶ gangrene of bowel

Intestinal ischaemia may also be due to arteritis (p.227), as a side effect of radiation therapy. Drug induced ulcers, e.g. potassium tablets and non-steroidal anti-inflammatory drugs, appear to be due to local ischaemia.

NEONATAL NECROTISING ENTEROCOLITIS

This lesion occurs in premature babies in their first week.

Necrosis and inflammation occur in bowel wall.

Gas bubbles in the submucosa and muscle give a characteristic X-ray appearance.

Bowel ischaemia appears to be the initial event, but there is then bacterial superinfection, especially by gas forming organisms.

INTESTINAL OBSTRUCTION

Intestinal obstruction can be caused by:
(a) Intraluminal blockage – e.g. gallstone ileus (p.367).
(b) Lesions of the bowel wall – e.g. tumours, inflammatory strictures, intussusception.
(c) External compression – e.g. hernias, volvulus.

The patient may present with colicky abdominal pain, vomiting and failure to pass flatus or faeces.

Acute obstruction

Immediately following the obstruction there is a period of very active peristalsis

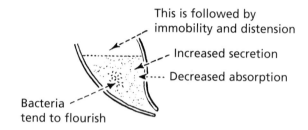

This is followed by immobility and distension

Increased secretion

Decreased absorption

Bacteria tend to flourish

Subacute obstruction

As the condition develops gradually, hypertrophy of the muscle is seen proximal to the obstruction.

Later, obstruction increases and muscle hypertrophy cannot compensate.

Dilatation of the bowel follows with accumulation of gas and fluid.

This gross distension has several effects:

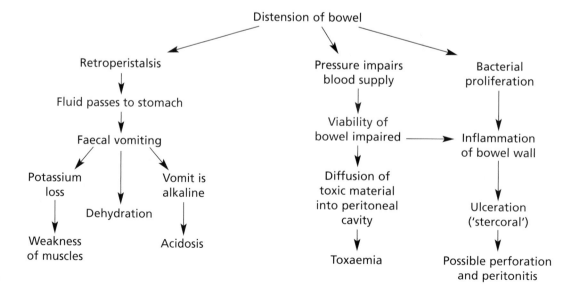

Distension of bowel

Retroperistalsis
↓
Fluid passes to stomach
↓
Faecal vomiting
↓
Potassium loss → Weakness of muscles
Dehydration
Vomit is alkaline → Acidosis

Pressure impairs blood supply
↓
Viability of bowel impaired ──→ Inflammation of bowel wall
↓
Diffusion of toxic material into peritoneal cavity
↓
Toxaemia

Bacterial proliferation
↓
Inflammation of bowel wall
↓
Ulceration ('stercoral')
↓
Possible perforation and peritonitis

HERNIA

HERNIA

This means the protrusion of peritoneum through an aperture.

When the hernial swelling appears on the surface of the body, it is termed 'external'; those which do not present on the body surface are 'internal'.

The main complication is protrusion of bowel through the aperture at:

1. Sites of potential weakness in the abdominal wall, e.g. inguinal canal, femoral canal, umbilicus, diaphragm. There may be congenital weakness in some individuals at these sites. In these cases a pouch of peritoneum protrudes through the aperture.
2. Normal peritoneal extensions, e.g. the foramen of Winslow leading to the lesser sac, jejunoduodenal fossa.
3. The abdominal wall following operation due to stretching of scar tissue.

Inguinal hernia

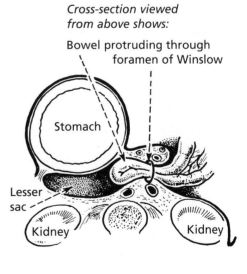

Cross-section viewed from above shows:

Bowel protruding through foramen of Winslow

HERNIA – COMPLICATIONS

Complications of hernia

Initially, when the herniated portion of bowel is small it can be pushed back into the abdominal cavity – *reducible*.

Increased intra-abdominal pressure, e.g. during muscular exertion, coughing or straining due to constipation, helps to induce the herniation, tends to make it progressive, and secondary changes occur.

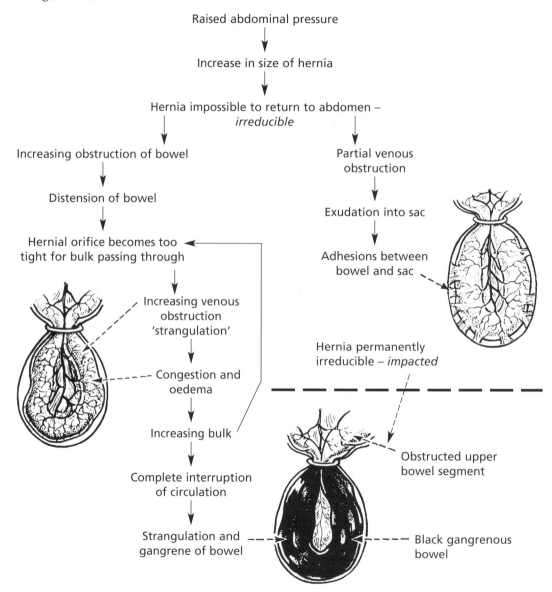

Raised abdominal pressure

↓

Increase in size of hernia

↓

Hernia impossible to return to abdomen –
irreducible

Increasing obstruction of bowel

↓

Distension of bowel

↓

Hernial orifice becomes too
tight for bulk passing through

↓

Increasing venous
obstruction
'strangulation'

↓

Congestion and
oedema

↓

Increasing bulk

↓

Complete interruption
of circulation

↓

Strangulation and
gangrene of bowel

Partial venous
obstruction

↓

Exudation into sac

↓

Adhesions between
bowel and sac

Hernia permanently
irreducible – *impacted*

Obstructed upper
bowel segment

Black gangrenous
bowel

INTUSSUSCEPTION

INTUSSUSCEPTION

This is a condition in which the bowel is invaginated into itself.

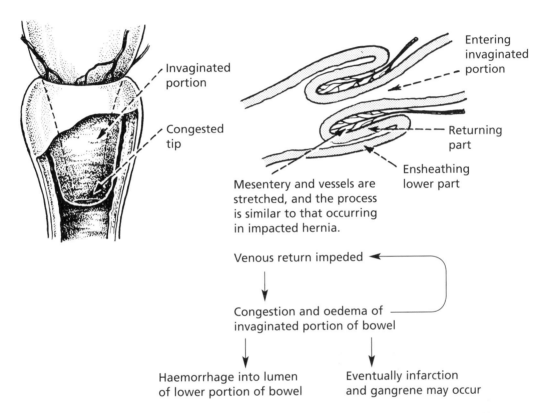

Invaginated portion

Congested tip

Entering invaginated portion

Returning part

Ensheathing lower part

Mesentery and vessels are stretched, and the process is similar to that occurring in impacted hernia.

Venous return impeded

Congestion and oedema of invaginated portion of bowel

Haemorrhage into lumen of lower portion of bowel

Eventually infarction and gangrene may occur

Sites

The commonest form is the ileocaecal type, the ileum being invaginated into the large intestine with the ileocaecal valve forming the apex. Less commonly, a portion of ileum may pass through the ileocaecal valve. Other sites are occasionally affected, e.g. small intestine or parts of colon.

Clinical manifestations

The patient presents with the signs and symptoms of acute obstruction, a mass in the abdomen and blood is passed per rectum.

Aetiology

It is thought that most cases arise as a result of a swelling in the intestinal wall which is pushed distally by peristalsis, dragging the wall of the bowel with it. Most cases arise in childhood due to swelling of lymphoid tissue produced by virus infection.

Polypoidal tumours of the intestine may cause intussusception in adults.

VOLVULUS AND HIRSCHSPRUNG'S DISEASE

VOLVULUS

As the name suggests, this is a rotation or revolving of the bowel. It affects bowel with a long mesentery. Another factor is the closeness of the ends of the affected loop.

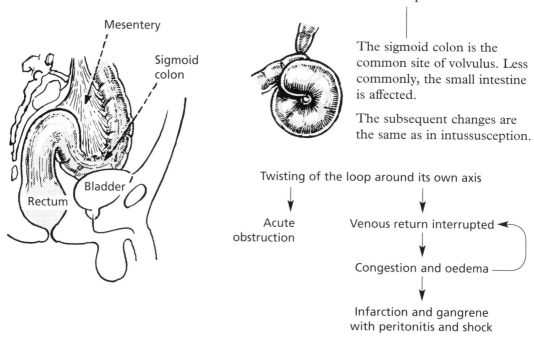

The sigmoid colon is the common site of volvulus. Less commonly, the small intestine is affected.

The subsequent changes are the same as in intussusception.

Twisting of the loop around its own axis

Acute obstruction

Venous return interrupted

Congestion and oedema

Infarction and gangrene with peritonitis and shock

HIRSCHSPRUNG'S DISEASE

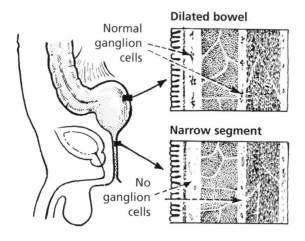

Hirschsprung's disease is a rare cause of chronic intestinal obstruction. It is due to a congenital absence of ganglion cells in the parasympathetic Auerbach and Meissner complexes of the rectum. Mutations in genes including the RETS gene are responsible.

The aganglionic rectal segment and anus cannot relax and the bowel above becomes grossly distended and hypertrophied.

TUMOURS OF THE COLON

The main tumours of the colon are epithelial – adenomas and carcinomas.

Adenomas – These are important because they may lead on to carcinoma.
(Adenoma–carcinoma sequence, p.143)

TUBULAR ADENOMA

The majority of tubular adenomas occur in the rectum and sigmoid colon. In the beginning it is a sessile swelling but soon becomes pedunculated.

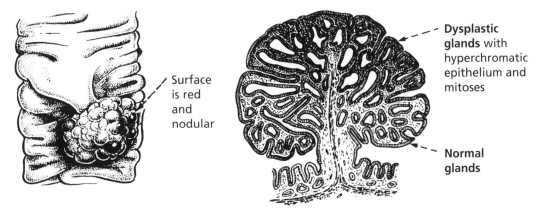

Surface is red and nodular

Dysplastic glands with hyperchromatic epithelium and mitoses

Normal glands

They are common in the older age groups and are frequently multiple.

VILLOUS ADENOMA

Villous adenomas are most commonly found in the rectum. They form a sessile mass which may be quite large and have a delicate frond-like structure.

Sessile mass

Epithelium usually of clear mucus-secreting type

Broad base with no pedicle

These often present with rectal bleeding.

Very rarely, there is an excessive production of mucus and fluid which may lead to marked loss of potassium, causing muscular weakness.

Many polyps are of mixed variety – part adenomatous, part villous. Both show a tendency to malignant change. If the tumour is of sessile variety invasion of the deeper tissues is immediate. In the pedunculated varieties, invasion of the intestinal wall is delayed – the stalk is first invaded.

TUMOURS OF THE COLON

ADENOMATOSIS COLI

This is an inherited condition (autosomal dominant: 50% of children affected) due to mutation of the APC gene, a tumour suppressor gene on chromosome 5.

Adenomatous polyps are found throughout the entire colon, appearing in late childhood. Carcinoma almost always occurs by the 3rd or 4th decade if colectomy is not carried out.

Tumours may also be seen in the stomach and small bowel.

Other Colonic Polyps

(1) METAPLASTIC POLYPS

These are usually multiple and present as a small sessile nodule showing unusual feathery metaplastic change in the epithelium. They are found in later life but seldom become malignant. Some polyps, known as serrated adenomas, have a mixture of adenomatous and metaplastic features.

(2) JUVENILE POLYPS

These are globular protrusions of the rectal mucosa in children who present with rectal bleeding. They are usually ulcerated and inflamed but probably represent a developmental abnormality. They are occasionally multiple, when there is a small risk of malignancy.

(3) **Inflammatory polyps** associated with chronic inflammatory bowel disease are described on page 310.

CARCINOMA OF THE COLON

This malignancy is the third commonest cancer world wide. Tumours in the right and left side tend to present differently.

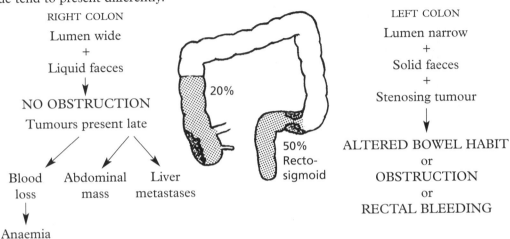

RIGHT COLON
Lumen wide
+
Liquid faeces
↓
NO OBSTRUCTION
Tumours present late

Blood loss → Abdominal mass → Liver metastases
↓
Anaemia

20%

50% Recto-sigmoid

LEFT COLON
Lumen narrow
+
Solid faeces
+
Stenosing tumour
↓
ALTERED BOWEL HABIT
or
OBSTRUCTION
or
RECTAL BLEEDING

Types of growth

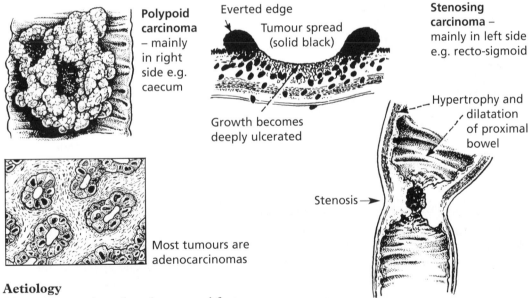

Polypoid carcinoma – mainly in right side e.g. caecum

Everted edge
Tumour spread (solid black)

Stenosing carcinoma – mainly in left side e.g. recto-sigmoid

Growth becomes deeply ulcerated

Most tumours are adenocarcinomas

Hypertrophy and dilatation of proximal bowel

Stenosis →

Aetiology
There are genetic and environmental factors.
(a) **Environmental:** Diets rich in animal fat and protein, especially low residue diets.
(b) **Genetic:** e.g. adenomatosis coli (APC gene); hereditary non-polyposis colorectal cancer syndrome (HNPCC) due to mutation of mismatch repair genes.
MOST CASES ARE SPORADIC.
(c) **Pre-existing lesions**
    1. Adenomatous polyps including adenomatosis coli.
    2. Inflammatory bowel disease (especially ulcerative colitis).

331

CARCINOMA OF THE COLON

SPREAD and STAGING (Dukes' staging)

Most carcinomas start
as an adenoma

Invasion through muscularis mucosae,
submucosa – into muscularis propria
but NOT through entire thickness.

Dukes' stage A – 5yr. survival >90%.

Spread in
peritoneum

Invasion of
adjacent
structures
e.g. bladder

Spread through wall to
serosa or perirectal fat.

Dukes' stage B – 5yr. survival 60%

Muscularis
mucosae

Lymphatic
spread to
mesenteric
lymph nodes

Local
lymph
node

Apical
lymph
node

Dukes' stage C – 5yr. survival 25%

Blood borne metastases to the liver usually occur later.

Carcinoembryonic antigen (CEA)
This is a glycoprotein normally produced by fetal endodermal tissues. It is also formed by a
number of cancers, among them a proportion of colonic carcinomas, and appears in the
blood. It cannot be used as a diagnostic test since it is found in non-neoplastic lesions such
as inflammation of the bowel. After treatment, however, changes in the blood concentration
of CEA may be used as an indication of recurrence of tumour growth.

Other tumours
Carcinoid tumour (p.334), lymphoma and connective tissue tumours e.g. gastro-intestinal
stromal tumours (GISTs) are occasionally found.

TUMOURS OF SMALL INTESTINE

BENIGN TUMOURS: adenomas, leiomyomas and lipomas are rare, but may cause intussusception (p.327).

Hamartomatous polyps, consisting of glands and muscle, occur in the Peutz–Jeghers syndrome, an autosomal dominant condition. Melanotic pigmentation of the lips and mouth is also seen.

CARCINOMA: adenocarcinoma is 50 times rarer in the small intestine than in the colon. About 40–50% occur in the duodenum, mainly around the ampulla of Vater and often arising from polyps. These present with obstructive jaundice. Tumours in the jejunum resemble those of the colon and may obstruct the lumen. An increased risk of carcinoma is seen in patients with Crohn's disease, coeliac disease and the Peutz–Jeghers syndrome.

LYMPHOMA: these are non-Hodgkin's lymphomas of 'B' or 'T' cell type.

Single or multiple tumours

| Ulceration and Haemorrhage | Perforation ↓ Peritonitis | Spread to lymph nodes or marrow | Stricture formation |

(a) **Enteropathy associated T-cell lymphoma.** These are seen in middle aged patients who often have had coeliac disease for many years.

(b) **B-cell lymphomas are usually of MALT type.** These may be of low or high grade.

Lymphoepithelial lesions – lymphoid cells infiltrate and destroy glands.

Diffuse infiltration of lymphoid cells

Reactive lymphoid follicle

(c) **Mediterranean lymphoma (α chain disease)**

? Infective origin (some cases respond to antibiotics).

Diffuse proliferation of lympho-plasmacytic cells (initially polyclonal)

MALABSORPTION   PRODUCTION OF EXCESS IgA

PROGRESSION TO MONOCLONAL B CELL LYMPHOMA

CONNECTIVE TISSUE TUMOURS

Gastrointestinal stromal tumours (GISTs) may present with bleeding, obstruction, or an abdominal mass. They often metastasise to the liver.

CARCINOID TUMOURS

These tumours arise from endocrine cells and can occur in the gut and lung. They are commonest in the appendix and small bowel.

APPENDICEAL CARCINOIDS
These may be incidental findings at appendicectomy or may cause appendicitis.

Yellow nodule

10% occur at base   70% occur at tip

SMALL BOWEL CARCINOIDS
These are commonest in the ileum.

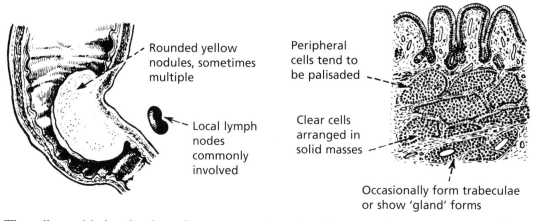

Rounded yellow nodules, sometimes multiple

Local lymph nodes commonly involved

Peripheral cells tend to be palisaded

Clear cells arranged in solid masses

Occasionally form trabeculae or show 'gland' forms

The cells can bind and reduce silver compounds and are known as 'ARGENTAFFIN CELLS'. They contain neurosecretory granules (E.M.) and express endocrine markers, e.g. chromogranin.

CARCINOID SYNDROME
These tumours may secrete a variety of neuroendocrine and paraendocrine substances, in many cases without any apparent clinical functional effects.

However, ileal carcinoids tend to produce peptides: such as 5-hydroxytryptamine (5HT) (serotonin). This is normally destroyed in the liver and lungs: when metastatic deposits are present in the liver the active agents enter the general circulation and produce the CARCINOID SYNDROME, characterised by episodic flushing, diarrhoea and right heart failure.

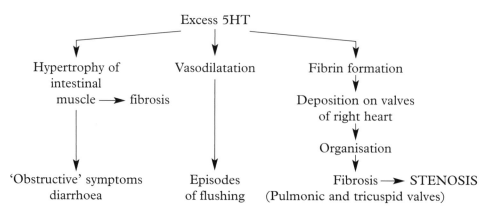

Excess 5HT

Hypertrophy of intestinal muscle → fibrosis

Vasodilatation

Fibrin formation

Deposition on valves of right heart

Organisation

'Obstructive' symptoms diarrhoea

Episodes of flushing

Fibrosis → STENOSIS (Pulmonic and tricuspid valves)

THE PERITONEAL CAVITY

PERITONITIS

Acute Peritonitis usually follows inflammation of a viscus,

e.g. 1. Appendicitis, cholecystitis, pancreatitis.
  2. Perforation e.g. duodenal ulcer, ruptured diverticulum.
  3. Ischaemia – vascular occlusion, volvulus, intussusception.

Patients on chronic ambulatory peritoneal dialysis (CAPD) are prone to episodes of peritonitis.

Primary Peritonitis

In the absence of visceral inflammation, primary peritonitis may occur in children with the nephrotic syndrome (pneumococcus) or in adults with cirrhosis (usually coliforms).

Peritonitis can be

LOCALISED
e.g. appendix abscess

GENERALISED

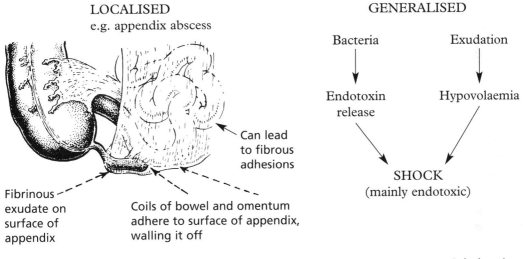

Bacteria → Endotoxin release

Exudation → Hypovolaemia

SHOCK
(mainly endotoxic)

Can lead to fibrous adhesions

Fibrinous exudate on surface of appendix

Coils of bowel and omentum adhere to surface of appendix, walling it off

Consequences of peritonitis.

(a) Shock ⟶ death.

(b) Recovery.

(c) Adhesions due to organisation of exudate ⟶ intestinal obstruction.

(d) Localised collections of pus. ⟶

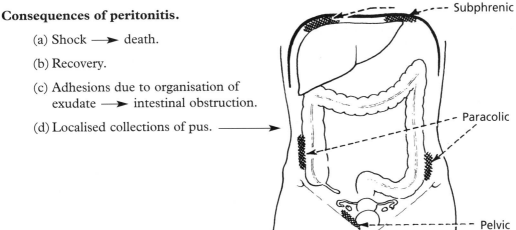

Subphrenic

Paracolic

Pelvic

THE PERITONEAL CAVITY

Chronic peritonitis

The most common type of chronic inflammation involving the peritoneum is that resulting from non-resolution of acute peritonitis.

A form of sclerosing peritonitis may complicate long term peritoneal dialysis.

Tuberculosis of the peritoneum is uncommon in Western countries, but frequent in developing countries. It commonly takes one of the following forms:

1. **Serous effusion.** Small grey tubercles are usually scattered over the peritoneal surface. In addition, the omentum is more extensively involved with the formation of a large fibrous mass in the upper abdomen.
2. **Caseation.** This can vary in extent, from isolated small masses to diffuse caseation involving most of the cavity.
3. **Adhesive peritonitis.** The cavity may be reduced to small pockets containing serous fluid. The source of infection may be caseous lymph nodes, tuberculous salpingitis or tuberculous ulcer of the intestine.

Ascites
Accumulation of serous fluid can occur:

1. As part of a general oedema from any cause such as cardiac or renal failure.
2. Portal venous obstruction as in hepatic cirrhosis, portal thrombosis or compression of the portal vein by tumour growth.
3. Tumours of the ovary.
4. Tumours of the peritoneum.

Tumours
Secondary tumours are common, due to spread of carcinoma from the stomach, ovary and large intestine.

Eventually loops of bowel are stuck together by tumour and adhesions resulting in 'frozen abdomen'.

Pseudomyxoma peritonei is seen when mucin secreting tumours e.g. of ovary or appendix spread widely throughout the peritoneum.

Primary tumours are rare. Mesothelioma is the most important. It is related to the inhalation of asbestos and the pathology is similar to that of mesothelioma of the pleura; large white plaques of solid tumour.

LIVER, GALL BLADDER AND PANCREAS

LIVER – ANATOMY

Conventionally the liver was considered to be composed of regular lobules, each arranged around a 'central vein' with portal tracts at the periphery.

Portal tract
Bile flow
Hepatic artery
Bile duct
Portal vein

Central vein (hepatic venule)   Blood flow

Histologically, it is evident that this is not quite true. The liver in section often has this appearance.

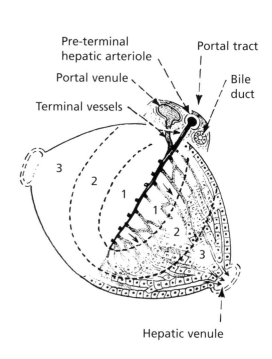

Portal tracts

'Central' venules

The portal tracts and hepatic venules appear to be distributed in a haphazard manner.

The acinar concept is now used.

The smallest unit is the simple acinus of varying shape.

The portal venule and hepatic arteriole both send terminal branches into the acinus (2/3 of the blood supply is portal and 1/3 arterial). They join to form a common trunk which will then contain partially oxygenated blood, and this percolates through the sinusoids to several 'terminal hepatic venules' (as in diagram).

In terms of oxygen supply and other nutrients, 3 zones exist.

Zone 1, with the best supply
Zone 2, with a reasonable supply
Zone 3, with the poorest supply which makes it most vulnerable to hypoxia.

In Zone 1, glycogen synthesis and glycogenolysis take place. It is also the main area of protein metabolism and formation of plasma proteins. Conjugation of certain drugs takes place.

Zone 3 is associated with glycogen storage, lipid and pigment formation and metabolism of certain drugs and chemicals. Zone 2 shares functions with the other zones.

Pre-terminal hepatic arteriole
Portal tract
Portal venule
Bile duct
Terminal vessels

Hepatic venule

LIVER – ANATOMY

A complex acinus consists of at least three simple acini organised around the terminal branches of a pre-terminal portal venule, hepatic arteriole and bile duct. The blood circulates through the parenchyma and drains into two or three hepatic venules.

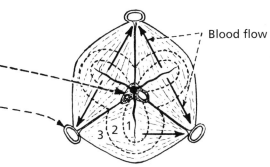

Zones 1, 2 and 3 form roughly concentric layers, zone 1 being the core of the complex acinus. Zone 3 is the outer layer at the periphery of the circulation and, at certain points, can come quite close to the preterminal vessels.

Complex acini (diagrammatic) – each consisting of three simple acini

Portal tract

'Central' hepatic venule

'Conventional' lobule, shown by shaded area, consisting of interdigitating acini

Pre-terminal hepatic arteriole

Portal venule

Bile duct

It must be realised that the acini interdigitate in a complex way so that masses of hepatic cells are of irregular shape and the apparent regularity shown in the diagram is merely schematic. This explains the difficulty in recognising the functional units in histological sections.

ANATOMY – HEPATIC LESIONS

The site of hepatic lesions is determined mainly by the microcirculation. Factors involved are:

1. PO_2 of blood
2. Enzyme functions of the zones
3. Filtration function.

LIVER NECROSIS

Perivenular necrosis

This form is a feature of many apparently unrelated conditions. It is brought about by damage in zone 3 of interdigitating acini (A in diagram). Thus it is a feature of shock due to circulatory collapse reducing the oxygen supply to zone 3. It also occurs in poisoning with chlorinated hydrocarbons (e.g. in chloroform) and drugs, e.g. paracetamol, substances metabolised in zone 3.

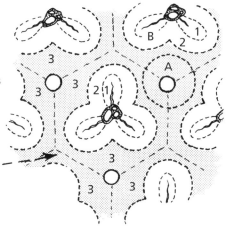

It is important to realise that zone 3, particularly, is continuous from one acinus to another, and in severe cases the hepatic venules are linked together by necrotic tissues. Microscopically, therefore, the lesions appear irregular in distribution due to differing planes of section.

Mid-zonal necrosis

This is uncommon. It is seen in yellow fever and injury affecting zones 2 and 1 (B in diagram).

Periportal necrosis
Rarely necrosis in zone 1 is due to its metabolism of drugs and chemicals; e.g. phosphorus poisoning causes marked fatty change in the periportal parenchyma, followed by necrosis.

Massive necrosis
This is an unusual lesion which can follow poisoning due to drugs, industrial chemicals or mushrooms. Rarely it is a complication of viral hepatitis.

JAUNDICE

If the serum bilirubin level exceeds 50 µmol/l, the patient becomes jaundiced.

Bilirubin is derived from the breakdown of effete red cells by the macrophage system, mainly in the spleen. It is conjugated to glucuronic acid in the liver and secreted in the bile.

Study of haemoglobin catabolism shows 3 main forms of jaundice:

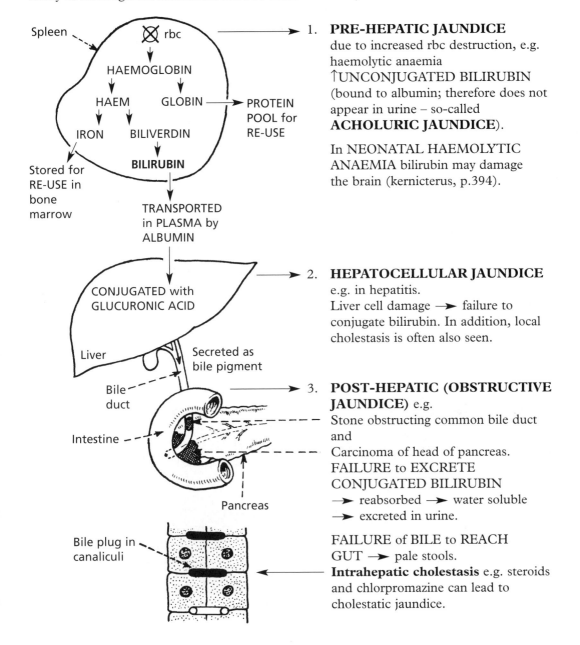

1. **PRE-HEPATIC JAUNDICE**
   due to increased rbc destruction, e.g. haemolytic anaemia
   ↑UNCONJUGATED BILIRUBIN
   (bound to albumin; therefore does not appear in urine – so-called
   ACHOLURIC JAUNDICE).

   In NEONATAL HAEMOLYTIC ANAEMIA bilirubin may damage the brain (kernicterus, p.394).

2. **HEPATOCELLULAR JAUNDICE**
   e.g. in hepatitis.
   Liver cell damage → failure to conjugate bilirubin. In addition, local cholestasis is often also seen.

3. **POST-HEPATIC (OBSTRUCTIVE JAUNDICE)** e.g.
   Stone obstructing common bile duct
   and
   Carcinoma of head of pancreas.
   FAILURE to EXCRETE CONJUGATED BILIRUBIN
   → reabsorbed → water soluble
   → excreted in urine.

   FAILURE of BILE to REACH GUT → pale stools.
   Intrahepatic cholestasis e.g. steroids and chlorpromazine can lead to cholestatic jaundice.

341

VIRAL HEPATITIS

ACUTE VIRAL HEPATITIS

Viral hepatitis is the most important form of hepatitis. It is seen worldwide. Viral hepatitis may be sporadic or epidemic and, depending on the responsible virus, transmitted by the faeco-oral or parenteral route.

Clinical features

Many episodes of viral hepatitis are subclinical; mild symptomatic cases are characterised by nausea, fever and anorexia. Severe attacks are characterised by jaundice and hepatic failure, and may be fatal.

Pathological features

EARLY stage

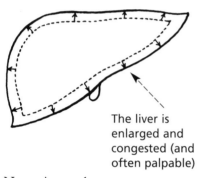

The liver is enlarged and congested (and often palpable)

Hepatic venule

Normal cells

Councilman body (apoptotic cell)

Swollen hepatocytes

Lymphocytic infiltrate in portal tract and in parenchyma

Liver cell necrosis is always present. It is most marked in Zone 3 (p.338).

Necrosis may be:
(a) focal (spotty) – scattered as single cells or
(b) more severe – forming areas of bridging between vessels (portal to hepatic venule) or
(c) panacinar – necrosis of complete acini up to massive necrosis of a large part of the liver occasionally occurs. When it does, it is most marked in the left lobe.

LATER stage

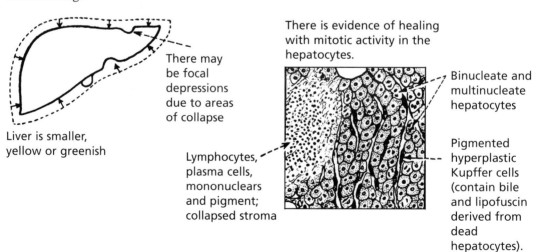

There may be focal depressions due to areas of collapse

Liver is smaller, yellow or greenish

Lymphocytes, plasma cells, mononuclears and pigment; collapsed stroma

There is evidence of healing with mitotic activity in the hepatocytes.

Binucleate and multinucleate hepatocytes

Pigmented hyperplastic Kupffer cells (contain bile and lipofuscin derived from dead hepatocytes).

VIRAL HEPATITIS

Biochemical changes

These changes result from liver damage

Disruption of bile canaliculi / interference with excretion
↓
Absorption of conjugated bile into blood (levels up to 300 µmol/l.)

Necrosis of hepatocytes
↓
Release of enzymes into blood
↓
Transferase enzymes (ALT, AST) greatly increased

Diminished production of proteins
↓
Coagulation mechanisms upset
↓
Prothrombin times increased

Clinical progress

1. In most cases, the disease is self-limiting and complete recovery occurs within 4–6 weeks.
2. Rarely death may occur due to massive (panacinar) liver necrosis.
   (a) In the early pre-icteric stage within 10 days – fulminant hepatic failure.
   (b) In 2–3 weeks. The liver is reduced in size.

Capsule is wrinkled

Loss of substance

Remaining liver tissue opaque, yellowish, without markings and is largely necrotic

Large necrotic area

Bile duct hyperplasia

This condition was often termed 'acute yellow atrophy'.

(c) Several weeks later.
   At this stage, regeneration is well advanced in places but function is inadequate and progressive failure occurs.

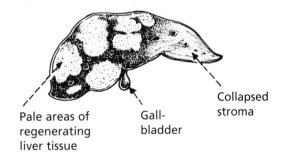

Pale areas of regenerating liver tissue

Gall-bladder

Collapsed stroma

Some types of hepatitis may progress to
3. Chronic hepatitis (p.347),
4. Cirrhosis,
5. Hepatocellular carcinoma.

343

VIRAL HEPATITIS

At least 5 viruses cause liver damage without significantly damaging other tissues (hepatitis A,B,C,D and E). The features are summarised and then discussed individually.

VIRUS	HAV	HBV	HCV	HDV	HEV
TYPE	PICORNA VIRUS	HEPADNA VIRUS	RNA FLAVIVIRUS	DEFECTIVE RNA VIRUS	RNA CALICIVIRUS
SPREAD	Faeco-oral	Parenteral	Parenteral	Parenteral	Faeco-oral
INCUBATION PERIOD (weeks)	2–4	4–20	2–25	6–9	3–9
SEVERITY of HEPATITIS	Usually mild	Often severe	Usually mild	Severe	Often mild. Severe in pregnancy
CHRONICITY	No	Approx 5% of adults, 90% of children	Approx 50%	Coinfection 5% Superinfection 95%	No
CARRIER STATE	No	Yes	Yes	Yes	No
VACCINE	Yes	Yes	No	Protected by HBV vaccine if HBV-ve	No

Other viruses which can affect the liver, but also affect other tissues include:
Yellow fever
Herpes viruses – Epstein–Barr, Cytomegalovirus, Herpes simplex
Coxsackie A and B
Lassa fever.

HEPATITIS B INFECTION

The **hepatitis B virus** is a member of the HEPA DNA virus group. Infection is by the parenchymal route – mainly IV drug abuse, blood products and sexual transmission.

The virus has several components:

A core containing
(a) DNA – partly double stranded
(b) DNA polymerase
(c) Core antigen HBcAg
(d) e antigen HBeAg

An **outer lipo-protein coat** (derived from the hepatocyte membrane) bearing Hepatitis B surface antigen (HBsAg)

42 μm diameter

The complete virion is known as the Dane particle. Spherical and tubular structures derived from the surface coat can also be found in the peripheral blood.

These antigens and antibodies to them are the basis for diagnosis of hepatitis B infection.

Dane particle

Spheres and tubules of HBsAg in blood

In **histological preparations**

HBsAg accumulates in the cytoplasm of cells – giving a 'ground glass' appearance.

HBcAg is found in the nuclei.

Uniform cytoplasm

'Sanded nuclei'

or can be stained by immunocytochemistry.

Positive staining with Anti-HBs

Positive staining with Anti-HBc

Serology: Antibodies to the various antigens appear in the blood.

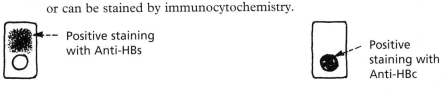

Six weeks after infection the surface antigen (HBsAg) appears in the blood, followed two weeks later by the e antigen (HBeAg), at the time of maximal viral replication.

345

VIRAL HEPATITIS

Outcome of Hepatitis B infection

In >90% of cases there is a vigorous immune reaction (cell mediated and humoral) to the virus resulting in its elimination. In the remaining patients, the illness pursues one of several courses:

HEPATITIS D

This is a defective RNA virus which requires HB virus for its release and infectivity. There are 2 patterns of infection:

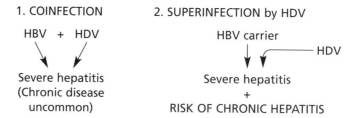

HEPATITIS C

This small RNA virus is transmitted parenterally and is seen in IV drug users or following infected blood transfusion. Acute hepatitis is mild and patients are rarely jaundiced. It is important because of the high risk of chronicity.

HEPATITIS A

This picornavirus is transmitted by the faeco-oral route, especially where hygiene is poor. Hepatitis is usually mild in children, but more severe in adults. IgM antibodies appear in the blood in the acute phase, and IgG during convalescence, thus conferring life long immunity. Chronic liver disease does not occur.

HEPATITIS E

This is most commonly seen in Africa and Asia. Although usually mild, it is particularly severe in pregnant women with a mortality of approximately 20%.

CHRONIC HEPATITIS

Inflammation of the liver which lasts for more than 6 months is regarded as chronic. (This definition excludes disorders such as alcoholic hepatitis.)

There are 4 main **causes:**

1. **Persistent viral infection** – hepatitis B, D and C.
2. **Autoimmune hepatitis.** This occurs especially in young women. In classic (type I) disease antinuclear and anti-smooth muscle antibodies are present in the serum. Liver specific autoantibodies e.g. to a sialoglycoprotein receptor (ASGP-R) on periportal hepatocyte cell surfaces can also be found. These patients often have other autoimmune diseases e.g. thyroiditis. A smaller subgroup, type II is defined by anti-Liver Kidney Microsomal antibodies (anti-LKM-1) and has a more aggressive disease.
3. **Drugs** – e.g. methyldopa, nitrofurantoin.
4. **In metabolic disorders** e.g. α_1-antitrypsin deficiency, Wilson's disease (p.357).

Pathologically, these are similar conditions, although subtle differences exist. The severity of the inflammation varies and a grading system devised by Ishak is commonly used – historically this was recognised by a division into 2 forms which are now recognised to be part of a spectrum.

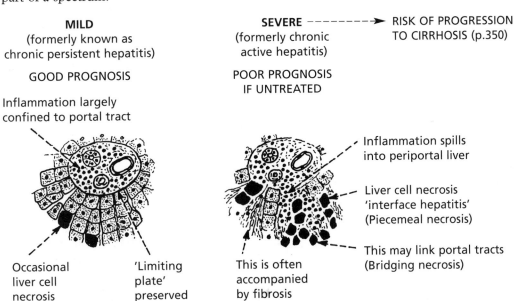

MILD
(formerly known as chronic persistent hepatitis)

GOOD PROGNOSIS

Inflammation largely confined to portal tract

Occasional liver cell necrosis

'Limiting plate' preserved

SEVERE ------> RISK OF PROGRESSION TO CIRRHOSIS (p.350)
(formerly chronic active hepatitis)

POOR PROGNOSIS IF UNTREATED

Inflammation spills into periportal liver

Liver cell necrosis 'interface hepatitis' (Piecemeal necrosis)

This may link portal tracts (Bridging necrosis)

This is often accompanied by fibrosis

347

ALCOHOLIC LIVER DISEASE

Excess consumption of alcohol is associated with liver disease in three main forms.

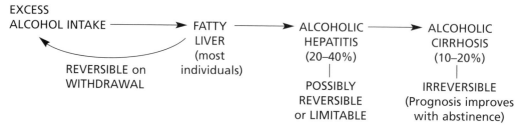

The progression from left to right does not occur in all patients: genetic predisposition, coexistant nutritional deficiencies, amount and duration of drinking and other factors determine the risk.

FATTY LIVER

This occurs in most heavy drinkers, even after a single episode of heavy intake. Fat accumulates in the hepatocytes due to abnormalities in the intermediate metabolism of lipids and carbohydrates.

Hepatic venule

Lipid droplets in hepatocytes (especially around hepatic venule)

Note: Fatty liver usually resolves within 2–4 weeks of abstinence.

Alcohol metabolism

ALCOHOLIC HEPATITIS

Fatty change is reversible even when extensive. In 20–40% of heavy drinkers, alcoholic hepatitis is superimposed. This varies from asymptomatic hepatitis to a life threatening condition with nausea, vomiting, abdominal pain and jaundice. Signs of liver failure and portal hypertension may be found.

Histologically, the main features are seen around hepatic venules:

1. Liver cell swelling – ballooning.
2. Accumulation of Mallory's hyaline – protein derived from intermediate filaments (mainly cytokeratin).
3. Liver cell necrosis.
4. Neutrophil polymorph reaction.
5. Pericellular fibrosis.

Acute Phase

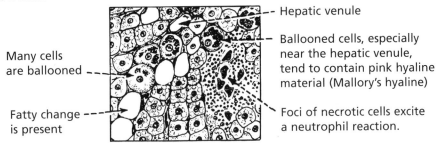

Many cells are ballooned

Fatty change is present

Hepatic venule

Ballooned cells, especially near the hepatic venule, tend to contain pink hyaline material (Mallory's hyaline)

Foci of necrotic cells excite a neutrophil reaction.

Progressing to pericellular fibrosis

Portal tracts

Fibrosis occurs mainly around hepatic venules which may be obliterated

Fibrosis may extend between adjacent hepatic venules

Perivenular fibrosis

Pericellular fibrosis

Alcoholic hepatitis is important as a cause of liver damage, especially because of the high risk of progression to cirrhosis.

Non-alcoholic steatohepatitis (NASH) is a histologically similar form of hepatitis seen in non-drinkers. Diabetes mellitus, severe obesity, jejuno-ileal bypass for obesity and certain drugs (e.g. tamoxiferin) appear to be responsible.

CIRRHOSIS

Cirrhosis is the end stage of many liver diseases. It is defined as:

A DIFFUSE process (i.e. the whole liver is affected) characterised by FIBROSIS and conversion of the liver architecture into abnormal NODULES.

Aetiology

There are very many causes including:

(i) Drugs and toxins e.g. alcohol, methotrexate, methyldopa.
(ii) Infections e.g. Hepatitis B and C.
(iii) Autoimmune diseases – chronic active hepatitis; primary biliary cirrhosis.
(iv) Metabolic conditions e.g. haemochromatosis, α_1-antitrypsin deficiency, Wilson's disease (excess accumulation of copper).
(v) Biliary obstruction e.g. gallstones, strictures, sclerosing cholangitis, cystic fibrosis.
(vi) Cryptogenic i.e. cause unknown.

The **mechanism** common to all cirrhosis is:

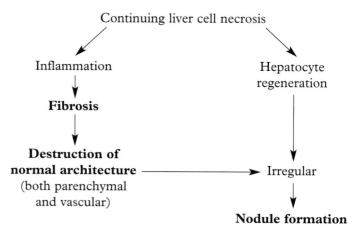

Hepatic stellate (fat-storing) cells found in the Space of Disse are activated and transformed into myofibroblast-like cells under the influence of cytokines such as TGFα, PDGF and TGF-β. The activated cells synthesise collagen leading to fibrosis.

The **major complications** of cirrhosis are:

1. Hepatocellular failure
2. Portal hypertension.
3. Hepatocellular carcinoma.

CIRRHOSIS

The initiating factor in the progression to cirrhosis is continuing hepatocellular damage. Its location within the acinus (p.338) and also its cause are reflected in the progression to irreversible damage.

The following contrasting diagrams illustrate this progression.

Alcoholic cirrhosis
develops from alcoholic hepatitis (p.349).

The initial damage is PERIVENULAR (Zone 3).

Secondary biliary cirrhosis
follows long-standing recurrent post-hepatic obstruction: the initial damage is PERIPORTAL (Zone 1).

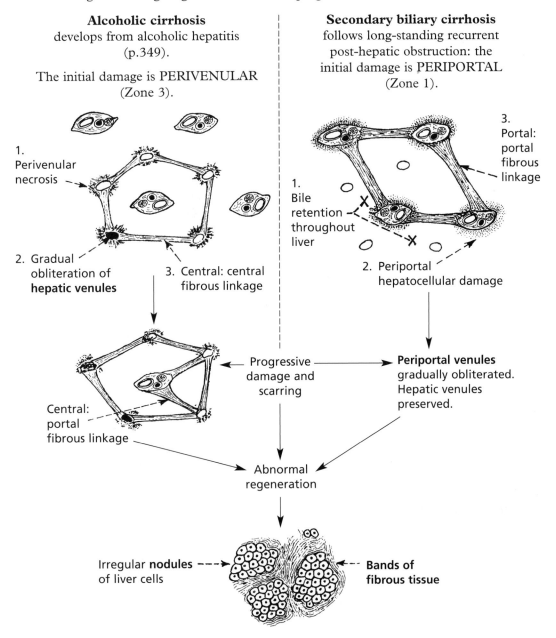

1. Perivenular necrosis

2. Gradual obliteration of **hepatic venules**

3. Central: central fibrous linkage

Central: portal fibrous linkage

1. Bile retention throughout liver

2. Periportal hepatocellular damage

3. Portal: portal fibrous linkage

Progressive damage and scarring

Periportal venules gradually obliterated. Hepatic venules preserved.

Abnormal regeneration

Irregular **nodules** of liver cells

Bands of **fibrous tissue**

351

CIRRHOSIS

PRIMARY BILIARY CIRRHOSIS (PBC)

This is a chronic disorder mainly affecting middle-aged women. Destruction of intra-hepatic bile ducts leads to scarring and eventually to cirrhosis. Patients typically present with fatigue, itching (from bile salt retention) or jaundice. Hyperlipidaemia is common.

Aetiology

This is an autoimmune disorder. Over 95% of patients have anti-mitochondrial antibodies in their serum. An overlap may be seen with autoimmune chronic hepatitis.

Pathology

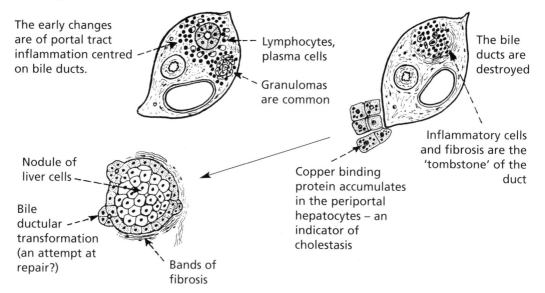

The early changes are of portal tract inflammation centred on bile ducts.

Lymphocytes, plasma cells

Granulomas are common

The bile ducts are destroyed

Inflammatory cells and fibrosis are the 'tombstone' of the duct

Copper binding protein accumulates in the periportal hepatocytes – an indicator of cholestasis

Nodule of liver cells

Bile ductular transformation (an attempt at repair?)

Bands of fibrosis

PRIMARY SCLEROSING CHOLANGITIS

This disease also attacks bile ducts, both intra- and extrahepatic. Men are usually affected and there is a strong association with ulcerative colitis.

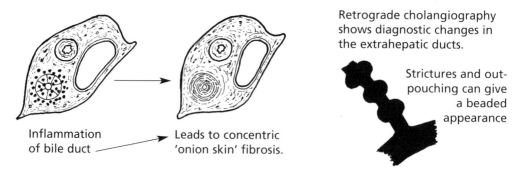

Inflammation of bile duct

Leads to concentric 'onion skin' fibrosis.

Retrograde cholangiography shows diagnostic changes in the extrahepatic ducts.

Strictures and out-pouching can give a beaded appearance

The late effects are similar to PBC. Liver failure and bile duct carcinoma are frequent complications.

HEPATOCELLULAR FAILURE

Failure of liver function can be:

1. Acute, with rapid onset (<8 weeks from onset of liver disease), e.g. in cases of massive necrosis due to poisoning e.g. paracetamol (or, less commonly, acute hepatitis).
2. Chronic and sometimes recurring, of slow onset, e.g. in cirrhosis or chronic hepatitis – representing decompensation.

The mechanism is different in the 2 types.

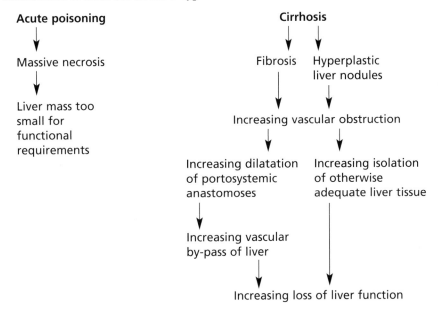

The **cardinal signs of hepatocellular failure are:**

    1. Jaundice.
    2. Hepatic encephalopathy.
    3. Ascites.
    4. Bleeding diathesis.

Other features include hypoglycaemia, acidosis and endocrine disturbances.

Jaundice

In acute liver failure, jaundice appears early and is related to the extent of liver damage. It arises as a result of lack of conjugation and excretion of bilirubin.

The time of appearance and type of jaundice in cases of chronic liver failure depend on the primary cause. In cases of biliary cirrhosis, the jaundice precedes other signs of liver failure and is of obstructive type, initially at least. Other forms of cirrhosis only give rise to jaundice at a late stage when it is of hepatic type, i.e. due to difficulties in bilirubin conjugation and excretion.

HEPATOCELLULAR FAILURE

HEPATIC ENCEPHALOPATHY

This term refers to the impaired mental state and neurological function due to liver failure. It takes the form of tremors, behavioural changes, convulsions, delirium, drowsiness and coma. In the acute form, severe symptoms such as convulsions, delirium and coma develop rapidly, while in chronic conditions milder changes are seen and coma is a late feature, unless a complication arises.

Acute

Brain

The basic cause is the same in both forms but the mechanism is somewhat different

Diminished detoxification of toxic intestinal nitrogenous compounds

Heart/lung

Increase in blood NH$_3$ etc.

Appearance of abnormal amines in systemic circulation

Necrosis ≡ Loss of detoxification

Toxic effect on brain

Interference with neurotransmission

Toxic N$_2$ compounds

Chronic

Brain

Heart/lung

Diversion through anastomotic channels

Cirrhosis ≡ Portal obstruction

Toxic N$_2$ compounds

Despite the serious disturbances of function, pathological changes in the brain of fatal cases are surprisingly slight.

Interstitial oedema

Perivascular oedema

Protoplasmic astrocytes enlarged and increased in number. Nuclei large with prominent nucleoli.

Aggravated by breakdown products of blood e.g. from bleeding varices.

HEPATOCELLULAR FAILURE

HEPATOCELLULAR FAILURE (*continued*)

1. **ASCITES** is usually due to a combination of **portal hypertension** and **hepatocellular failure**.

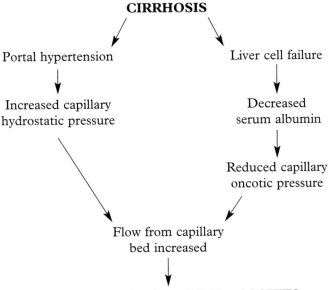

CIRRHOSIS

Portal hypertension

Liver cell failure

Increased capillary hydrostatic pressure

Decreased serum albumin

Reduced capillary oncotic pressure

Flow from capillary bed increased

Accumulation of peritoneal fluid = **ASCITES**

2. **ANAEMIA** usually of normocytic/normochromic type (p.408) is common – splenomegaly may cause hypersplenism and pancytopenia (p.430)

3. **Metabolic disorders**

   (a) Reduced protein synthesis e.g. fibrinogen, prothrombin, factors V, VII, IX, X ⟶ bleeding diathesis.

   (b) Reduced liver glycogen storage ⟶ hypoglycaemia.

   (c) Reduced elimination of endogenous oestrogen ⟶ gynaecomastia, testicular atrophy and spider naevi (small skin capillary telangiectasia).

4. **Hepato-renal failure** is an important complication of a major haemorrhage from oesophageal varices.

Liver transplantation is increasingly used to treat acute and chronic hepatocellular failure, as well as some small hepatocellular carcinomas. As with other transplanted organs, acute and chronic rejection are seen.

PORTAL HYPERTENSION

In cirrhosis of the liver, **portal hypertension** is important in addition to any hepatocellular deficiency.

Causes

By far, the most important cause is cirrhosis, but there are many others broadly classified as (1) pre-hepatic, (2) intra-hepatic and (3) post-hepatic.

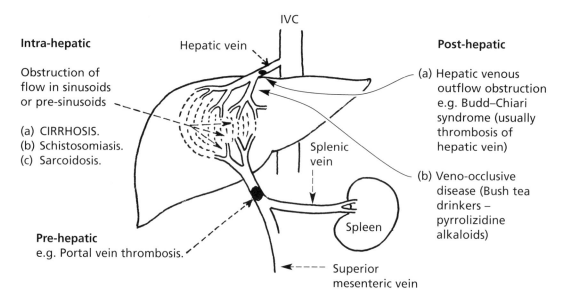

Intra-hepatic

Obstruction of flow in sinusoids or pre-sinusoids

(a) CIRRHOSIS.
(b) Schistosomiasis.
(c) Sarcoidosis.

IVC

Hepatic vein

Post-hepatic

(a) Hepatic venous outflow obstruction e.g. Budd–Chiari syndrome (usually thrombosis of hepatic vein)

(b) Veno-occlusive disease (Bush tea drinkers – pyrrolizidine alkaloids)

Splenic vein

Spleen

Pre-hepatic
e.g. Portal vein thrombosis.

Superior mesenteric vein

Effects

The main consequences are:

Portal hypertension

Splanchnic congestion

Porto-systemic shunting

Splenomegaly ± hypersplenism

Ascites

e.g. oesophageal varices

Blood flow bypassing liver

aggravated by hypoalbuminaemia due to hepatocellular failure

Haemorrhage

Toxic effects e.g. **encephalopathy** (p.354)

Simple clinical examination may show swollen abdomen due to ascites and caput medusae – engorged subcutaneous veins around the umbilicus.

METABOLIC DISORDERS AND THE LIVER

HAEMOCHROMATOSIS

This is due to a mutation on chromosome 6, encoding the HFE protein which regulates iron absorption.
Heterozygotes absorb excess iron, but homozygotes develop the disease.

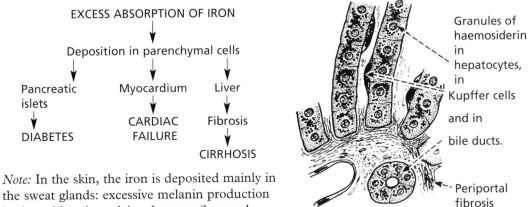

EXCESS ABSORPTION OF IRON

↓

Deposition in parenchymal cells

Pancreatic islets → DIABETES

Myocardium → CARDIAC FAILURE

Liver → Fibrosis → CIRRHOSIS

Granules of haemosiderin in hepatocytes, in Kupffer cells and in bile ducts.

Periportal fibrosis

Note: In the skin, the iron is deposited mainly in the sweat glands: excessive melanin production in the epidermis explains the term 'bronzed diabetes' for these cases.

HAEMOSIDEROSIS – Excess dietary iron and repeated blood transfusions may overload the body iron stores but cause less liver damage.

WILSON'S DISEASE (HEPATO-LENTICULAR DEGENERATION)

A rare autosomal recessive condition (due to mutation of the ATP7B gene on chromosome 13 which encodes a copper transporting enzyme). This is characterised by accumulation of copper in the liver, brain (basal ganglia) and cornea (Kayser–Fleischer rings). Serum levels of caeruloplasmin (a copper binding protein) are reduced. The liver can show an acute hepatitis, chronic hepatitis or cirrhosis.

α_1-ANTITRYPSIN DEFICIENCY

This enzyme is a protease inhibitor (Pi) produced mainly by the liver. Reduced levels or activity of the enzyme (abnormal forms coded by allelic variants) may result in liver damage.

Liver disease is found in most **homozygotes** (PiZZ) and presents as neonatal hepatitis, chronic active hepatitis or cirrhosis. Heterozygotes are rarely badly affected.

The abnormal enzyme is not secreted by liver cells and accumulates as globules in the periportal hepatocytes.

Note: α_1-antitrypsin deficiency is an important factor in the development of emphysema (p.261).

357

INFECTIONS AND INFESTATIONS

PYOGENIC INFECTIONS
These are now much less common due to the efficient use of antibiotics. Abscess of the liver occurs mainly in two conditions:

1. **Ascending cholangitis**

2. **Suppurative pylephlebitis**
   This arises from suppurative lesions in the abdominal cavity such as:

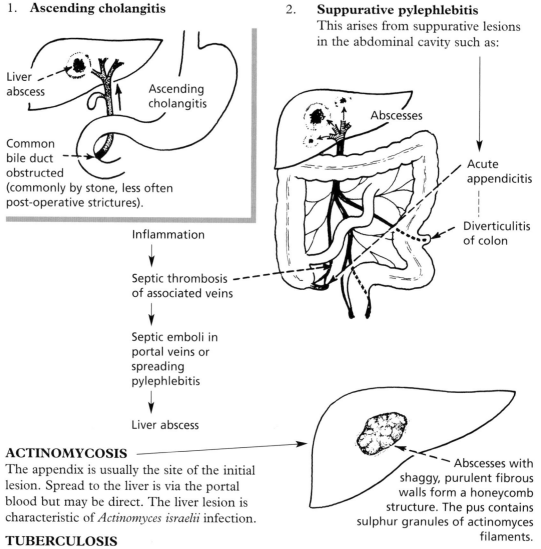

Inflammation

↓

Septic thrombosis of associated veins

↓

Septic emboli in portal veins or spreading pylephlebitis

↓

Liver abscess

ACTINOMYCOSIS
The appendix is usually the site of the initial lesion. Spread to the liver is via the portal blood but may be direct. The liver lesion is characteristic of *Actinomyces israelii* infection.

Abscesses with shaggy, purulent fibrous walls form a honeycomb structure. The pus contains sulphur granules of actinomyces filaments.

TUBERCULOSIS
This is rare. Miliary tubercles may be seen in generalised infection.

HEPATIC GRANULOMAS (Tuberculoid reactions)
Giant cell granulomas are also common in sarcoidosis and may also occur in brucellosis, histoplasmosis and primary biliary cirrhosis, among many other causes.

INFECTIONS AND INFESTATIONS

SPIROCHAETAL INFECTIONS

Three spirochaetal infections can involve the liver.

1. Leptospira icterohaemorrhagica (Weil's Disease)

This organism is associated with the presence of rats and working in wet conditions. It is prevalent among workers in sewers and abbatoirs, miners and agricultural workers.

The rat is a reservoir of infection, and rat excreta contain the organism. The disease is characterised by fever, jaundice, haemorrhages into and from various organs, e.g. lungs, kidneys, and renal damage. The liver lesion is characteristic. Death may occur from intrapulmonary haemorrhage or renal failure.

Proliferation of hepatocytes

Focal necrosis with inflammation

Separation of liver cells (a post-mortem artefact – not seen in biopsies)

2. *Treponema pallidum*

Syphilitic lesions of the liver are now uncommon in the U.K.

(a) *Congenital infection.* This usually produces a diffuse interstitial fibrosis which isolates individual liver cells and causes ischaemic atrophy. It is accompanied by a striking mononuclear infiltration and tiny areas of coagulative necrosis – miliary gummata. Spirochaetes are often plentiful.

(b) *Acquired infection.* Lesions can occur in the secondary and tertiary stages. In the secondary stage, a diffuse, inflammatory reaction with miliary gummata can occur. Large gummata may be seen in tertiary syphilis. Gross scarring with distortion follows healing – hepar lobatum.

3. Borrelia

Borrelia occur in many parts of the world and several species exist e.g. *B. recurrentis*. They are transmitted by lice and ticks from animals acting as reservoirs, especially rodents. The infections produce peri-venular necrosis of the liver. Jaundice may be severe and liver failure can result in death.

INFECTIONS AND INFESTATIONS

PROTOZOAL DISEASES

Amoebic 'abscess'

This is a complication of amoebic dysentery due to *Entamoeba histolytica*. The 'abscess' is usually single, in the upper right lobe of liver. An irregular fibrous wall encloses what appears to be brownish pus. The 'pus' consists of necrotic liver cells, debris and red cells. Amoebae may be found in the inner wall. There are no pus cells. It may remain localised or track through the diaphragm into the lung, pleural or pericardial cavities.

Malaria

On initial infection, the parasites develop within the hepatocytes but produce little damage. In chronic malaria, red cells containing parasites are engulfed by Kupffer cells which become hyperplastic and contain brown malarial pigment.

In benign tertian malaria, the parasite can survive for long periods within the liver cells (exoerythrocytic cycle).

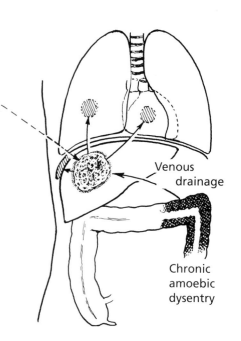

Venous drainage

Chronic amoebic dysentry

Kala-azar (Visceral Leishmaniasis)

The liver is enlarged due to hyperplasia of the Kupffer cells which phagocytose many Leishman–Donovan bodies, the protozoan responsible.

METAZOAL DISEASES Trematodes (flukes)

Schistosomiasis (Bilharzia)

S. mansoni is common in Egypt and other parts of Africa. *S. japonicum* is found in China, Japan and the Philippines. Both infections involve the liver.

The schistosomes colonise the intestinal tract. They invade the intestinal veins; ova are released into the blood stream and embolise the portal venules of the liver. There is a focal granulomatous reaction which may lead to extensive portal fibrosis without cirrhosis. Portal hypertension can result with its associated complications.

S. mansoni

INFECTIONS AND INFESTATIONS

METAZOAL DISEASES (*continued*)

Two other varieties of fluke disease exist —
clonorchiasis (Chinese fish fluke) and
fascioliasis (sheep fluke). Both produce an
ascending cholangitis. Clonorchiasis can cause
biliary obstruction and marked proliferation of
bile ducts. Cholangiocarcinoma may develop.
Infestation in both cases is due to eating raw
or insufficiently cooked food.

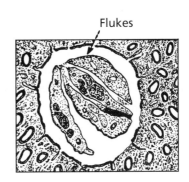
Flukes

Hydatid disease

This is a cystic condition caused by the embryos of *Echinococcus granulosus*, a small
tapeworm. The condition is commonest in sheep and may occur in humans in close contact
with them. Cattle and pigs may also be affected. Adult worms are found in dogs fed on the
infected tissues of sheep, cattle or pigs. Ova
are excreted by the dogs and are ingested
by other animals including humans. The
disease is commonest in Australia, New
Zealand, South America and the Middle
East.

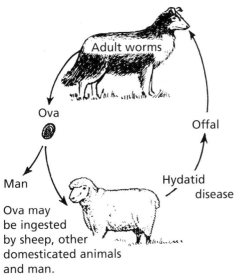

Adult worms

Ova

Offal

Man

Hydatid
disease

Ova may
be ingested
by sheep, other
domesticated animals
and man.

Digestion of the chitinous membrane by
gastric juice liberates the embryos which
invade the intestinal veins and reach the
liver. Sometimes they pass into the systemic
circulation and cysts form in the lungs,
muscles, kidneys, spleen or brain.

The cyst may be very large, usually
multilocular, due to budding of daughter
cysts.

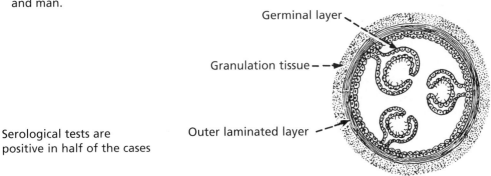

Germinal layer

Granulation tissue

Outer laminated layer

Serological tests are
positive in half of the cases

TUMOURS OF LIVER

PRIMARY BENIGN TUMOURS
Very few varieties are recognised.

1. **Cavernous haemangioma.** This is the commonest type. It forms a dark purple, sharply demarcated geometric patch on the liver surface. It has the usual structure of a cavernous angioma (see p.132).

2. **Liver cell adenoma.** These small tumours are rare, but an increased incidence has been associated with the use of contraceptive and anabolic steroids. They consist of normal liver trabeculae without normal portal tracts. Intraperitoneal bleeding may occur.

3. **Bile duct adenoma.** These small tumours are usually incidental findings at laparotomy. They consist of tiny bile duct structures set in loose connective tissue. Occasionally bile duct cystadenomas form large tumours.

SECONDARY TUMOURS
The liver is by far the most frequent site, of all organs, of secondary tumour deposits and they form the commonest type of liver tumour. Apart from the gastrointestinal tract, the lung and breast are the most frequent sites of primary growth. Melanoma, leukaemic infiltration and involvement by lymphoma are also common.

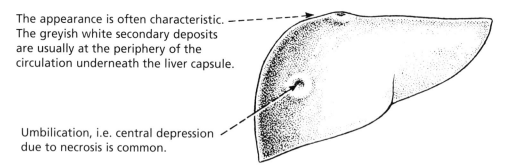

The appearance is often characteristic. The greyish white secondary deposits are usually at the periphery of the circulation underneath the liver capsule.

Umbilication, i.e. central depression due to necrosis is common.

Variations in appearance are produced by haemorrhage, necrosis and the type of tumour, e.g. mucus-secreting carcinomas.

The secondary tumours grow rapidly and are frequently the main cause of death. An exception is the secondary deposits from a carcinoid tumour which grow slowly over a period of years (p.334).

Increasingly metastases, e.g. from colorectal cancers, are treated by radio frequency ablation or surgical resection.

PRIMARY CARCINOMA OF LIVER

HEPATOCELLULAR CARCINOMA (HCC)

This, the commonest primary malignancy of the liver, is unusual in Western Europe, but is very common in Africa and commonest in Mozambique and in South-East Asia. Males are particularly affected.

Three main types of growth are described:

Solitary large tumour   Multifocal form   Diffuse growth

In all three forms the liver is often cirrhotic (80%) (particularly in the West).

Histological structure: The cells grow in columns resembling normal liver.

Branching trabeculae

Functional activity is often displayed:
(a) bile secretion,
(b) fat formation,
(c) glycogen storage

Spread

In addition to diffuse growth within the liver, **invasion of hepatic veins** occurs early and there may be metastases to lung, bone and also the draining lymph nodes.

The proximate **cause of death** may be (i) liver failure, (ii) the complications of portal hypertension (especially in cirrhotic patients) and (iii) massive intraperitoneal haemorrhage.

Systemic manifestations include hypoglycaemia, hypercalcaemia and polycythaemia (due to production of erythropoietin).

Diagnosis

Liver biopsy is usually required. High levels of alpha-fetoprotein (normally produced in the fetal liver), >500 μg/l are strong supportive evidence (not all tumours produce this protein). This can be demonstrated in tumour cells by immunostaining. In-situ hybridisation can show mRNA for albumin in αFP-negative tumours.

Increased levels of αFP are also seen in:
1. Cases of testicular teratoma (p.526) or ovarian yolk sac tumour (p.512).
2. Liver damage (the levels are much lower).

PRIMARY LIVER CELL TUMOURS

HEPATOCELLULAR CARCINOMA (HCC) *(continued)*

Aetiology

The aetiological agents vary in low and high incidence areas.

WESTERN EUROPE

ALCOHOLIC LIVER DISEASE

Also chronic active hepatitis including HBV + HCV, haemochromatosis

S.E. ASIA and AFRICA

HEPATITIS B + C VIRUSES

Aflatoxins (aspergillus flavus toxins)

In a minority of cases **no cirrhosis** is found

CIRRHOSIS

HEPATOCELLULAR CARCINOMA

FIBROLAMELLAR CARCINOMA

This uncommon variant (<5%) occurs especially in children and young adults. It is important because the prognosis is much better following surgical resection.

Histologically

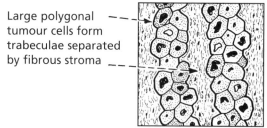

Large polygonal tumour cells form trabeculae separated by fibrous stroma

Other differences from conventional HCC are:
(1) Usually no cirrhosis
(2) AFP not raised
(3) Hepatitis B infection rare
 – aetiology uncertain.

CHOLANGIOCARCINOMA

These tumours arise from bile ducts at both intra- and extrahepatic sites.

They are usually adenocarcinomas: some show excess mucus secretion and evoke a dense fibrous response.

Cirrhosis is rarely present.

There is an increased incidence in association with ulcerative colitis and primary sclerosing cholangitis, and in the Far East there is a clear association with liver fluke (clonorchis) infestation.

Cells resemble bile duct epithelium.

GALLBLADDER AND BILE DUCT – ANATOMY

Anatomy

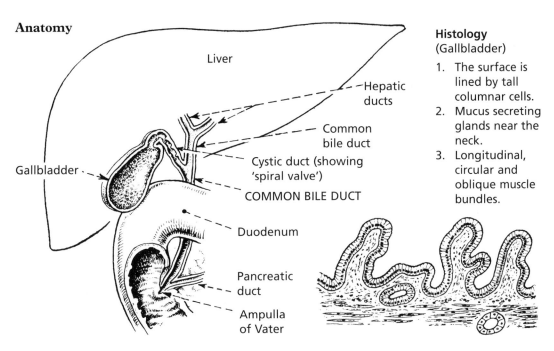

Histology
(Gallbladder)

1. The surface is lined by tall columnar cells.
2. Mucus secreting glands near the neck.
3. Longitudinal, circular and oblique muscle bundles.

The function of the gallbladder is to concentrate and store bile.

GALLSTONES

Gallstones are the principal cause of gallbladder disease and its consequences.
There are 3 main types:

1. **Mixed stones** account for 80% of all gallstones. They are always **multiple** and **faceted** due to contact with one another.

On section

Thin shell of calcium salts

They have a laminated structure – layers of cholesterol, bile pigment and calcium salts.

2. **Cholesterol stone**
   – is usually solitary, oval and up to 2–3 cm in length.
   They are associated with excessive cholesterol in the bile.

Radiating glistening cholesterol crystals (pale yellow)

Often has a tiny dark central deposit

3. **Bile pigment stones** – are always multiple and are usually due to chronic haemolysis with excess bilirubin production.

Rarely more than 1 cm in diameter, black and irregular.

365

GALLSTONES

Clinical manifestations and complications

Many subjects are asymptomatic or have only mild dyspepsia – most symptoms are attributable to the complications.

1. **ACUTE CHOLECYSTITIS**

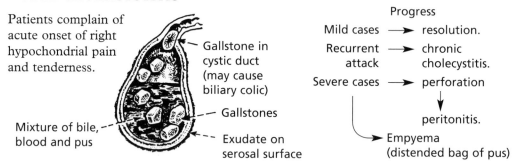

Patients complain of acute onset of right hypochondrial pain and tenderness.

Gallstone in cystic duct (may cause biliary colic)

Gallstones

Mixture of bile, blood and pus

Exudate on serosal surface

Progress

Mild cases ⟶ resolution.

Recurrent attack ⟶ chronic cholecystitis.

Severe cases ⟶ perforation
⟶ peritonitis.

Empyema (distended bag of pus)

2. **CHRONIC CHOLECYSTITIS**

In the majority of cases the symptoms are of vague 'indigestion ', intolerance of fatty foods and vague right hypochondrial pain: in some cases there is a history of acute attacks.

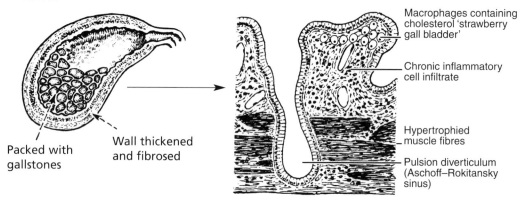

Packed with gallstones

Wall thickened and fibrosed

Macrophages containing cholesterol 'strawberry gall bladder'

Chronic inflammatory cell infiltrate

Hypertrophied muscle fibres

Pulsion diverticulum (Aschoff–Rokitansky sinus)

3. **MUCOCELE** – can occur when the cystic duct is blocked.

This occurs when there has been long-standing obstruction of the cystic duct.

Stone blocking cystic duct

Bile absent, clear, watery fluid distends sac (mucocele)

Mucosa flattened

Thin wall

Villi tiny

Inflammatory cells

Muscle almost absent: thin fibrous wall

GALLSTONES

GALLSTONES (*continued*)

4. COMMON DUCT GALLSTONES

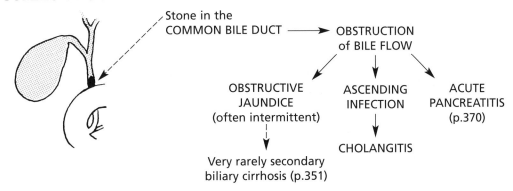

Stone in the
COMMON BILE DUCT ⟶ OBSTRUCTION
of BILE FLOW

OBSTRUCTIVE   ASCENDING   ACUTE
JAUNDICE   INFECTION   PANCREATITIS
(often intermittent)   (p.370)

CHOLANGITIS

Very rarely secondary
biliary cirrhosis (p.351)

Note: In addition to jaundice, persistent skin itching, due to retention of bile salts, may occur.

5. GALLSTONE ILEUS

Very rarely a stone may ulcerate through the gallbladder into the intestine and cause obstruction.

Contracted, inflamed gallbladder

Large barrel-shaped stone

Intestine or duodenum drawn
up by inflammatory fibrosis

Impaction in ileum

Intestinal obstruction

6. CARCINOMA of the GALLBLADDER

This is uncommon, but almost always associated with gallstones.

Most cases are adenocarcinomas which spread directly to the liver.

Less commonly
at neck

CARCINOMAS of the
BILIARY TRACT are
also found ...

... at junction of the
cystic and common ducts.

... at ampulla of Vater.

These are not always
associated with gallstones.

Most tumours
are at fundus

367

GALLSTONES – AETIOLOGY

Although gallstones are found in 10–20% of the population, the prevalence increasing with age, the exact mechanisms of their formation remain incompletely understood. Risk factors include (a) female gender, (b) obesity, (c) pregnancy, (d) drugs such as the cholesterol lowering drug clofibrate now seldom used and (e) gastrointestinal disease e.g. Crohn's disease.

The principal constituents of bile are **cholesterol, phospholipids** and **bile acids** (cholic acid and chenodeoxycholic acid).

The **stability of cholesterol** depends on adequate amounts of bile acids. Micelles are formed.

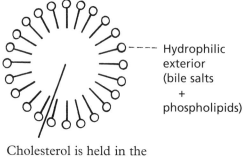

Hydrophilic exterior (bile salts + phospholipids)

Cholesterol is held in the hydrophobic interior

Their **enterohepatic circulation** is essential to maintain adequate concentrations of bile salts.

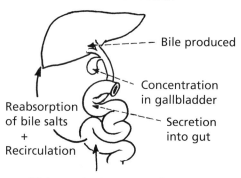

Bile produced

Concentration in gallbladder

Reabsorption of bile salts + Recirculation

Secretion into gut

This can be interrupted by mucosal disease e.g. Crohn's disease

The ratio of cholesterol:bile salts is very important.

Increased biliary cholesterol secretion
or
Increased cholesterol synthesis
or
Decreased bile salts (e.g. in Crohn's disease)

Ratio increased

$$\dfrac{\text{Cholesterol} \uparrow}{\text{Bile salts} \downarrow} \longrightarrow$$ Precipitation of CHOLESTEROL → NUCLEATION (formation of tiny stones)

↓

Progressive accumulation of cholesterol and pigment

↓

ENLARGING STONES

Stones often lead to infection: it is likely that infection promotes further stone production.

These mechanisms are responsible for cholesterol and mixed stones. Pigment stones are seen in haemolytic anaemia, but also in relation to infection e.g. of *E. coli*. The mechanisms are poorly understood.

PANCREAS

The exocrine glandular portion of the pancreas produces its digestive secretion which is delivered to the second part of the duodenum.

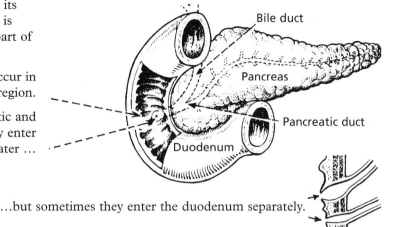

Bile duct

Pancreas

Pancreatic duct

Duodenum

Anatomical variations occur in this region.

Commonly the pancreatic and bile ducts fuse as they enter the ampulla of Vater …

…but sometimes they enter the duodenum separately.

Microscopically, the exocrine tissue is similar to salivary glands.

In addition, foci of endocrine islet tissue occur throughout the pancreas (islets of Langerhans)

Exocrine secretory granules

Function: The exocrine pancreas produces an alkaline secretion containing digestive enzymes.
Sodium bicarbonate – gives a pH 7.5–8.0
Amylase – splits starches. Lipase – digests lipids.
Trypsinogen ⎱ converted to active proteolytic
Chymotrypsinogen ⎰ enzymes, trypsin, chymotrypsin.

The islet tissue produces insulin and glucagon (and other neuropeptides). Disorders of the islets e.g. diabetes, are discussed on page 643.

An understanding of the microcirculation is important. The gland has a lobular structure. The larger arteries, veins and ducts course in the fibrous septa between the *lobules*.

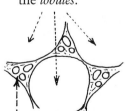

Interlobular artery, vein and duct

This diagram shows the circulation and duct system within the lobule (intralobular).

This watershed zone at the *periphery* of the lobule is susceptible when there is a circulatory perfusion deficit

This zone at the centre of the lobule is susceptible if there is damage to the intralobular duct

ACUTE PANCREATITIS

There is evidence that mild pancreatitis is not uncommon but, in a significant number of cases, progression to a severe fatal disease occurs. Clinically, there is an acute abdominal emergency with pain and shock.

The essential pathological changes are due to tissue necrosis caused by the action of liberated enzymes on the pancreatic tissues. The severity of the lesion depends on the amount of enzyme set free, the distance it diffuses, anti-proteolytic factors and the structures affected. The pancreatic damage occurs in two forms:

1. **Periductal necrosis** – in the centre of each affected lobule.

2. **Perilobular necrosis** – affecting the periphery of lobules.

Damage to the epithelial lining of the duct allows diffusion of active enzymes into the adjacent tissues

Small areas of necrosis appear around the ducts of some of the lobules

This type is associated with gallstones and alcohol.

Ischaemic necrosis occurs at the periphery of the lobules and is further complicated by liberation of enzymes

This type is associated with circulatory perfusion failure; e.g in severe shock; prolonged operations and hypothermia.

Both types of damage, if not inhibited by antitrypsins and $\alpha 2$ macroglobulins derived from the blood and pancreas itself, will progress, often very rapidly, to the very severe form –

PANLOBULAR PANCREATITIS

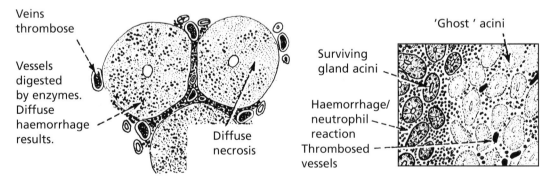

Veins thrombose

Vessels digested by enzymes. Diffuse haemorrhage results.

Diffuse necrosis

Surviving gland acini

'Ghost' acini

Haemorrhage/ neutrophil reaction

Thrombosed vessels

The initial damage is severe, and large quantities of enzymes are liberated, including trypsin, chymotrypsin, lipase, elastase and phospholipase. Locally, these set up a progressive pathological process.

ACUTE PANCREATITIS

SEVERE PANCREATITIS (*continued*)

Damage to pancreas

↓

Release of enzymes – especially activation of TRYPSIN

↓

Digestion of cell membranes

↓   ↓

Necrosis of gland tissue   Necrosis of interstitial tissue

↓   ↓

Further release of enzymes   Thrombosis and necrosis of vessels

↓   ↓

Extension of pancreatic damage

The released enzymes spread beyond the exocrine tissues of the pancreas:

1. *Via lymphatics to abdominal tissues* especially the omentum and mesenteries

Naked eye appearance

Opaque white patches of necrotic fatty tissue containing free fatty acids – due to action of phospholipase and proteolytic enzymes – lipase splits fat.

2. *Locally causing destruction of islet tissue* – hyperglycaemia may occur.

3. *Via blood stream.*

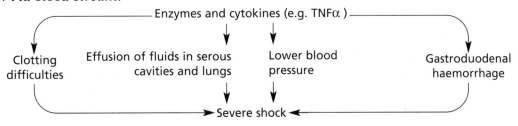

Enzymes and cytokines (e.g. TNFα)

Clotting difficulties   Effusion of fluids in serous cavities and lungs   Lower blood pressure   Gastroduodenal haemorrhage

→ Severe shock ←

These effects are largely due to activation of thromboplastins and formation of vasoactive kinins. Hypoxia due to pulmonary oedema intensifies the shock.

Hypocalcaemia giving rise to tetany may occur due to deposition of calcium soaps in the necrotic fat cells of the omentum and peritoneum. Commonly hypocalcaemia merely reflects low serum albumin levels.

Raised serum amylase levels are used as a diagnostic test.

ACUTE PANCREATITIS

Aetiology
Two factors are important: (1) gallstones and (2) alcohol.

Gallstones
Between 40 and 60% of all cases of severe pancreatitis are associated with gallstones. Recurrent attacks are common.

A likely mechanism postulated is of

Bile reflux
In most patients, the bile duct and pancreatic duct have a common entrance to the ampulla of Vater. Stones passing down the bile duct could, by blocking the ampulla, cause reflux of bile along the pancreatic duct.

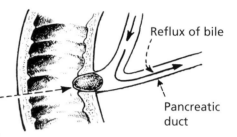

Note: Pancreatitis may also occur in those patients whose common bile duct and pancreatic duct enter the ampulla separately (p.369).

Alcohol
Acute pancreatitis is common in alcoholics and the incidence of this association is directly related to the consumption of alcohol by the local population.

The causal relationship is obscure, but it is possible that in both gallstone and alcoholic pancreatitis there is a common pathogenic mechanism. Alcohol may cause ampullary spasm.

Other causes include:
Trauma, including surgery.
Viruses e.g. mumps, coxsackie B.
Hypercalcaemia e.g. in hyperparathyroidism.
Drugs e.g. steroids.

Complications
(i)   Shock is common, leading to death in 10% of patients.
(ii) Recurrent attacks may lead to chronic pancreatitis.
(iii) Collections of fluid may be surrounded by fibrous tissue – pancreatic pseudocyst (p.374).

CHRONIC PANCREATITIS

Chronic pancreatitis predominantly affects alcoholic men. The pathological changes are similar in all cases.

The process begins in the finer ductules and the associated acini → Protein rich plugs appear in the ductules → Ductules and acini become dilated behind the obstructing protein

Normal

Epithelium of acini becomes low cubical

Duct epithelium necrotic at site of obstruction

Epithelium degenerates and disappears

Acini eventually atrophy and collapse

Round cell infiltration appears around the degenerating glandular unit

Glandular tissue is replaced by fibrosis

The change is focal. More and more protein plugs form, some in larger ducts. Obstruction of these may lead to production of cysts.

Ultimately, a large proportion of the exocrine tissue is destroyed.

Fibrosis with lymphocytic infiltrate

Cystic dilatation of ducts Epithelial lining usually atrophic and incomplete

Small ducts, possibly reactive hyperplasia } This may mimic carcinoma in biopsy material

Eosinophilic protein plug in duct

Islet tissue initially survives

CHRONIC PANCREATITIS

With progress of the disease, two other developments take place:

1. *Calcification.* This occurs mainly in the protein plugs in the ducts, resulting in the formation of calculi.

2. *Rupture of the duct cysts into the surrounding tissues.* A granulation tissue reaction is set up with formation of a pseudocyst. The result depends on the site of the pseudocyst.

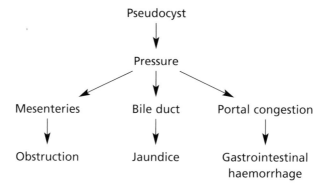

Rupture into the peritoneal cavity causes ascites, frequently haemorrhagic.

Progressive destruction of the parenchyma with fibrosis may ultimately convert the pancreatitis into a thin hard cord.

Effects
Patients typically complain of abdominal pain.

Apart from the complications due to cyst rupture, destruction of pancreatic tissue may lead to:

1. Insufficiency of exocrine secretion → steatorrhoea and wasting.

2. Diabetes mellitus. 30% of patients eventually develop this due to destruction of islet tissue.

Aetiology
1. The main factor in 75% of cases in Western civilisation is alcohol. Patients have generally consumed more than 150 g daily over a long period of time.

2. Some cases may follow recurrent attacks of acute pancreatitis.

3. A peculiar type of chronic pancreatitis occurs in Africa and South East Asia. It is related to chronic malnutrition with particular deficiency of protein, from infancy. Extensive calcification of the pancreatic tissue occurs. It has been suggested that there is a genetic predisposition to the disease.

CYSTIC FIBROSIS (Mucoviscidosis)

This is a common autosomal recessive inherited disease due to genetic mutation on chromosome 7; a high percentage (about 4%) of the population are carriers.

The gene involved is called cystic fibrosis transmembrane conductance regulator (CFTR). Its essential function is the control of the transfer of chloride across cell membranes. Many mutations of the gene have been recorded, each being responsible for subtle variations in the evolution of the disorder.

All the exocrine secretory tissues are affected to a greater or lesser degree: the pathological results vary according to which organ is mainly affected – pancreas, bronchi, bowel, biliary tree, testis.

The essential change is as follows:

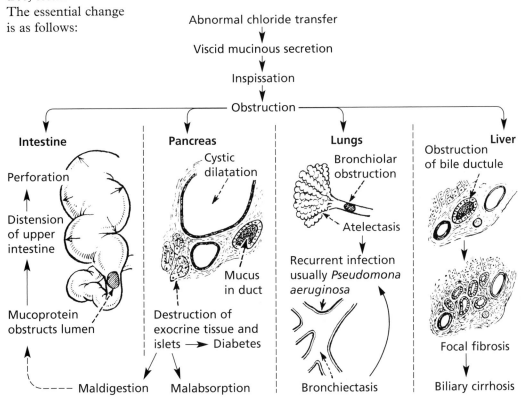

Abnormal chloride transfer
↓
Viscid mucinous secretion
↓
Inspissation
↓
Obstruction

Intestine

Perforation

Distension of upper intestine

Mucoprotein obstructs lumen

Maldigestion

Pancreas

Cystic dilatation

Mucus in duct

Destruction of exocrine tissue and islets → Diabetes

Malabsorption

Lungs

Bronchiolar obstruction

Atelectasis

Recurrent infection usually *Pseudomona aeruginosa*

Bronchiectasis

Liver

Obstruction of bile ductule

Focal fibrosis

Biliary cirrhosis

Clinical features

Neonatal

Intestinal obstruction (meconium ileus) may lead to intestinal perforation and fatal peritonitis.

Childhood:

There is failure to thrive due to maldigestion and malabsorption, and steatorrhea is common – all features of pancreatic insufficiency. The lungs are affected, with recurrent episodes of infection often leading to death in early adult life. Lung transplantation and gene therapy offer hope of improved survival. Liver lesions are of late development.

There is increase of sodium chloride in the sweat of patients and their heterozygote siblings. This provides a diagnostic test which is now supplemented by genetic screening.

TUMOURS OF PANCREAS

Benign tumours of the pancreas such as cystadenomas are rare. They may produce symptoms due to pressure on other structures.

CARCINOMA
This affects 15 per 100 000 in Western countries.

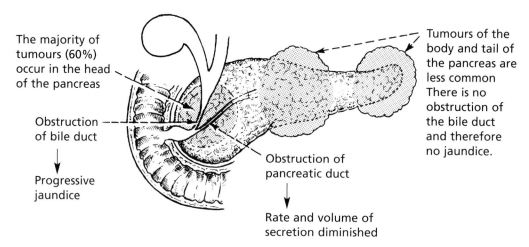

The majority of tumours (60%) occur in the head of the pancreas

Tumours of the body and tail of the pancreas are less common There is no obstruction of the bile duct and therefore no jaundice.

Obstruction of bile duct

↓

Progressive jaundice

Obstruction of pancreatic duct

↓

Rate and volume of secretion diminished

Local spread and/or distant metastases are found in 85% of cases at the time of diagnosis and the 5 year survival rate is 3–5%.

The tumour arises from the duct epithelium and in almost all cases it is an adenocarcinoma. Papillary cystadenocarcinoma, adenosquamous carcinoma and giant cell carcinoma are forms occasionally encountered.

Tumours in the body and tail are commonly larger than tumours of the head, probably due to later diagnosis in the relative absence of symptoms.

Thrombosis of unknown cause and at distant sites, e.g. femoral vein, is apt to occur when the tumour is in the body or tail.

Aetiology
1. Pancreatic carcinoma is most frequent in males in the 5th–7th decades.
2. There is a statistical association with alcohol, cigarette smoking, a diet high in fat and carbohydrate and chronic pancreatitis.
3. In the U.S.A., the incidence is higher in the black population and a similar situation is true of the Maoris in New Zealand.

Endocrine Tumours
Islet cell tumours are described on page 647.

CHAPTER 11

HAEMOPOIETIC AND
LYMPHO-RETICULAR TISSUES

HAEMOPOIESIS

The derivation of blood cells

In the **bone marrow** a '**pluripotent**' stem cell gives rise to **all blood cells.**

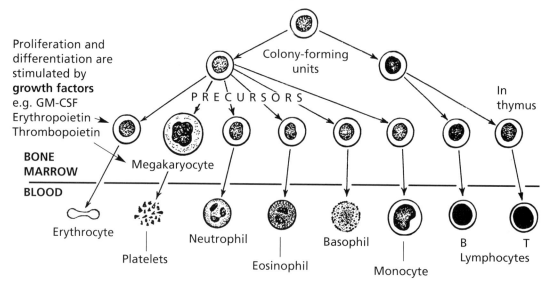

Proliferation and differentiation are stimulated by **growth factors** e.g. GM-CSF Erythropoietin Thrombopoietin

Colony-forming units

PRECURSORS

In thymus

BONE MARROW

BLOOD

Megakaryocyte

Erythrocyte

Platelets

Neutrophil

Eosinophil

Basophil

Monocyte

B T
Lymphocytes

Haemopoiesis in bone marrow

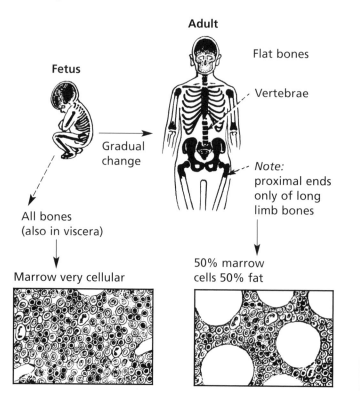

Fetus

Adult

Flat bones

Vertebrae

Gradual change

Note: proximal ends only of long limb bones

All bones (also in viscera)

Marrow very cellular

50% marrow cells 50% fat

When extra blood cells are required MARROW HYPERPLASIA occurs

Extension down long bones

Increased cellularity – obliteration of fat spaces

HAEMATOLOGY – LABORATORY TESTS

Investigation of blood diseases depends on examination of 1. PERIPHERAL BLOOD and 2. BONE MARROW.

1. PERIPHERAL BLOOD

Blood count: this is normally done by sophisticated electronic machines.
The main parameters are:

(i) **HAEMOGLOBIN (Hb) CONCENTRATION** (g/dl whole blood)
Normal values: Male 15.5±2.5: Female 14.0±2.5

(ii) **CELL COUNT**
Red Cell count: Males $5.5±1.0 \times 10^{12}/l$.
Females $4.8±1.0 \times 10^{12}/l$.
White Cell Count: $4–11 \times 10^9/l$.
Neutrophils – $2.0–7.5 \times 10^9/l$.
Lymphocytes – $1.5–4.0 \times 10^9/l$.
Monocytes – $0.2–0.8 \times 10^9/l$.
Eosinophils – $0.04–0.4 \times 10^9/l$.
Basophils – $0.01–0.1 \times 10^9/l$.
Platelets – $150–400 \times 10^9/l$.

(iii) **MEAN RED CELL VOLUME (MCV)**
Normal – 85±8 fl (femtolitres)

Also measured are:
MEAN CELL HAEMOGLOBIN
Normal = 29.5±2.5 picograms.
MEAN CELL HAEMOGLOBIN CONCENTRATION (MCHC)
Normal = 33±3 g/dl.

BLOOD FILM – stained by a Romanowski method.

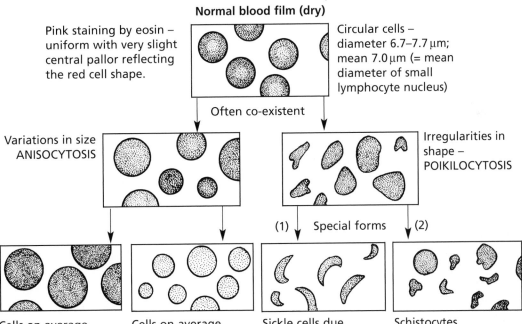

Normal blood film (dry)

Pink staining by eosin – uniform with very slight central pallor reflecting the red cell shape.

Circular cells – diameter 6.7–7.7 μm; mean 7.0 μm (= mean diameter of small lymphocyte nucleus)

Often co-existent

Variations in size ANISOCYTOSIS

Irregularities in shape – POIKILOCYTOSIS

(1) Special forms (2)

Cells on average LARGER – MACROCYTIC

Cells on average SMALLER – MICROCYTIC and often paler staining (hypochromic)

Sickle cells due to abnormal haemoglobin (p.407)

Schistocytes (Fragments of red cells damaged in the flowing blood, e.g. through abnormal vessels or cardiac prostheses.)

379

HAEMATOLOGY – LABORATORY TESTS

Another useful test is the measurement of the **PACKED CELL VOLUME (PCV)** or haematocrit.

This is obtained by centrifuging anticoagulated whole blood in a haematocrit tube.

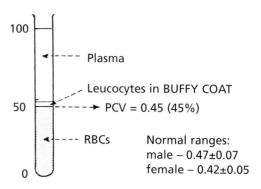

- - - - Plasma

Leucocytes in BUFFY COAT

PCV = 0.45 (45%)

- - - - RBCs

Normal ranges:
male – 0.47±0.07
female – 0.42±0.05

2. BONE MARROW EXAMINATION

Examination of bone marrow is important in explaining abnormalities of the peripheral blood.

In the past, aspiration of marrow from the sternum was commonly performed. Now the posterior iliac crest is used – it is safer and allows marrow to be **aspirated** and a **trephine** biopsy to be taken.

Film of aspirate allows detailed observation of **cell morphology**.

Marrow cells

Fat spaces

Bone

Histological preparation of trephine material allows assessment of **architecture**.

ERYTHROPOIESIS

Normal marrow erythropoiesis is said to be NORMOBLASTIC.

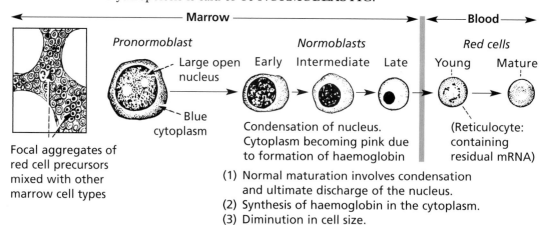

◄─────────────── Marrow ───────────────► ◄── Blood ──►

Pronormoblast   *Normoblasts*   *Red cells*

Large open nucleus   Early Intermediate Late   Young   Mature

Blue cytoplasm

Focal aggregates of red cell precursors mixed with other marrow cell types

Condensation of nucleus. Cytoplasm becoming pink due to formation of haemoglobin

(Reticulocyte: containing residual mRNA)

(1) Normal maturation involves condensation and ultimate discharge of the nucleus.
(2) Synthesis of haemoglobin in the cytoplasm.
(3) Diminution in cell size.

When the essential factors vit. B_{12} or folic acid are deficient, the red cell precursors show clear morphological changes – erythropoiesis is said to be MEGALOBLASTIC (p.388).

ANAEMIA

The most important function of the red cell is the transport of oxygen bound to haemoglobin. The most common and important disorder associated with disease of the red cells is ANAEMIA, which is defined as a reduction below normal of the concentration of haemoglobin in the blood.

Anaemia in men – Hb < 13 g/dl: in women – < 11.5 g/dl.

Effect of anaemia

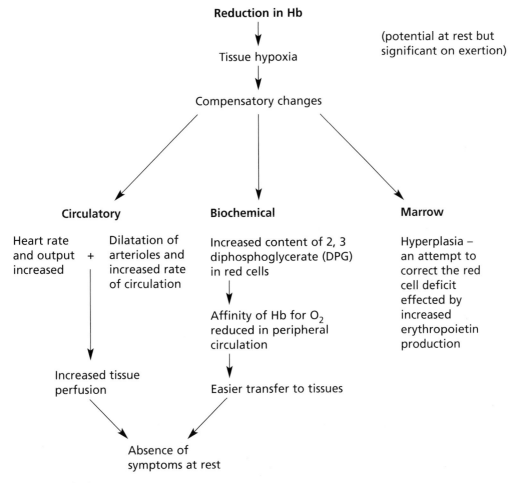

Reduction in Hb

↓

Tissue hypoxia

(potential at rest but significant on exertion)

↓

Compensatory changes

Circulatory

Heart rate and output increased + Dilatation of arterioles and increased rate of circulation

↓

Increased tissue perfusion

Biochemical

Increased content of 2, 3 diphosphoglycerate (DPG) in red cells

↓

Affinity of Hb for O_2 reduced in peripheral circulation

↓

Easier transfer to tissues

Marrow

Hyperplasia – an attempt to correct the red cell deficit effected by increased erythropoietin production

Absence of symptoms at rest

Clinical associations

1. Diminished exercise tolerance, i.e. dyspnoea on exertion.
2. Rapid, full, bounding pulse: decreased circulation time.

Note: Pallor is not a reliable sign of anaemia – it may be obscured by the circulatory changes.

ANAEMIA

The effects of anaemia are greatly influenced by its severity, duration and rate of development.

In moderate anaemias of slow evolution, symptoms such as dyspnoea only appear on exertion, and even when the haemoglobin falls as low as 6–7 g/dl, clinical indications may be slight.

Pathological complications of anaemia

1. Effects of degenerative arterial disease are aggravated, e.g. symptoms of ANGINA PECTORIS and lower limb CLAUDICATION are increased.
2. In severe anaemias effects are seen in organs.

Note: Therefore blood transfusion used in the treatment of anaemia is given *slowly* and as *packed cells* to avoid fluid overload.

In very rapidly developing anaemias, the compensatory mechanisms cannot adjust adequately – the condition merges into SHOCK.

ANAEMIA

Aetiology

Although in the last analysis any anaemia is due to the failure of the bone marrow to produce sufficient red cells in any particular circumstance, an understanding of the role of various aetiological agents and of the **four main mechanisms** by which anaemia develops depends on a knowledge of the basic facts of the life cycle of the red blood cells.

Assets **The 'RED CELL BALANCE SHEET'** *Liabilities*

Production *Losses*

BONE MARROW — RBC life span is about 120 days in the circulation

SPLEEN

LIVER
LYMPH NODES
BONE MARROW

Young cells (reticulocytes) released – about 1% of total RBCs per day

Worn out cells removed by macrophage system – about 1% loss per day

Mechanisms

(A) in the marrow

(i)	(ii)
Actual diminution in productive marrow (hypoplasia or aplasia) or marrow replacement by tumour.	Marrow unable to produce sufficient normal red cells, usually due to deficiency of an essential factor. e.g. iron: Vit B_{12}.
↓	↓
HYPOPLASTIC ANAEMIAS	DYSHAEMOPOIETIC ANAEMIAS

(B) in the circulation

(iii)	(iv)
Excessive loss of RBCs due to acute haemorrhage.	Excessive destruction of RBCs by the macrophage system particularly in the spleen (a) of normal RBCs e.g. in hypersplenism or autoimmunity. (b) of abnormal cells e.g. in hereditary spherocytosis.
↓	↓
ACUTE POST-HAEMORRHAGIC ANAEMIA	HAEMOLYTIC ANAEMIAS

Note: Many forms of anaemia have more than one component.

e.g. 1. The abnormal cells produced in the hypoplastic and dyshaemopoietic anaemias usually have a shortened life span so that a haemolytic element is superimposed.

2. The anaemia of chronic blood loss is almost wholly dyshaemopoietic in type due to the external loss of iron.

ANAEMIA

HYPOPLASTIC and APLASTIC ANAEMIAS

These are rare conditions and, as the names imply, are due to marrow failure with diminished numbers or absence of haemopoietic cells. Usually all three marrow cell lines are affected, resulting in pancytopenia in the peripheral blood.

Marrow failure of this type is dealt with in detail on page 409.

Marrow failure due to extensive tumour infiltration or fibrosis also occurs.

The anaemias associated with miscellaneous chronic diseases ('Secondary' anaemias) are dealt with on page 408.

DYSHAEMOPOIETIC ANAEMIAS

The usual cause of these anaemias is deficiency of an essential factor required for proper haemoglobin synthesis or erythroblast maturation and development. They are associated with a hypercellular marrow and are divided into two main groups:

(1) normoblastic and (2) megaloblastic, depending on the type of erythroblastic maturation in the marrow.

Deficiency of essential factor

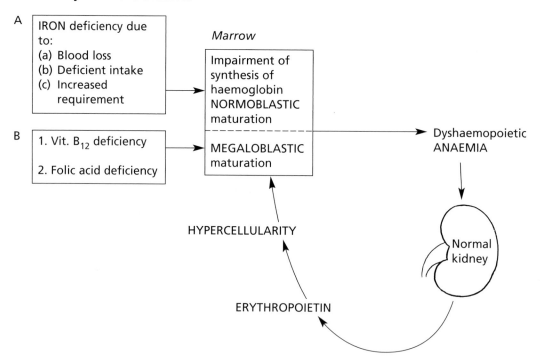

Note: In severe renal failure, deficiency of erythropoietin may contribute to anaemia.

IRON DEFICIENCY ANAEMIA

IRON DEFICIENCY ANAEMIA is the commonest anaemia on a world basis due to (a) poor nutrition, (b) intestinal parasites (esp. hookworm) causing bleeding and (c) multiple pregnancies.

In Western countries, in the adult male and post-menopausal women, iron deficiency anaemia is nearly always due to alimentary blood loss and reflects the incidence of the causative diseases, e.g. cancer, peptic ulceration, hiatus hernia, aspirin ingestion, etc. Without IRON the haem moiety of the haemoglobin molecule cannot be synthesised.

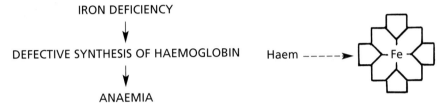

Changes in the blood are mainly in the red cells which become:

MICROCYTIC (cells smaller — mean diameter < 6.7 μm)

HYPOCHROMIC (contain less haemoglobin ∴ less well stained).

Normal

Fairly uniform red cells – size and shape (mean diameter 7.2 μm)

Definite central pallor – ring staining
Variation in size – anisocytosis
Variation in shape – poikilocytosis

MCV (mean cell volume) is . . . . LOW (< 80)
(Normal: 80–92 fl)

MCH (mean cell haemoglobin) is . . . . LOW (< 27)
(Normal: 27–32 pg)

MCHC (mean corpuscular haemoglobin concentration) is . . . . LOW (< 30)
Normal mean: (33 g/dl)

Serum IRON (normal 10–30 μmol/l) is . . . . LOW

Serum FERRITIN (normal 15–300 μg/l) is . . . . LOW

Serum IRON BINDING CAPACITY (45–70 μmol/l) is . . . . RAISED

Serum IRON SATURATION $\left[\dfrac{\text{IRON}}{\text{Binding capacity}}\right] \times 100$ [Normal 16–60%] . . . LOW

The reticulocyte count is NORMAL except following episodes of haemorrhage. Usually there are no changes in the leucocytes and platelets.

The **bone marrow** is hypercellular and contains many small poorly haemoglobinised normoblasts; no stainable iron is present.

IRON DEFICIENCY ANAEMIA

IRON METABOLISM

Iron is normally conserved and is recycled so that absorption of iron from the diet, which occurs maximally in the duodenum and upper jejunum, is required to replace only the small inevitable losses. Since the diet contains iron in excess of requirements, the intestinal mucosal apoferritin mechanism exists to control absorption.

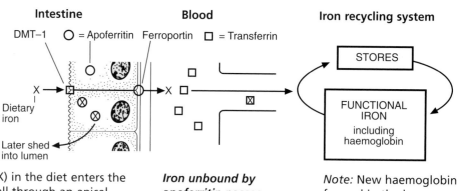

The iron (X) in the diet enters the mucosal cell through an apical uptake transporter (DMT-1) and having combined with apoferritin (O) is retained in the cell as ferritin (⊗).

Note: This bound iron is subsequently shed along with the cell into the lumen.

Iron unbound by apoferritin passes through the cell through a basolateral transporter (ferroportin) and is transported in the blood to join the iron recycling system.

Note: New haemoglobin formed in the bone marrow contains 95% iron from recycling system, 5% from diet.

The state of the iron stores controls the apoferritin (a form of intracellular transferrin) content of the intestinal mucosal cell by a feed-back mechanism, thus:

APOFERRITIN LOW
∴ Decreased binding (ferritin)
∴ Increased absorption

APOFERRITIN HIGH
∴ Increased binding
∴ Decreased absorption

ACUTE IRON OVERLOAD

If a large dose of medicinal iron preparations is taken (particularly by children in error) the absorption and transport mechanisms are overwhelmed and free iron radicles exert very toxic effects.

IRON DEFICIENCY ANAEMIA

The iron balance may be summarised as follows.

INPUT
(Adult male)

Average: 1 mg/day
derived from foods
(a) animal muscle
(b) vegetables.
The average diet contains
10–20 mg iron, of which
about 10% is absorbed.
In the adult female, the
average daily input is
about 2 mg.

BODY IRON
Total 3–6 g

(a) *Functional iron*
 in haemoglobin,
 myoglobin,
 enzyme systems,
 transferrin
⎫ 70% at
⎬ least

(b) *Storage iron*
 in liver, spleen,
 bone marrow
 as ferritin,
 haemosiderin
⎫ 30% or
⎬ less

OUTPUT

Average: 1 mg/day
Skin desquamation and
miscellaneous secretions

Menstruation
This extra loss of about
0.5 to 1 mg requires
extra input in the
female

Anaemia results when this delicate balance is upset in one of three main ways.

1. *Increased output* This almost always is caused by blood loss – often small in amount and chronic (1 ml blood = 0.5 mg iron). In the female, uterine bleeding is a common cause, and in both sexes bleeding from the alimentary tract is important.
2. *Decreased input*
   (a) Poor diet (including diets containing substances antagonistic to iron absorption, e.g. phytates, phosphates)
   (b) Malabsorption – due to bowel disease e.g. coeliac disease, or post-surgical e.g. post-gastrectomy.
3. *Increased body requirement*
   (a) During rapid growth in childhood
   (b) In pregnancy.

Usually anaemia develops slowly (except in cases of serious haemorrhage).

(1) ———————→ (2) ———————→ (3) ———————→ (4)
Iron   Mobilisation   Exhaustion   Deficient synthesis
deficiency   of reserves   of reserves   of haemoglobin

                                    Increased absorption
                                    if available in diet may
                                    postpone (4)

                                                       (5) Anaemia

THE MEGALOBLASTIC ANAEMIAS

These dyshaemopoietic anaemias are almost always caused by deficiency of either vitamin B_{12} or folic acid which are intracellular co-enzymes, particularly important for the synthesis of DNA.

The effects of deficiency occur in most organs of the body but are prominent where cell turnover is rapid, e.g. in the **marrow**.

Results in organs particularly affected

1. MUCOUS MEMBRANES of alimentary tract and genitalia → Regenerative activity cannot balance surface cell losses → THINNING (atrophy) often with functional deficiencies

2. BONE MARROW blood cell precursors of all series affected → Many immature red cells are destroyed in the marrow. Red cells released into blood have a shortened life span. → Megaloblastic

Increased growth factors cause increased cellularity. → Hypercellular

Note:

(a) Vit B_{12} (but not folic acid) has a separate function in the maintenance of the integrity of myelin. Therefore deficiency leads to neuropathies – particularly **subacute combined degeneration** (p.391).

(b) The marrow and blood appearances are essentially similar in deficiency of vit B_{12} and folic acid from any cause. The classic disease of this type is **pernicious anaemia**.

PERNICIOUS ANAEMIA (PA)

This serious and severe anaemia was first described by the English physician Addison in the mid 19th century. At that time it was invariably fatal, but nowadays it can be treated with complete success. It is due to vitamin B_{12} deficiency and is always associated with achlorhydria and gastric mucosal atrophy, due to autoimmune gastritis.

Vitamin B_{12} metabolism and causes of deficiency:

	Deficiency of vitamin B_{12}	
Normal	**In PA**	**Other causes**
Source: Food – vit B_{12} in animal products, e.g. meat, eggs. Daily requirement = 1 µg	Normal	Dietary deficiency, e.g. strict vegans – takes many years to develop.
Secretion of intrinsic factor (IF) by parietal cells of gastric mucosa. IF: B_{12} complex formed	Gastric atrophy No IF ∴ No IF: B_{12} complex	Surgical operations on stomach, e.g. gastrectomy.
Passage through intestine to terminal ileum	Normal	Loss during passage in intestine, e.g. utilised by tape worms or bacteria (blind loop syndrome).
Absorption site – can only be absorbed if complexed with IF	No absorption	Disease of ileum, e.g. Crohn's disease: ileal resection.
Storage in liver – over 3 years' supply		Gradual depletion of liver stores over several years

Released into blood stream bound to transcobalamin to act as important co-enzyme in several intercellular synthetic pathways but particularly of DNA.

Especially important to:

(1) Bone marrow . . . . ANAEMIA (MEGALOBLASTIC)
(2) Nervous system . . . . . ± NERVE CHANGES
(3) Epithelial coverings . . ± TONGUE MUCOSAL ATROPHY

PERNICIOUS ANAEMIA (PA)

Blood changes

There is a pancytopenia, i.e. reduction in RBCs, granulocytes and platelets but the red cells are larger (macrocytosis).

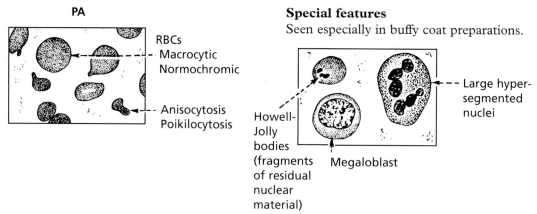

PA

RBCs
- Macrocytic
  Normochromic

- Anisocytosis
  Poikilocytosis

Special features

Seen especially in buffy coat preparations.

Large hyper-segmented nuclei

Howell-Jolly bodies (fragments of residual nuclear material)

Megaloblast

Marrow changes

Hyperplasia – often complete cellularity in flat bones and extension down length of femur.

Normal

Total cellularity

In PA

Megaloblastic change

All marrow elements affected

Mechanism of production of gastritis

PA is an autoimmune disease. The gastric atrophy is caused by an immune reaction against parietal cell cytoplasmic constituents and specifically by antibodies to intrinsic factor (IF).

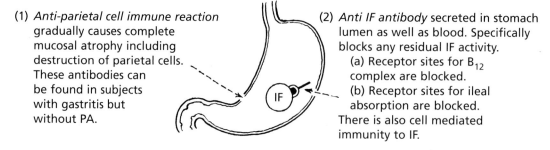

(1) *Anti-parietal cell immune reaction* gradually causes complete mucosal atrophy including destruction of parietal cells. These antibodies can be found in subjects with gastritis but without PA.

IF

(2) *Anti IF antibody* secreted in stomach lumen as well as blood. Specifically blocks any residual IF activity.
  (a) Receptor sites for B_{12} complex are blocked.
  (b) Receptor sites for ileal absorption are blocked.
There is also cell mediated immunity to IF.

There is an increased familial incidence of PA and other organ specific autoimmune diseases, e.g. Hashimoto's thyroiditis.

PERNICIOUS ANAEMIA (PA)

Associated changes

1. *Nervous system*

(a) Subacute combined degeneration of spinal cord.

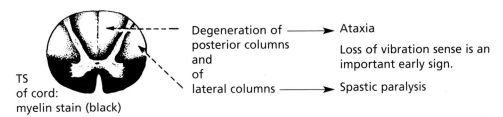

TS
of cord:
myelin stain (black)

Degeneration of ⟶ Ataxia
posterior columns
and
of   Loss of vibration sense is an
     important early sign.
lateral columns ⟶ Spastic paralysis

Note: This serious degeneration may occur before clinical anaemia is present, and is aggravated by the administration of folic acid.

(b) Peripheral neuropathy – both sensory and motor loss.

2. *Epithelial surfaces*

Atrophy is common especially in the tongue and vagina – where senile atrophy is aggravated.

Smooth

Thin
easily
damaged
mucosa

Vaginal smear

Normal
squamous
cells

Cells with
large open
nuclei

3. *Effects of long continued haemolysis*

The abnormal cells have a shortened life cycle.
(a) Mild/moderate splenic enlargement.
(b) Iron deposition in liver, kidney, spleen and marrow.
(c) Increased bilirubin in blood (mild jaundice).

FOLIC ACID DEFICIENCY

FOLIC ACID (Pteroyl-glutamic acid) DEFICIENCY

Normal metabolism

Source
Polyglutamines in
green vegetables, cereals,
meat, fish and eggs
(not milk)

Minimum daily requirement
50 µg

Body reserves 50–100 days

Absorption
As mono-
glutamate
in jejunum

Utilisation
For DNA synthesis. Vit B_{12} is
necessary for synthesis of the active
tetrahydrofolate form (FH4)

Deficiency

Dietary
Low intake of vegetables.
Anorexia, alcoholism, poverty (elderly),
infants (late weaning)

Increased requirements
Pregnancy (fetal growth)
Infancy and childhood (rapid growth)
Haemolysis
Malignancy

Malabsorption
Coeliac disease
Surgical by-pass

Utilisation block
Drugs e.g. methotrexate in
cancer chemotherapy
also anti-convulsants
e.g. phenytoin.

Note:
(1) Since the marrow and blood changes in folic acid and vitamin B_{12} deficiency are similar, the differential diagnosis has to be obtained by other laboratory tests – particularly the measurement of vit B_{12} in the serum and of folic acid in RBCs. Special tests of absorption of vit B_{12} (e.g. Schilling test) are available.
(2) Since the causes of vit B_{12} and folic acid deficiency are often non-specific and associated with malabsorption, other deficiencies (e.g. iron) may occur at the same time.
(3) All megaloblastic anaemias are macrocytic, but *not all* macrocytic anaemias are megaloblastic.
(4) There is a strong association between folic acid deficiency in PREGNANCY and congenital neural tube defects.

THE HAEMOLYTIC ANAEMIAS

HAEMOLYTIC ANAEMIAS

In all haemolytic anaemias, the basic pathological change is a reduction in the life span of the red cells; another way of expressing this is that there is an increased rate of red cell destruction – haemolysis.

The balance between the increased haemolysis and the consequent increased production of red cells by the bone marrow may be illustrated in three main situations:

1. Shortened red cell life span –   ⇌   Marrow production increased × 6
   e.g. 1/6 normal (20 days)

   Balance maintained – – – – – – ∴ → No anaemia
   (compensated erythropoiesis)

2. Shortened red cell life span –   ⇌   Marrow production increased
   e.g. 1/12 normal (10 days)   maximally × 8 to 10 normal

   Balance not maintained – – – – – – ∴ → ANAEMIA

3. Shortened red cell life span –   ⇌   The hyperplastic marrow is susceptible to deficiency of essential factors; thus infections, pregnancy may limit the marrow response

   (a) e.g. 1/6 normal   (b) e.g. 1/12 normal   e.g. to × 3

   Compensated haemolysis   Haemolytic anaemia

   Precipitated into haemolytic anaemia   Serious aggravation (crisis)

Red cells may be destroyed

(a) in the spleen, liver – extravascular haemolysis.

(b) in the blood stream – intravascular haemolysis, with release of haemoglobin into plasma (p.395).

THE HAEMOLYTIC ANAEMIAS

Effects of the increased degradation of haemoglobin

In most haemolytic conditions, the red cells are removed and the haemoglobin degraded in the usual way, i.e. by phagocytosis by the macrophage system.

Note: 1. The bilirubin is unconjugated and is attached to protein so that renal excretion does not occur – **acholuric jaundice.**

2. Unconjugated bilirubin is toxic to the central nervous system of neonates; **kernicterus** (see p.398) is a serious complication of haemolytic disease of the newborn.

THE HAEMOLYTIC ANAEMIAS

Effects of liberation of haemoglobin

In all haemolytic processes, small amounts of haemoglobin are liberated into the blood stream. The free haemoglobin rapidly forms a complex with **haptoglobin** – an α globulin.

Free Hb in blood $\xrightarrow{\text{Rapid}}$ Hb/Haptoglobin complex $\longrightarrow$ to macrophage system – disposal as above

The complex is protective against damaging effects of the free haemoglobin, particularly on the kidneys.

In severe intravascular haemolysis, e.g. severe malaria, incompatible blood transfusion and with the toxic action of chemicals and bacteria, the mechanism may be overloaded.

Excess Hb in blood $\longrightarrow$ SATURATION OF HAPTOGLOBIN RESERVES

Hb remains free in plasma

KIDNEY – tubular damage

HAEMOGLOBINAEMIA   HAEMOGLOBINURIA   HAPTOGLOBIN in blood – LOW

REACTIVE BONE MARROW CHANGES

There is a marked hyperplasia ———— Extension of RED MARROW into long bones

Marrow packed with well haemoglobinised normoblasts

± Haemosiderin depending on rate of iron utilisation

Blood appearances   Release into blood of many young red cells
         20–30% RETICULOCYTES – occasional normoblasts.
Film – normocytic: may be mild macrocytosis due to young cells.
   – normochromic: may be polychromasia due to young cells.

The blood film may of course reflect the specific red cell abnormality responsible for the anaemia, e.g. spherocytosis.

EXTRINSIC HAEMOLYTIC ANAEMIAS

The causes of shortened red cell survival are divided into 2 main groups.

1. EXTRINSIC (factors outside the red cells) and 2. INTRINSIC (defects of red cells).
Extrinsic haemolytic anaemias fall into 4 groups due to:

(a) **ANTIBODIES** (either auto-immune or iso-antibodies, (b) **Infections**,
(c) **Chemical damage** to the red cell and (d) **Physical damage** to the cell.

(1a) AUTO-IMMUNE HAEMOLYTIC ANAEMIA

Auto-immune haemolytic anaemias are classified according to the temperature at which the
reaction occurs and the presence of an underlying cause.

WARM (37°C – usually IgG)	COLD (< 30°C – usually IgM)
Primary – so-called idiopathic haemolytic anaemia: usually in adults.	Idiopathic cold agglutination disease

WARM (37°C – usually IgG)

Primary – so-called idiopathic
haemolytic anaemia:
usually in adults.

Secondary – associated with
(i) **lymphomas** e.g. chronic
lymphocytic leukaemia,
Hodgkin's disease.
(ii) **other cancers.**
(iii) **connective tissue diseases**
e.g. systemic lupus
erythematosus,
rheumatoid arthritis.
(iv) **drugs** e.g. methyl dopa.

Mechanism:
Coating of RBC
with IgG
antibodies
often
against
Rhesus
'e' antigens.

Destruction in
spleen which is
often enlarged.

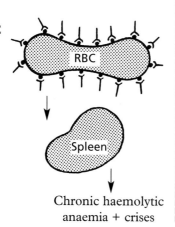

Chronic haemolytic
anaemia + crises

COLD (< 30°C – usually IgM)

Idiopathic cold agglutination disease
(i) lymphomas.
(ii) *Mycoplasma pneumoniae.*
(iii) viral infections e.g. measles.

Mechanism
IgM
antibody

combines
with RBC

Agglutination
↓
Blockage of
peripheral
vessels
↓
**Painful hands
and feet**

**Complement
activation**
↓
Intravascular lysis
↓
**Paroxysmal cold
haemoglobinuria**

INCOMPATIBLE BLOOD TRANSFUSION/
HAEMOLYTIC DISEASE OF THE NEWBORN

(1b) DESTRUCTION of RBCs is due to ISO-ANTIBODIES

In these, the antibodies act against antigens which are derived from another individual of the same species.

Incompatible ABO blood transfusion is a classic example.

e.g. **Donor Blood**
Group A
i.e. cells contain
A antigen

Recipient
Group O (cells contain neither A nor B antigen)
Plasma contains *Anti-A* (iso-antibody) (and Anti-B)

→ Agglutination

Haemolysis

Clinical and pathological effects

Rigor: loin pain
Haemoglobinuria
Jaundice (after 12 hours)
SHOCK → maybe DEATH

Perhaps later:
Haemostatic failure ────→ maybe DEATH
Renal failure

(1c) HAEMOLYTIC DISEASE OF THE NEWBORN (HDN). This occurs in Rhesus positive fetuses conceived by Rh-negative mothers. The usual mechanism is as follows:

First pregnancy: Rh-positive fetus in Rh-negative mother – no antibodies present;
∴ *Healthy Baby*

But during this pregnancy, iso-immunisation of the mother may occur.

Towards term and particularly during labour the placental barrier is breached and fetal RBCs enter the maternal circulation.

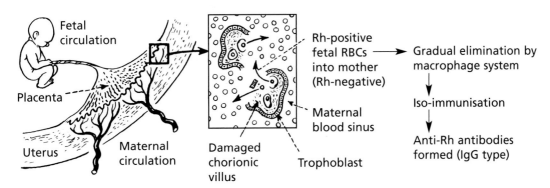

Fetal circulation

Placenta

Uterus

Maternal circulation

Damaged chorionic villus

Rh-positive fetal RBCs into mother (Rh-negative)

Maternal blood sinus

Trophoblast

Gradual elimination by macrophage system

Iso-immunisation

Anti-Rh antibodies formed (IgG type)

HAEMOLYTIC DISEASE OF THE NEWBORN

The basic mechanism is influenced by three important factors:

(a) The maternal immune response tends to be proportional to the number of fetal cells entering the circulation.

(b) The maternal immune response is boosted in successive Rh incompatible pregnancies – the highest maternal antibody titres are found in the latest of multiple pregnancies.

(c) Fetal/maternal ABO compatibility influences the Rh immune response.

e.g. ABO compatible		ABO incompatible	
Fetus	*Mother*	*Fetus*	*Mother*
Group O Rh+	Group O Rh−	Group A Rh+	Group O Rh−
Gradual elimination of fetal cells		Rapid destruction of fetal cells	
∴ *Maximum* immune response		∴ *Minimum* immune response	

Subsequent pregnancies: All Rh-positive fetuses conceived by a mother who has acquired anti-Rh antibodies either during previous pregnancies or by blood transfusion (in this case the first fetus also) are at risk.

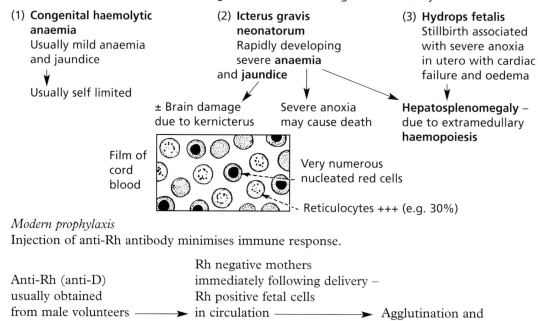

Uterus

Placenta

Maternal anti-Rh antibodies IgG type
↓
Pass placental barrier
↓
Enter fetal circulation and **destroy fetal red cells** (agglutination and haemolysis)

The effects are graded into three categories of severity:

(1) **Congenital haemolytic anaemia**
Usually mild anaemia and jaundice
↓
Usually self limited

(2) **Icterus gravis neonatorum**
Rapidly developing severe **anaemia** and **jaundice**

± Brain damage due to kernicterus

Severe anoxia may cause death

(3) **Hydrops fetalis**
Stillbirth associated with severe anoxia in utero with cardiac failure and oedema
↓
Hepatosplenomegaly – due to extramedullary **haemopoiesis**

Film of cord blood

Very numerous nucleated red cells

Reticulocytes +++ (e.g. 30%)

Modern prophylaxis
Injection of anti-Rh antibody minimises immune response.

Anti-Rh (anti-D) usually obtained from male volunteers ⟶ Rh negative mothers immediately following delivery – Rh positive fetal cells in circulation ⟶ Agglutination and rapid elimination
Minimal or no immune response

EXTRINSIC HAEMOLYTIC ANAEMIAS

2. INFECTIONS

There are three mechanisms by which infections cause haemolysis:

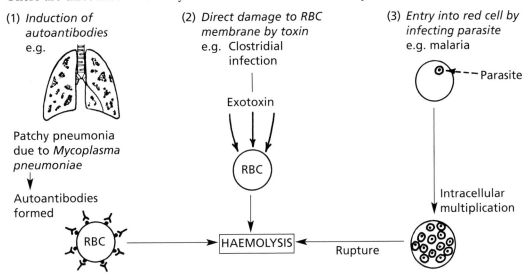

(1) *Induction of autoantibodies* e.g.

Patchy pneumonia due to *Mycoplasma pneumoniae*
↓
Autoantibodies formed

(2) *Direct damage to RBC membrane by toxin* e.g. Clostridial infection

Exotoxin
RBC
↓

(3) *Entry into red cell by infecting parasite* e.g. malaria

Parasite

Intracellular multiplication

Rupture

HAEMOLYSIS

3. DRUGS AND CHEMICALS

The three main mechanisms by which drugs and chemicals cause haemolysis are:

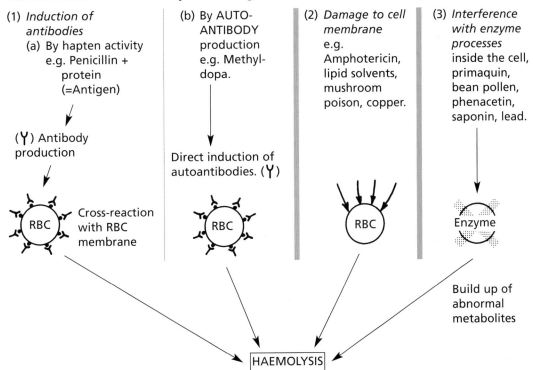

(1) *Induction of antibodies*
  (a) By hapten activity e.g. Penicillin + protein (=Antigen)
↓
(Y) Antibody production
↓
RBC — Cross-reaction with RBC membrane

(b) By AUTO-ANTIBODY production e.g. Methyl-dopa.
↓
Direct induction of autoantibodies. (Y)

(2) *Damage to cell membrane* e.g. Amphotericin, lipid solvents, mushroom poison, copper.

RBC

(3) *Interference with enzyme processes* inside the cell, primaquin, bean pollen, phenacetin, saponin, lead.
↓
Enzyme

Build up of abnormal metabolites

HAEMOLYSIS

399

EXTRINSIC HAEMOLYTIC ANAEMIAS

4. MECHANICAL TRAUMA

The results of damage to red cells within the circulation are:

(1) Intravascular haemolysis

↓

Haemoglobinuria

(2) Formation of red cell fragments (schistocytes)

seen in blood film as 'burr', 'triangle', 'helmet' cells

The main circumstances in which red cells are damaged are:

(a) In the **heart and great vessels**

When the blood flow is subjected to undue turbulence or jet effect. An important example nowadays is with prosthetic valves in the left side of the heart.

RBCs damaged by shearing stresses where valve seating is defective or through the valve itself.

(b) In the **microcirculation**

(i)   When the blood flow in arterioles is impeded by strands of fibrin.

(1) Liberation of haemoglobin
(2) Emergence of fragments

RBCs being distorted and cut by fibrin sieve

This condition is called MICROANGIOPATHIC HAEMOLYTIC ANAEMIA and occurs in many disease states involving small blood vessels e.g. malignant hypertension and/or intravascular coagulation.

(ii) When blood vessels are subjected to direct trauma. This is seen classically in military recruits marching long distances in hard soled boots, when the blood vessels of the soles of the feet are squeezed with every step – **march haemoglobinuria.**
The haemolysis is usually not severe enough to be of clinical significance, but haemoglobinuria may cause alarm.

EXTRINSIC HAEMOLYTIC ANAEMIAS

Other causes of haemolysis include:

1. Hypersplenism

In enlargement of the spleen from any cause, the sequestration of red cells is increased so that haemolytic anaemia may result.

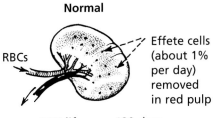

Normal

RBCs

Effete cells (about 1% per day) removed in red pulp

RBC life span 120 days

Hypersplenism

RBCs

RBCs removed in greater numbers and before they are completely effete

RBC life span reduced

2. Burns

Large burn

Tissue destruction including blood vessels and red blood cells

In severe burns haemolysis is an important component of the acute anaemia which develops.

3. Inadvertent use of intravenous hypotonic solutions

Hypotonic solution

Blood vessel

RBCs swell and burst

Intravascular haemolysis

This is a very rare accident but can have catastrophic consequences.

EXTRINSIC HAEMOLYTIC ANAEMIAS – MALARIA

Malaria is an endemic disease in many parts of Africa, Asia, Central and South America. Many millions of cases occur each year and the mortality is at least 1%. The disease is particularly severe in non-immune subjects from temperate climates; in endemic areas where the 'herd' immunity is high, a low grade chronic illness is common.

Female anopheline mosquitos act as intermediate hosts in the life cycle of the parasite, a protozoon (genus *Plasmodium*).

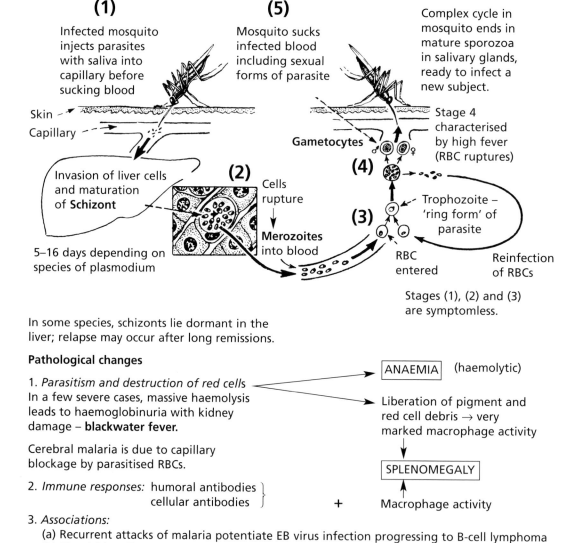

(1)

Infected mosquito injects parasites with saliva into capillary before sucking blood

Skin

Capillary

Invasion of liver cells and maturation of **Schizont**

5–16 days depending on species of plasmodium

(2) Cells rupture

Merozoites into blood

(5)

Mosquito sucks infected blood including sexual forms of parasite

Complex cycle in mosquito ends in mature sporozoa in salivary glands, ready to infect a new subject.

Gametocytes

Stage 4 characterised by high fever (RBC ruptures)

(4)

(3) Trophozoite – 'ring form' of parasite

RBC entered

Reinfection of RBCs

Stages (1), (2) and (3) are symptomless.

In some species, schizonts lie dormant in the liver; relapse may occur after long remissions.

Pathological changes

1. *Parasitism and destruction of red cells*
In a few severe cases, massive haemolysis leads to haemoglobinuria with kidney damage – **blackwater fever.**

Cerebral malaria is due to capillary blockage by parasitised RBCs.

2. *Immune responses:* humoral antibodies ⎱
                   cellular antibodies ⎰

3. *Associations:*
   (a) Recurrent attacks of malaria potentiate EB virus infection progressing to B-cell lymphoma
   (b) The sickle cell gene protects against falciparum malaria

ANAEMIA (haemolytic)

Liberation of pigment and red cell debris → very marked macrophage activity

SPLENOMEGALY

+ Macrophage activity

INTRINSIC HAEMOLYTIC ANAEMIAS

INTRINSIC DEFECTS – Usually hereditary.

In (i) cell membrane   (ii) enzymes   (iii) molecular structure of haemoglobin
(haemoglobinopathies).

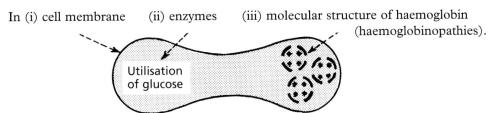

1. Cell membrane defects

(a) ***Hereditary spherocytosis:*** the majority of cases are familial (autosomal dominant).

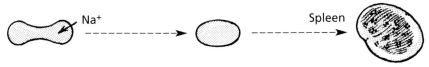

The primary defect is in the proteins which support the plasma membrane – SPECTRIN and ANKYRIN.

The cells assume a spherical shape due to instability of the plasma membrane.

Premature sequestration and destruction in splenic pulp. Splenomegaly is common.

Note: Splenectomy is usually 'curative' but the red cell defect remains.

The severity of the haemolysis is variable; many cases are compensated and not anaemic, but crises are common e.g. if folate deficiency supervenes. Intercurrent infections may precipitate increased red cell destruction with jaundice or temporary bone marrow hypoplasia, e.g. parvovirus infection, with severe anaemia.

The laboratory diagnosis depends on:
    (1) typical blood film with spherocytes,
    (2) high reticulocyte count and
    (3) increased osmotic fragility of RBCs.

(b) ***Hereditary elliptocytosis*** is similar to spherocytosis in many respects, but it is usually not severe enough to cause anaemia or jaundice. Haemolysis is usually mild.

(c) ***Hereditary abetalipoproteinaemia***: a rare disease in which the red cell membranes are abnormal and the cells become spiky (acanthocytes).

(d) ***Paroxysmal nocturnal haemoglobinuria*** – a rare, acquired condition in which anchorage of proteins to the red cell membrane is abnormal. The cells are particularly susceptible to the action of complement (usually activated by the alternative pathway) at low pH. Intravascular haemolysis results.

INTRINSIC HAEMOLYTIC ANAEMIAS

INTRINSIC DEFECTS of the RED CELLS (*continued*)

2. Enzyme defects

Usually hereditary. Glucose is the source of energy with which the red cell metabolism is maintained. Glycolysis is effected by two classic enzyme pathways.

The following simplified diagram outlines the pathways and indicates only the main enzymes and substrates.

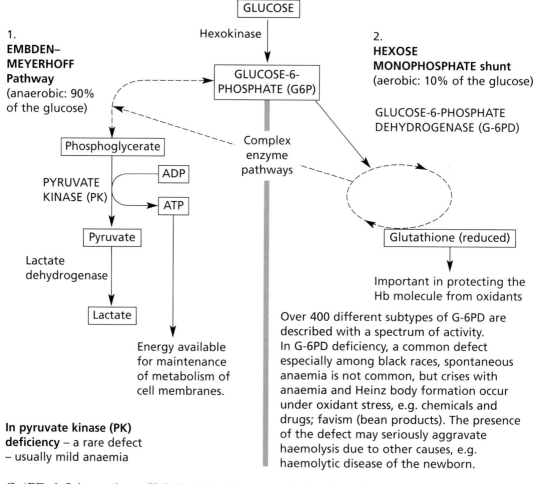

1.
EMBDEN–MEYERHOFF Pathway
(anaerobic: 90% of the glucose)

GLUCOSE

Hexokinase

GLUCOSE-6-PHOSPHATE (G6P)

Phosphoglycerate

PYRUVATE KINASE (PK)

ADP

ATP

Pyruvate

Lactate dehydrogenase

Lactate

Complex enzyme pathways

Energy available for maintenance of metabolism of cell membranes.

In pyruvate kinase (PK) deficiency – a rare defect – usually mild anaemia

2.
HEXOSE MONOPHOSPHATE shunt
(aerobic: 10% of the glucose)

GLUCOSE-6-PHOSPHATE DEHYDROGENASE (G-6PD)

Glutathione (reduced)

Important in protecting the Hb molecule from oxidants

Over 400 different subtypes of G-6PD are described with a spectrum of activity. In G-6PD deficiency, a common defect especially among black races, spontaneous anaemia is not common, but crises with anaemia and Heinz body formation occur under oxidant stress, e.g. chemicals and drugs; favism (bean products). The presence of the defect may seriously aggravate haemolysis due to other causes, e.g. haemolytic disease of the newborn.

G-6PD deficiency shows X-linked inheritance so that in the male the defect is fully expressed, while in the female heterozygote there are two populations of red cells in the blood (1) normal cells and (2) defective cells.

In both these defects and in the rare defects of other enzymes in the pathways which have been described the expression of the abnormal gene is very variable from case to case.

DISORDERS OF HAEMOGLOBIN SYNTHESIS

3. Haemoglobinopathies

Varieties of normal haemoglobin are illustrated:

Normal haemoglobin molecule

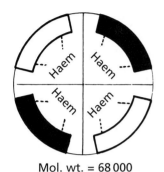

Mol. wt. = 68 000

4 subunits each consisting of a haem core with a polypeptide chain attached. The haem core is constant while the polypeptide chains occur in pairs. 4 different polypeptide chains occur normally.

■ α chain   ▨ γ chain

☐ β chain   ▨ δ chain

There are 3 types of normal haemoglobin.

97% adult Hb – – Haemoglobin A = 2α + 2β chains

3% adult Hb – – Haemoglobin A$_2$ = 2α + 2δ chains

Fetal Hb – – Haemoglobin F = 2α + 2γ chains

Fetal haemoglobin is replaced by adult haemoglobin during the first year ('haemoglobin switching'). Note that the α chain occurs in all normal haemoglobins.

Two copies of the α chain genes (αα/αα) are present on chromosome 16; β, γ and δ genes are found in a complex on chromosome 11. A number of globin-like genes are also present but are omitted for simplicity.

In the **thalassaemias** and **haemoglobinopathies** there are abnormalities in the production and structure of haemoglobin chains due to mutation of these genes.

THE THALASSAEMIAS

These are inherited disorders in which synthesis of globin chains is diminished or absent. They are common in the Mediterranean, Middle East and India.

α-thalassaemia – reduction of α chain synthesis.
β-thalassaemia – reduction of β chain synthesis.

Diminished production of α or β chains
Imbalance of α and β chains

Reduced Hb synthesis
'Ineffective erythropoiesis'

Abnormal aggregation of globin chains

Abnormal RBCs

Reduced RBC production

Haemolysis

ANAEMIA
(hypochromic microcytic)

The severity of the disease depends on (i) the degree of globin chain abnormality and (ii) whether the patient is homozygous or heterozygous for the defect.

There are normally 4 α genes (αα/αα).

In the **α-thalassaemias** the genetic defects are illustrated as follows:

1. **Hb-Barts hydrops syndrome** (– – / – –)
   All 4 genes for the α chain are absent. Fetal Hb cannot be formed and the fetus dies in utero.
2. **Hb-H disease** (– α / – –): only one α gene is present. This leads to an excess of β chains which form tetramers called Hb-H.
   There is a moderate microcytic hypochromic anaemia with splenomegaly.
3. **α-thalassaemia** traits (– α / – α): even if two α genes are absent, the remaining two are active and the symptoms and anaemia are usually mild.

β-thalassaemia

β-thalassaemia major – two defective β genes.
   The excess of α genes leads to severe anaemia with haemolysis. The marrow becomes hyperplastic and there is atrophy of bones. The main form of haemoglobin is HbF – which persists into adult life.

β-thalassaemia minor – one defective β gene.
   The anaemia is mild. The red cells are microcytic and hypochromic and a mistaken diagnosis of iron deficiency anaemia can be made. These subjects act as carriers for β-thalassaemia major.

SICKLE CELL DISEASE

This disorder is very common in Central Africa but also occurs in the Mediterranean, Middle East and India. It affects the black population of USA and the Caribbean.

It is due to a mutation in the β chain of haemoglobin (the amino-acid glutamic acid is substituted by valine) and is inherited as an autosomal recessive trait.

The effects are *mild* in heterozygotes (Hb AS) = **sickle cell trait**; they are severe in homozygotes (Hb SS) = **sickle cell anaemia**.

The effects are summarised as follows:

1. **At molecular level** HbS becomes less soluble in low levels of oxygen tension.

2. **In the red cell** this causes distortion (sickling).

3. **In tissues**

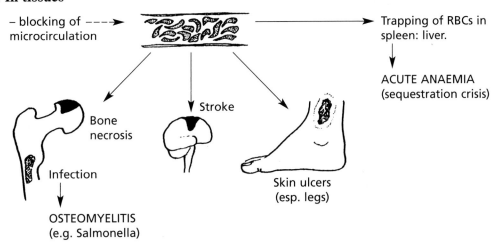

Acute sickle cell crises are often provoked by:

(1) infection, (2) cold, (3) low pO_2 e.g. flying in unpressurised aircraft.

In addition, infection, especially by **parvoviruses in childhood**, may provoke an **aplastic anaemia** crisis.

Note: HbS confers resistance to malaria: in terms of evolution this confers a survival benefit to those carrying the HbS gene.

ANAEMIA OF CHRONIC DISORDERS

This term describes the anaemias seen commonly in patients with chronic diseases
e.g. (ia) Chronic inflammation e.g. rheumatoid arthritis, SLE
     (ib) Chronic infection e.g. T.B.
     (ii) Malignancy.

The anaemia is usually mild (Hb > 9 g/dl).
The mechanism is not fully understood.

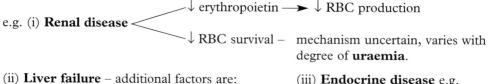

Shortened life span e.g. 80
days (i.e. mild haemolysis)

RBC

effects of
cytokines
e.g. IL-I, TNF

CHRONIC
DISEASE

Erythropoietin
depression

BONE
MARROW

Diminished
RBC production

usually
NORMOCYTIC
NORMOCHROMIC

ANAEMIA

Diminished
iron utilisation

Diminished
iron utilisation

May be
HYPOCHROMIC

Blocks iron release
from macrophages.
Serum iron ↓
Ferritin ↑

The components have varying
significance from case to case.

In addition, malignant tumour growth may cause anaemia by 2 more specific mechanisms.

(a) Chronic bleeding from the surface of
an ulcerated tumour – especially from
the alimentary tract ⟶ iron deficiency.

(b) Replacement of the bone marrow
by malignant tumour.

Normocytic Normochromic Anaemias are also found in other systemic diseases.

e.g. (i) **Renal disease** ⟨ ↓ erythropoietin ⟶ ↓ RBC production

↓ RBC survival – mechanism uncertain, varies with
degree of **uraemia**.

(ii) **Liver failure** – additional factors are:

Liver ⟨ — Bleeding varices,
— Deficiency of coagulation factors,
— Hypersplenism,
— Alcoholic – other nutritional
deficiencies.

(iii) **Endocrine disease** e.g.

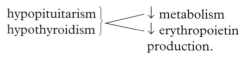

hypopituitarism ⎫ ⟨ ↓ metabolism
hypothyroidism ⎭ ↓ erythropoietin
production.

APLASTIC ANAEMIA

In this rare disorder there is:

A reduction in bone marrow stem cells ⟶ Failure of production of mature cells ⟶ Pancytopenia (of varying severity)

Bone marrow is hypoplastic ⟶

Fat spaces

Occasional surviving haemopoietic cells

There are a number of different types
(a) **Idiopathic** – in 2/3 of cases no cause is found.
(b) **Drug induced** – this may be:
  (i) Predictable e.g. Cytotoxic chemotherapy.
  (ii) Idiosyncratic e.g. Chloramphenicol (1 in 25 000–60 000 affected).
    Phenylbutazone.
(c) **Virus induced** e.g. Hepatitis, Epstein–Barr Virus.
(d) **Autoimmune.**
(e) **Inherited** e.g. Fanconi's anaemia – Autosomal recessive.

Treatment This consists of:
(a) Supportive therapy e.g. blood transfusion.
(b) Attempts to restore haemopoiesis   e.g. bone marrow transplantation,
    – anabolic steroids,
    – immunosuppressive therapy,
    – withdrawal of causative drugs.

The sideroblastic anaemias

In these rare anaemias, failure of synthesis of the haem component of the haemoglobin molecule is indicated by the presence of a ring of iron granules around the normoblast nucleus.

 Ringed sideroblast

Iron granules (in mitochondria) stained by Prussian blue reaction

In a few cases, pyridoxine allows haem synthesis to proceed normally

The condition arises secondarily in many of the chronic disease states mentioned on the previous page, or as a result of drug treatment or chemical poisoning (e.g. lead). Some cases are 'primary' – representing a form of myelodysplasia.

The anaemia is usually *dimorphic*; i.e. showing hypochromic and macrocytic features combined.

POLYCYTHAEMIA

POLYCYTHAEMIA

Polycythaemia (erythrocytosis) is defined by a haemoglobin level above the normal range: in true polycythaemia the red cell mass is increased and the haematocrit is always elevated.

Note: **Relative Polycythaemia** is the result of fluid loss with a decrease in plasma volume and a normal red cell mass.

Aetiology

There are two types:

SECONDARY POLYCYTHAEMIA

The red cell increase is the result of increased stimulation of marrow by erythropoietin. Two main groups of conditions are associated with this:

1. (Commonly) Conditions causing tissue HYPOXIA:
   (a) Living at high altitudes
   (b) Chronic cardiac disease especially R → L shunts
   (c) Chronic respiratory disease
   (d) Presence of abnormal haemoglobin causing defective release of O_2 to tissues – usually hereditary.

2. (Rarely) Renal tumours and ischaemia; occasionally tumours of other organs.

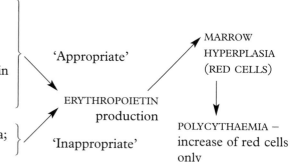

PRIMARY POLYCYTHAEMIA (*Polycythaemia Rubra Vera*)

This is a myeloproliferative disorder with increased red cell production. It may be associated with an increase in other marrow elements. Splenomegaly is usually present. A minority of patients develop acute leukaemia.

Effects of polycythaemia

(a) There is usually a distinctly florid complexion.
(b) Increased blood viscosity causes arterial and venous thrombosis.
(c) Increased marrow activity → increased uric acid metabolism → tendency to gout.

NEUTROPHIL GRANULOCYTES

NEUTROPHIL Neutrophil Granulocyte (Polymorphonuclear Leucocyte)

The essential function of these cells is protection against microbial infection by phagocytosis and killing. They are produced alongside red blood cells, platelets and monocytes from a common stem cell in the marrow.

Marrow Production – stained by a Romanowski method

Stem cell (Primitive – multipotential)	Myeloblast (committed)	Promyelocyte	Myelocyte	Metamyelocyte	Neutrophil in marrow and blood

Note the nuclear changes progressing from large open nucleus and several nucleoli to the mature condensed multi-lobed state. The cytoplasm matures with the acquisition of specific granules.

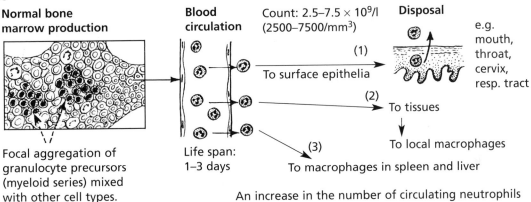

Normal bone marrow production

Focal aggregation of granulocyte precursors (myeloid series) mixed with other cell types. Myeloid/Erythroid ratio 3 to 8:1

Blood circulation

Life span: 1–3 days

Count: $2.5–7.5 \times 10^9/l$ (2500–7500/mm³)

(1) To surface epithelia

(2) To tissues

(3) To macrophages in spleen and liver

Disposal

e.g. mouth, throat, cervix, resp. tract

To local macrophages

An increase in the number of circulating neutrophils reflects an increased activity in the tissues at the site of an acute inflammatory reaction.

Neutrophil activation

TISSUES

INFECTION or NECROSIS — PHAGOCYTOSIS and KILL

CHEMICAL MEDIATORS (granulocyte) e.g. G-CSF. GM-CSF (granulocyte/monocyte)

COMPLEMENT ACTIVATION

CHEMOTAXIS

Blood stream

Marrow (normal)

Hyperplastic

Increased number of neutrophils

Neutrophil leucocytosis (count over $7.5 \times 10^9/l$)

411

DISORDERS OF NEUTROPHILS

Neutrophil leucocytosis does not occur in: (a) some acute bacterial infections, e.g. typhoid fever, brucellosis, (b) many chronic bacterial infections, (c) most virus infections unless acute bacterial infection or necrosis occurs, (d) overwhelming infections with severe toxaemia.

In the **absence (agranulocytosis)** or **diminished numbers** of neutrophils
$- < 2.5 \times 10/1$ ($2500/mm^3$) increased susceptibility to infection results.
There are 2 **main mechanisms** which often co-exist.

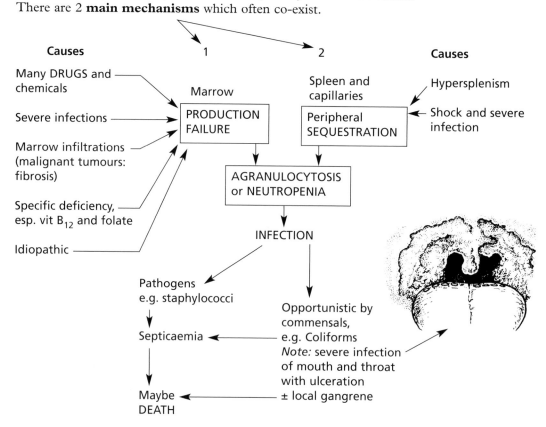

Causes 1 2 Causes

Many DRUGS and chemicals

Severe infections

Marrow infiltrations (malignant tumours: fibrosis)

Specific deficiency, esp. vit B_{12} and folate

Idiopathic

Marrow
PRODUCTION FAILURE

Spleen and capillaries
Peripheral SEQUESTRATION

Hypersplenism

Shock and severe infection

AGRANULOCYTOSIS or NEUTROPENIA

INFECTION

Pathogens e.g. staphylococci

Septicaemia

Maybe DEATH

Opportunistic by commensals, e.g. Coliforms
Note: severe infection of mouth and throat with ulceration
± local gangrene

Drugs may act in the following ways:

1. By direct dose related toxic effect, e.g. modern chemotherapeutic agents.

2. By an immunological reaction, the drug acting as a **hapten**, e.g. amidopyrine.

Marrow failure

Drugs and chemicals may affect the production of all three marrow cell types together or in various combinations.

3. By an idiosyncratic action in sensitive subjects small doses are effective, e.g. chloramphenicol (compare aplastic anaemia, page 409).

DISORDERS OF NEUTROPHILS

Disorders of neutrophil function

Divided into 3 groups: (1) chemotaxis, (2) microbial phagocytosis and (3) microbial kill.

Chemotaxis and phagocytosis may be defective due to:

(a) an intrinsic defect of the neutrophils e.g. leucocyte adhesion deficiency – reduction of B_2 integrin expression.
(b) plasma deficiency of chemotactic factors and opsonins – seen especially when there are deficiencies in the complement cascade.

Microbial kill fails when there is an intracellular enzyme defect e.g. in *chronic granulomatous disease* (CGD) and the Chediak–Higashi syndrome where the neutrophils contain abnormal giant granules.

The normal sequence following phagocytosis is:

(1) Bacterium in phagosome

The act of phagocytosis rapidly triggers a burst of intracellular enzyme activity ...

(2)

Powerful bactericidal effect

. . . with rapid production of H_2O_2
+
Myeloperoxidase
+
Halogen (I or Cl)

(3)

(a) Bacterium digested by acid hydrolases and other enzymes
(b) Neutrophil degranulated

CHRONIC GRANULOMATOUS DISEASE (CGD)

It is a rare hereditary disorder in which the neutrophils have normal phagocytic function but are unable to kill certain bacteria. The disease is fully expressed only in males. It presents as multiple chronic abscesses and granulomas affecting skin, lungs, bones, spleen and liver.

The rapid production of H_2O_2 is defective (in the neutrophils and also in macrophages due to deficiency of NADPH-oxidase).

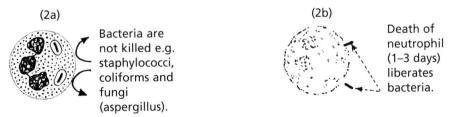

(2a)

Bacteria are not killed e.g. staphylococci, coliforms and fungi (aspergillus).

(2b)

Death of neutrophil (1–3 days) liberates bacteria.

About 2/3 of cases are X-linked (fully expressed in males): the remainder are recessive. The neutrophils are unable to reduce nitroblue tetrazolium (used as a diagnostic slide test).

PLATELETS AND COAGULATION

These small, non-nucleated discs, derived from the cytoplasm of the bone marrow megakaryocytes, are released into the blood stream by a budding process.

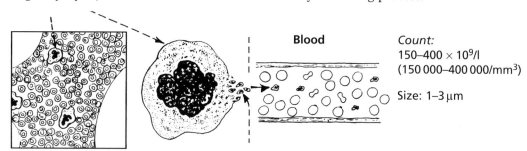

Blood

Count:
$150–400 \times 10^9/l$
($150\,000–400\,000/mm^3$)

Size: $1–3\,\mu m$

Platelets contain von Willebrand factor, adenosine diphosphate (ADP), vasoactive amines including serotonin (5HT) and histamine and phospholipid

Their main role is in preventing blood loss after injury.

e.g. skin wound.

Free flow of blood

Rapid **activation** of **clotting mechanism**

Release of ADP and thromboxane

Further platelet aggregation and adherence.

(a) Contraction of blood vessel

(b) **Aggregation of platelets** at site of endothelial damage – triggered by contact with collagen.

Activation of clotting cascade

Formation of fibrin network – reinforces platelet plug.

ABNORMALITIES OF COAGULATION

Blood may (a) CLOT INSUFFICIENTLY or (b) CLOT EXCESSIVELY

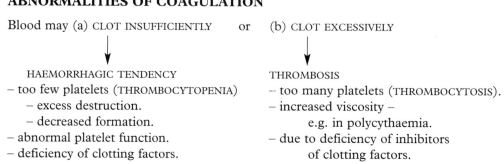

HAEMORRHAGIC TENDENCY
– too few platelets (THROMBOCYTOPENIA)
  – excess destruction.
  – decreased formation.
– abnormal platelet function.
– deficiency of clotting factors.

THROMBOSIS
-- too many platelets (THROMBOCYTOSIS).
– increased viscosity –
    e.g. in polycythaemia.
– due to deficiency of inhibitors
    of clotting factors.

DISORDERS OF PLATELETS

Disorders of the platelets include:
(a) deficiencies of number – thrombocytopenia – lead to bleeding tendency.
(b) defective function.

THROMBOCYTOPENIA

Although the normal platelet count ranges from $150–400 \times 10^9/l$, a risk of dangerous spontaneous haemorrhage is unusual unless the count falls below $30 \times 10^9/l$.
The causes of thrombocytopenia fall into two main groups:

1. **Deficient marrow production**	2. **Increased destruction**
Hypoplasia or aplasia ⎫	Platelets damaged by *drugs,*
⎬ of marrow	*immune mechanisms*
Replacement	
(e.g. leukaemia, fibrosis) ⎭	Platelets sequestered in *hypersplenism*
Dyshaemopoiesis	Platelets utilised in *coagulation*
(e.g. Vit B_{12} deficiency)	*disorders* (e.g. DIC)

Note: Marrow examination throws light on the possible mechanism.

In (1) megakaryocytes are reduced in number (except in vit. B_{12} deficiency)	In (2) megakaryocytes are increased and immature in an attempt to make good the platelet loss

PURPURA is the term used for disorders involving bleeding from capillaries, with the production of small petechial spots. Mild to moderate thrombocytopenia or defective platelet formation are the usual causes. Two examples are illustrative:

1.**Idiopathic thrombocytopenic purpura** is due to **auto-immune** destruction of platelets. Antibodies are directed against platelet membrane glycoproteins.
(a) **Acute:** mainly in children, provoked by viral infection: it is usually self-limiting in a few weeks.
(b) **Chronic:** mainly in young women with an insidious onset and lasting many years: splenectomy is often required (the spleen is the major site of platelet destruction).

2. **Defective platelet function** has many forms – **von Willebrand's disease** (vWD) is the commonest. The gene encoding vWF is located on chromosome 12.
vWF is a large protein which potentiates the binding of platelets to subendothelial collagen and also acts as a carrier for coagulation factor VIII.

Diminished function or lack of vWF
↓ ↓
Diminished platelet adhesion Diminished factor VIII activity
↓ ↓
HAEMORRHAGE

THROMBOCYTOSIS (increased platelet numbers) may occur in a mild form (with no clinical significance) reactive to a variety of disorders of chronic inflammation and cancer. Larger counts are seen as a concomitant of myeloproliferative disorders (e.g. essential thrombocytosis, chronic myeloid leukaemia) and are of serious clinical significance due to thrombosis.

415

THE COAGULATION CASCADE

The coagulation of blood is essentially the result of conversion of **FIBRINOGEN** to **FIBRIN**, but the chemical pathway leading to this final phase is a complicated cascade in which inert coagulation factors are serially activated. At each step augmentation takes place.

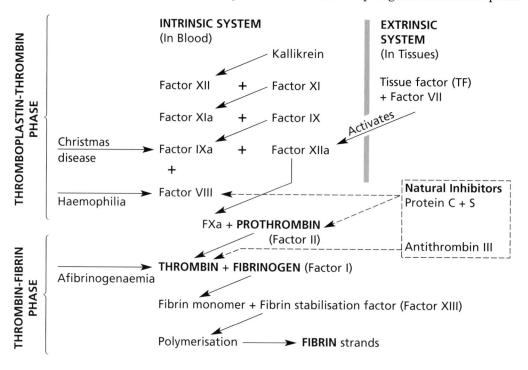

Note: 'a' denotes activated form

The system contains several feed-back loops (not illustrated) which can inhibit the cascade at various levels.

Anti-thrombin III and the protein C/protein S system are powerful inhibitors preventing uncontrollable coagulation.

Vitamin K is required for the production of factors II, VII, IX and X. CALCIUM ions and phospholipids (mainly derived from platelets) are essential for many of the steps in thrombin production. Once thrombin is formed, it appears to stimulate several of the preceding reactions and also the polymerisation of fibrin.

Fibrinolytic System – following fibrin deposition this is operative.

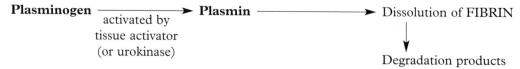

INHERITED DEFECTS OF COAGULATION

These are less common than acquired abnormalities, but are of considerable importance.

HAEMOPHILIA A

Haemophilia is due to deficiency of Factor VIII – an essential cofactor in the activation of Factor X in the intrinsic system.

Factor VIII is encoded by a gene on the long arm of the X chromosome – haemophilia is inherited as an X-linked recessive, i.e. almost all patients are male. Their mothers are usually carriers, but about 30% of cases are due to new mutations. Around 1 in 10 000 is affected.

Clinical Features

The severity depends on the levels of Factor VIII.

		Level of Factor VIII
Severe:	Frequent spontaneous bleeding.	<2% of normal
Moderate:	Bleeding after minor trauma – rarely spontaneous.	2–10%
Mild:	Bleeding severe only after major trauma or surgery.	10–50%

Important sites of bleeding are:

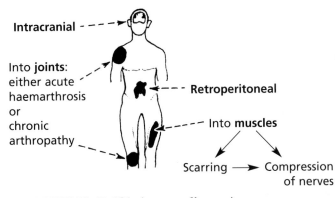

Note: In the past, the use of virus infected Factor VIII in treatment has caused HIV (AIDS) and Hepatitis C infection. Similar concerns apply to variant CJD (p.559).

HAEMOPHILIA B (Christmas disease)

This is due to deficiency of Factor IX – also carried by a gene on the X chromosome. The clinical features are similar, but the prevalence is lower (1 in 30 000 males).

Rarely deficiencies of other coagulation factors are seen e.g. fibrinogen, Factor XI and Factor V.

They are treated by infusion of the appropriate factors.

417

ACQUIRED DEFECTS OF COAGULATION

This large and heterogeneous group of conditions includes:

VITAMIN K DEFICIENCY

Vitamin K, a fat soluble vitamin, is essential for synthesis of Factors II, VII, IX and X in the liver. Deficiency leads to spontaneous bleeding e.g. into skin and mucous membranes, and failure of blood clotting.

In **adults**, deficiency may be due to

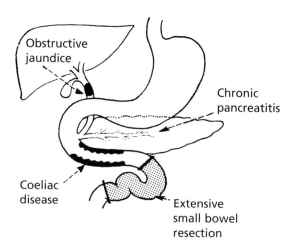

(a) MALABSORPTION
    (particularly of fat)

(b) DIETARY DEFICIENCY – rare
    – Vitamin K is widely distributed
    e.g. in green vegetables, oils.

(c) INHIBITION – by COUMARIN
    anticoagulants e.g. WARFARIN.

In **neonates**, vitamin K deficiency leads to bleeding – from GI tract (melaena neonatorum) and bruising. Breast milk contains little vitamin K – the disorder is uncommon in those receiving bottled milk. A severe deficiency may be seen in infants whose mothers took anticoagulants or anticonvulsants.

LIVER DISEASE

The bleeding tendency in these patients is multifactorial.

This complicates bleeding e.g. from OESOPHAGEAL varices.

'ACQUIRED HAEMOPHILIA'

Rarely, antibodies develop which block the effects of serum coagulation factors, especially Factor VIII. This may be idiopathic or follow auto-immune disease or drug treatment.

Disseminated Intravascular Coagulation (DIC) (see next page).

DISSEMINATED INTRAVASCULAR COAGULATION

In this disorder the coagulation system is activated, but the consumption of platelets and clotting factors which follows leads to a paradoxical bleeding tendency.

There are numerous causes:

(a) SEPTICAEMIA – especially gram negative septicaemia,
          – in meningococcal infections.
(b) SHOCK e.g. following severe burns.
(c) OBSTETRIC DISORDERS e.g. abruptio placentae, amniotic embolism, eclampsia.
(d) MALIGNANCY – especially acute promyelocytic leukaemia and mucin secreting
          adenocarcinomas (e.g. of stomach).
(e) IMMUNOLOGICAL DISORDERS e.g. autoimmune diseases,
          – incompatible blood transfusion.

The basic mechanism is as follows:

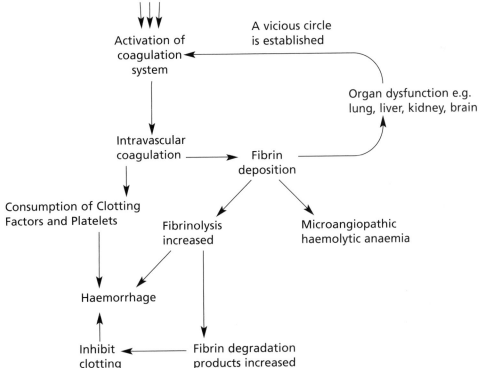

Patients frequently develop renal and hepatic failure and 'shock lung' [e.g. in the haemolytic uraemic syndrome (HUS) which is often associated with toxigenic *E.coli* infection – especially *E.coli* 0157 (see p.314)].

THROMBOPHILIA – THROMBOTIC DISORDERS

The major types, causes and effects of thrombosis are discussed on pages 157–161.

Recently, a group of inherited disorders has been discovered where deficiency of NATURAL ANTICOAGULANTS leads to an increased risk of venous thrombosis. This may be deep venous thrombosis in the lower limbs or visceral e.g mesenteric veins. There is also an increased risk of pulmonary embolism.

The main forms are:

(a) **ANTITHROMBIN DEFICIENCY**
Antithrombin, a member of the SERPIN group of **Ser**ine **p**rotease **in**hibitors, is synthesised in the liver. It blocks the action of F IXa, F Xa, F XIa and thrombin. Deficiency is due to mutation of a gene on the long arm of chromosome 1 – the effects depend on the exact type of mutation. The prevalence is around 1 in 20 000.

Note: **Heparin**, the anticoagulant, acts by enhancing the action of antithrombin.

(b) **PROTEIN C DEFICIENCY**
This is a Vitamin K dependent protein, synthesised in the liver. Together with protein S it blocks the action of Factor Va and Factor VIIIa. Around 1 in 15–30 000 is affected. In addition to deep thrombosis, patients also get superficial thrombophlebitis.

(c) **PROTEIN S DEFICIENCY**
This protein is secreted by the liver, platelets and endothelial cells. Its function is to bind with protein C to inhibit Factors Va and VIIIa.

(d) **ACTIVATED PROTEIN C RESISTANCE**
This is an inherited disorder where a mutation affects the Factor V gene. The protein is resistant to the effects of protein C – simulating protein C deficiency.

The possible role of minor deficiencies of these genetic factors in the more common forms of thrombosis is not yet established. The well known risk factors for thrombosis are listed below.

Acquired risk factors for thrombosis include:

Arterial	Venous
ATHEROMA	IMMOBILITY
SMOKING	TRAUMA/SURGERY
HYPERTENSION	MALIGNANCY
MYELOPROLIFERATIVE DISORDERS	ORAL CONTRACEPTIVES
	OBESITY

THE LYMPHOID SYSTEM

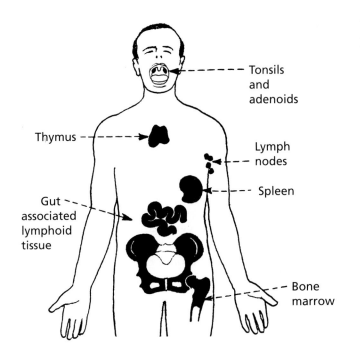

The lymphoid organs are principally involved in:

(a) Production and maturation of lymphocytes – thymus (T cells) and bone marrow (B cells).

(b) Antigen presentation and the immune response.

(c) 'Filtration' and phagocytosis of micro-organisms and particulate material.

LYMPH NODES

The basic structure reflects the main functions.

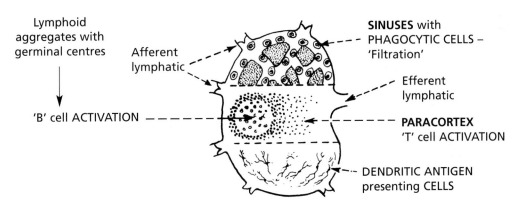

LYMPHADENOPATHY

Lymph node enlargement may be **localised** or **generalised**. It may be due to:

(a) reactive hyperplasia e.g. – infection by bacteria or viruses,
                        – particulate material,
                        – immune stimulation e.g. Rheumatoid arthritis,
                        – draining degradation products from a cancer.
(b) due to neoplasia e.g. – secondary deposits of carcinoma,
                     – primary lymphoid tumours.

REACTIVE HYPERPLASIA

The changes include three basic and several subsidiary:

Normal small inactive lymph node

Small, ill-defined germinal centres

Rather sparse scattering of lymphocytes in reticular framework. Very narrow peripheral sinus

Sinuses not prominent

Macrophages not prominent

ACTIVATION

Basic changes

(1) Increased lymph flow

(2) Activation of Macrophages and antigen presenting cells

(3) 'B' and 'T' Lymphocyte activation

Node enlarged

Widening of sinuses

Macrophages lining and filling sinuses

(a) Numerous well-formed germinal centres

(b) packed 'T' lymphocytes in paracortex (incl. 'blast' cells)

Subsidiary changes
1. Infiltration by neutrophils (in acute inflammation)
2. Increased blood flow (prominent venules)
3. Increased plasma cells ⎫
4. Increased eosinophils ⎬ → Chronic inflammation

The qualitative and quantitative variations and combinations of these changes are very numerous; in most reactive states the appearances are non-specific. In only a few instances do particular patterns of response reflect a specific stimulus.

LYMPHADENOPATHY – INFECTIONS

ACUTE BACTERIAL LYMPHADENITIS
This is seen draining an infected area.

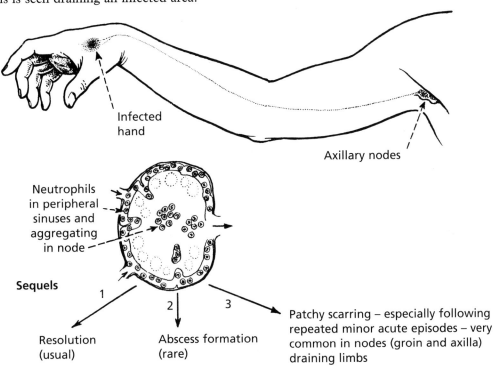

Infected hand

Axillary nodes

Neutrophils in peripheral sinuses and aggregating in node

Sequels

1 — Resolution (usual)

2 — Abscess formation (rare)

3 — Patchy scarring – especially following repeated minor acute episodes – very common in nodes (groin and axilla) draining limbs

In **LYMPHOGRANULOMA VENEREUM (LGV)**, the enlarged lymph nodes show a striking histological appearance.
LGV is an infection by *Chlamydia trachomatis*. The portal entry is by venereal contact and the disease runs a subacute course.

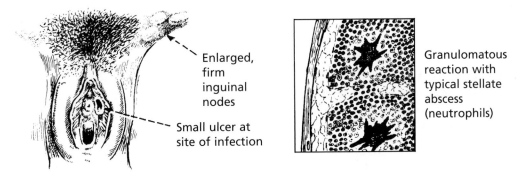

Enlarged, firm inguinal nodes

Small ulcer at site of infection

Granulomatous reaction with typical stellate abscess (neutrophils)

The diagnosis has to be confirmed by a skin test (Frei test) or a complement fixation test.

In **CAT SCRATCH FEVER**, the nodes draining the scratched area show similar histological changes. The organism *Bartonella henselae* is responsible.

LYMPHADENOPATHY

TUBERCULOSIS is associated with a granulomatous response (p.42), often with caseation due to delayed type sensitivity.

Granuloma – activated macrophages

Langhans' giant cell

Bacilli identified on Ziehl–Neelsen stain

Caseation

VIRAL LYMPHADENITIS – Many infections induce paracortical hyperplasia – with activation of T cells.

In **GLANDULAR FEVER** (Infectious mononucleosis), an infection by Epstein–Barr virus of young adults, the cervical lymph nodes are particularly involved.

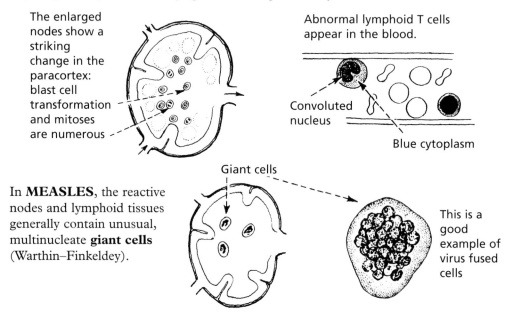

The enlarged nodes show a striking change in the paracortex: blast cell transformation and mitoses are numerous

Abnormal lymphoid T cells appear in the blood.

Convoluted nucleus

Blue cytoplasm

In **MEASLES**, the reactive nodes and lymphoid tissues generally contain unusual, multinucleate **giant cells** (Warthin–Finkeldey).

Giant cells

This is a good example of virus fused cells

In **TOXOPLASMOSIS**, a protozoal disease (*Toxoplasma gondii*) which may cause serious damage to the fetus or neonate and present with lymph node enlargement in the adult, the histological appearances in the node may indicate the aetiology. The diagnosis is confirmed by serological tests.

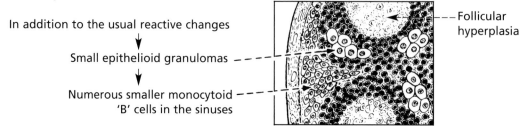

In addition to the usual reactive changes
↓
Small epithelioid granulomas
↓
Numerous smaller monocytoid 'B' cells in the sinuses

Follicular hyperplasia

LYMPHADENOPATHY – NON-INFECTIVE CAUSES

FOREIGN MATERIAL

Lymph nodes to which foreign particulate material drains often show marked enlargement due to accumulation of macrophages which have ingested the foreign material.

For example: – carbon and silica in hilar lymph nodes
              – silicone e.g. in axillary lymph nodes in patients with prosthetic joints and breast implants.

CHRONIC SKIN DISEASE (so-called dermatopathic lymphadenopathy) e.g. psoriasis, eczema and mycosis fungoides (p.440).

The following may be seen lying free and in macrophages:
    Fat
    Melanin – from damaged skin
    Haemosiderin – from minor bleeding in skin

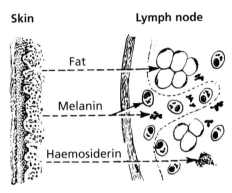

SARCOIDOSIS

In this disease of unknown aetiology (possibly infective?) non-caseating granulomas are seen.

The appearances clearly resemble tuberculosis, but the granulomas remain discrete and there is no caseation.

Sarcoid type granulomas are also seen in the lymph nodes of patients with other granulomatous diseases e.g. Crohn's disease and in lymph nodes draining tumours.

SPLEEN

The anatomy of the spleen reflects both its basic function, which is filtration of the blood, and sequential functions of phagocytosis and the immune response.
Normal average weight – 150 g.

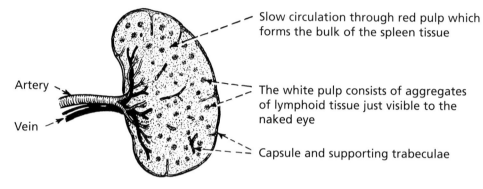

Slow circulation through red pulp which forms the bulk of the spleen tissue

Artery

Vein

The white pulp consists of aggregates of lymphoid tissue just visible to the naked eye

Capsule and supporting trabeculae

Microscopic appearance

Lymphoid aggregate – mediates IMMUNE RESPONSE.

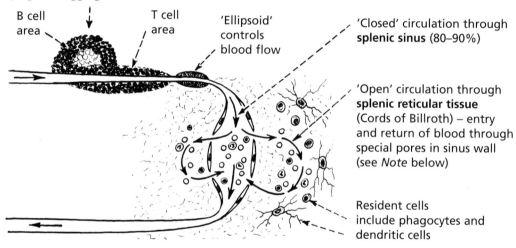

B cell area

T cell area

'Ellipsoid' controls blood flow

'Closed' circulation through **splenic sinus (80–90%)**

'Open' circulation through **splenic reticular tissue** (Cords of Billroth) – entry and return of blood through special pores in sinus wall (see *Note* below)

Resident cells include phagocytes and dendritic cells

The red pulp is the site of filtration and phagocytosis of the following:

1. Effete cells and cell debris – especially blood cells but also cell debris derived from the body generally

2. Microbes and their toxins

3. Abnormal or excess material derived from metabolic processes.

Note: The special pores allowing re-entry of RBCs to the circulation have a 2 μm aperture: abnormal RBCs (e.g. spherocytes) cannot pass through and are trapped.

SPLENOMEGALY

Enlargement of the spleen is an important and common clinical sign. Increase in the red pulp due to increased numbers of phagocytes and/or increased numbers of blood cells is the major component, in chronic infections particularly, hyperplasia of the lymphoid tissue contributes.

An aetiological classification under 5 broad headings is convenient.

Enlargement associated with: 1. INFECTIONS
2. CIRCULATORY DISTURBANCES
3. STORAGE DISEASES and DEGENERATIONS
4. NEOPLASIA – primary and secondary
5. DISORDERS OF THE BLOOD.

1. INFECTIONS

In acute systemic bacterial infections the spleen shows slight to moderate enlargement (200–400 g).

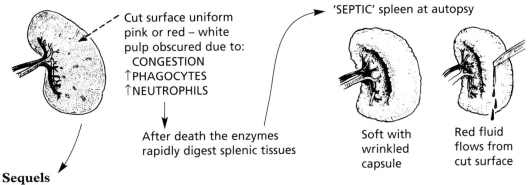

Cut surface uniform pink or red – white pulp obscured due to:
CONGESTION
↑PHAGOCYTES
↑NEUTROPHILS

After death the enzymes rapidly digest splenic tissues

'SEPTIC' spleen at autopsy

Soft with wrinkled capsule

Red fluid flows from cut surface

Sequels

(a) Resolution as infection resolves.
(b) Occasionally spreads through capsule to adjacent tissues, with or without abscess formation.
(c) Only extremely rarely does abscess formation occur within the spleen.

In non-pyogenic and chronic infections, there may be moderate enlargement.

Firm

Cut surface shows lymphoid aggregates

Red pulp contains increased PHAGOCYTES often PLASMA CELLS

Examples: Subacute infective endocarditis
Tuberculosis
Typhoid fever
Infectious mononucleosis
Brucellosis
In protozoal diseases – malaria and kala-azar – there is often massive enlargement

SPLENOMEGALY

2. CIRCULATORY DISTURBANCES

Congestive splenomegaly occurs in two main conditions:

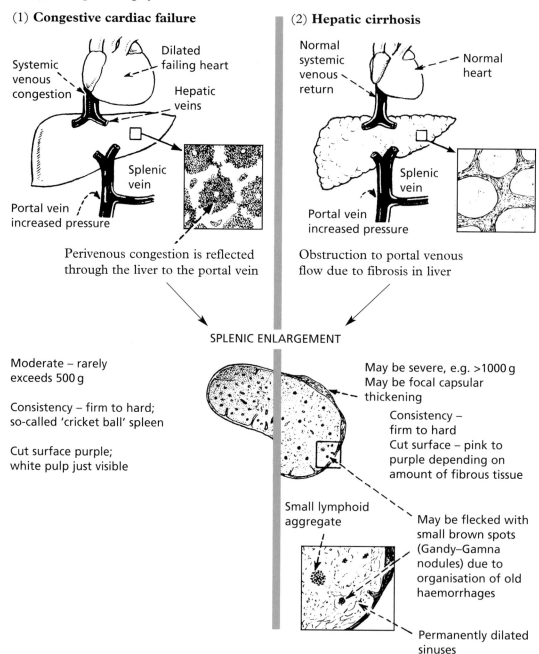

(1) Congestive cardiac failure

Dilated failing heart

Systemic venous congestion

Hepatic veins

Splenic vein

Portal vein increased pressure

Perivenous congestion is reflected through the liver to the portal vein

(2) Hepatic cirrhosis

Normal systemic venous return

Normal heart

Splenic vein

Portal vein increased pressure

Obstruction to portal venous flow due to fibrosis in liver

SPLENIC ENLARGEMENT

Moderate – rarely exceeds 500 g

Consistency – firm to hard; so-called 'cricket ball' spleen

Cut surface purple; white pulp just visible

May be severe, e.g. >1000 g
May be focal capsular thickening

Consistency – firm to hard
Cut surface – pink to purple depending on amount of fibrous tissue

Small lymphoid aggregate

May be flecked with small brown spots (Gandy–Gamna nodules) due to organisation of old haemorrhages

Permanently dilated sinuses

The type of splenomegaly associated with portal venous hypertension may have serious haematological effects (see Hypersplenism).

SPLENOMEGALY

3. STORAGE DISEASES AND DEGENERATIONS

The diseases associated with this type of enlargement are rare.

Examples are:

Amyloidosis (see pp.22–24)
Lipid storage diseases (see p.21) including Gaucher's disease,
Niemann–Pick disease and Tay–Sachs disease.

Some disorders of glycogen storage.

4. NEOPLASIA

(a) PRIMARY –   the spleen is rarely the seat of primary tumour growth, although occasional primary splenic lymphomas occur.

(b) SECONDARY –   the spleen is rarely affected by secondary tumour, e.g. carcinoma and sarcoma, but it is commonly involved during the systematised spread of **lymphomas** and **leukaemias**.

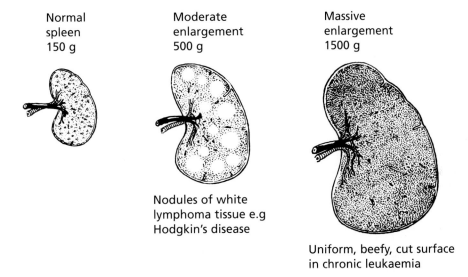

Normal
spleen
150 g

Moderate
enlargement
500 g

Massive
enlargement
1500 g

Nodules of white
lymphoma tissue e.g
Hodgkin's disease

Uniform, beefy, cut surface
in chronic leukaemia

Splenic enlargement may be a feature of histiocytosis-X (Langerhans cell histiocytosis).

SPLENOMEGALY

5. DISORDERS OF THE BLOOD

Splenic enlargement is associated with blood disorders in two main circumstances:

1. Splenic enlargement causing blood disorders (hypersplenism).

ENLARGED SPLEEN ⟶ Increased capacity ⟶ Reduction in circulating
from any cause, but   for sequestration of   blood cells, i.e.
particularly in cases   blood cells   *anaemia,*
of **portal hypertension**   *leucopenia,*
                                                           thrombocytopenia,
                                        Marrow ⟵   separately or together,
                                        hyperplasia   i.e. **pancytopenia**

2. Blood disorder causing splenic enlargement

(a) Production of abnormal blood ⟶ Increased demand ⟶ Increase
cells, e.g. in haemolytic anaemias: on sequestration   in spleen
idiopathic thrombocytopenia   function of spleen   size
(antibody coated platelets)

                                    Infiltration of spleen
                                    by neoplastic cells
(b) leukaemias   Increase in
and lymphomas   spleen size
                                    Increased sequestration
                                    of abnormal cells

(c) In chronic marrow ⟶ Resumption by spleen of ⟶ Increase in spleen
failure due to fibrosis   fetal blood forming role   size – may be massive
or secondary tumour   (extramedullary   (500–2 000 g)
infiltration   haemopoiesis)

Note: When a blood disorder initiates splenic enlargement the disability may be
compounded by superimposed hypersplenism, e.g.

MALARIA
(haemolysis of
parasitised red cells)

ANAEMIA ⟶ SPLENIC ENLARGEMENT

Anaemia   INCREASED
aggravated   SEQUESTRATION of RBCs

HYPERSPLENISM

DISEASES OF THE SPLEEN – MISCELLANEOUS

HYPOSPLENISM

Hyposplenism is not usually a cause of major disability. It occurs following splenectomy and in cases of splenic atrophy.

The effects are considered under two main headings:

1. On the cells of the blood

Loss of splenic sequestration function

↓

Deficiency in disposal of abnormal cells

Red cell series:
(a) increased acanthocytes
(b) increased Howell–Jolly bodies
(c) increased number of iron-containing cells

Neutrophils: may be leucocytosis

Platelets: may be thrombocythaemia

Seen especially after splenectomy – usually not permanent

2. On resistance to infection

Loss of filtration of bacteria from blood ⟶ Occasional cases of **septicaemia** – especially caused by *Streptococcus pneumoniae* – young children are particularly susceptible

CIRCULATORY AND VASCULAR CHANGES

(a) *Infarction*
(i) Embolism causing infarction is not uncommon but usually clinically unimportant.

(ii) Enlarged spleens are particularly susceptible to infarction without embolism.

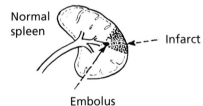

Normal spleen

Infarct

Embolus

Thrombosis of artery

Infarct especially in terminal illness

(b) *Hyalinisation of splenic arterioles*

This is an almost invariable concomitant of ageing and is not related to systemic arteriosclerosis or hypertension.

Hyaline thickening of arteriolar wall

THYMUS

This 'primary' lymphoid organ is concerned with the development and processing to maturation of the long-lived T lymphocytes which are then distributed to the lymphoid tissues and to the circulating pool of T lymphocytes.

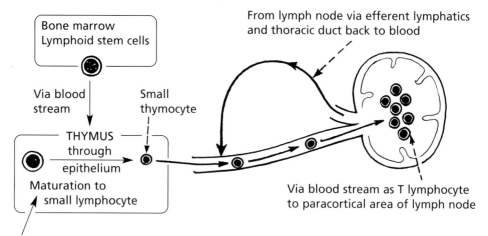

Mechanism – stimulation by hormones formed locally by thymic epithelial cells.

This activity is maximal in the fetal and childhood stages. Involution is rapid after puberty.

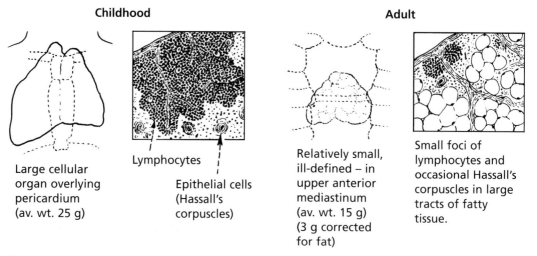

Congenital thymic aplasia or hypoplasia
The resulting T cell deficiency is associated with disordered cell-mediated immune response.

Note: Thymectomy in adult life has little pathological significance since the T lymphocytes produced in childhood are long enough lived to obviate serious immune deficiency.

THYMUS

Thymic hyperplasia

Assessment by weight alone is unsatisfactory due to the variability of the fat content in adult life. A weight over 35 g probably represents hyperplasia, but the appearance of lymphoid follicles with germinal centres is a more reliable indication.

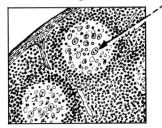

Associated conditions:
    Auto-immune disorders,
      e.g. Systemic lupus erythematosus
        Addison's disease
        Thyrotoxicosis
        Pancytopenia
        and *NB* MYASTHENIA GRAVIS

Thymic tumours

Thymomas are rare tumours: they are essentially low-grade carcinomas with an admixture of lymphoid cells: they rarely metastasise. They may have auto-immune associations similar to thymic hyperplasia.

The bulk of these lobulated and nodular tumours compresses adjacent mediastinal structures

(a) Compression of respiratory passages → dyspnoea and cough.

(b) Oesphagus → dysphagia.

(c) Great veins → cyanosis and suffusion of face.

Other primary tumours arising in the thymus are;
    (1) T cell lymphoblastic lymphomas (adolescent males)
    (2) Hodgkin's disease.
    (3) Mediastinal large 'B' cell lymphoma
    (4) Germ cell tumours (e.g. teratoma).
    (5) Carcinoids.

The thymus in Myasthenia Gravis (MG)

MG is a disease of voluntary muscles in which weakness is the main feature. The association with the thymus is striking in that 80% of all patients with MG have either thymic hyperplasia or thymoma.

Follicular hyperplasia (80%) – seen especially in young females.
Thymoma (20%) – seen especially in middle aged males.
The results of thymectomy in MG patients are very unpredictable.

The detailed pathological changes in MG and the mechanisms by which the thymus is linked with the disease are described on pages 109, 593.

NEOPLASTIC LYMPHADENOPATHY

Lymph node enlargement may be due to
  (a) Invasion by SECONDARY TUMOURS – especially CARCINOMAS –
or (b) Primary lymphoid tumours – LYMPHOMAS.

SECONDARY TUMOUR invasion
Carcinoma of the breast is taken as an example.

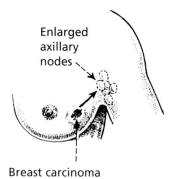

Enlarged
axillary
nodes

Breast carcinoma

Note:

(i) The nodal enlargement is not necessarily due to secondary tumour.

   Reactive hyperplasia is also common in nodes draining tumours especially if there is ulceration. The distinction between these 2 causes of node enlargement can only be made with certainty by **histological examination.**

(ii) The invasion of a group of nodes occurs in a step-wise fashion: a single node (the SENTINEL node) is invaded initially and spread to adjacent nodes follows.

(a)

Tumour cells are
first seen in the
capsular sinus.

Eventually much
of the node is
replaced

(b)

lymphatic

Primary
tumour

Sentinel
node is
invaded

Spread to
adjacent
nodes

Identification of the sentinel node may
be required in the investigation of
breast cancer and malignant melanoma.

LYMPHOMAS
Lymphomas are malignant tumours derived from lymphoid cells. They may arise within lymph nodes or at other sites (extra-nodal lymphomas).

Classically, they are divided into 2 main groups.

  (a) Hodgkin's disease 20–25%
    – almost always of lymph node origin.
    – characterised by the presence of Reed–Sternberg cells.

  (b) Non-Hodgkin's disease 75–80%

    – three-quarters arise in lymph nodes

In recent years, modern immunocytochemical, molecular biological and cytogenetic techniques have been applied to the study of lymphomas. The traditional division between Hodgkin's and non-Hodgkin's lymphoma has been challenged but remains of major clinical importance.

NON-HODGKIN'S LYMPHOMAS

These solid tumours mainly affect middle aged to elderly patients.

They may arise

      (a) Within lymph nodes   or   (b) in extra-nodal sites.

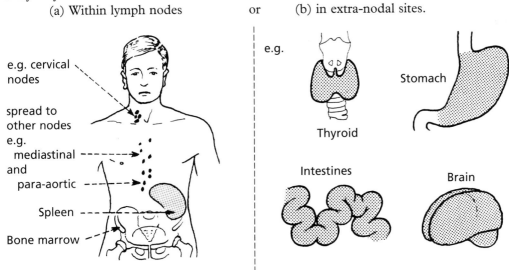

Eventually a generalised spread with involvement of liver, lungs and heart may occur.

DEGREE OF MALIGNANCY

The natural history tends to separate lymphomas into two main groups which have links with the morphological appearances.

1. Low grade malignancy associated with well differentiated relatively inactive cell types,
– progress of years.

2. High grade malignancy associated with primitive actively proliferating cells,
– progress over weeks or months.
Tend to respond well to chemotherapy.

PATHOLOGICAL COMPLICATIONS

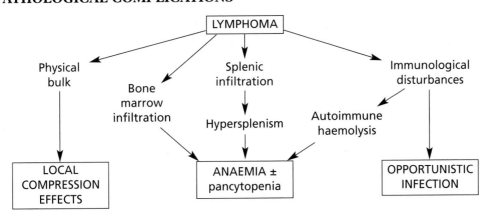

NON-HODGKIN'S LYMPHOMAS

Classification

This is a confusing area. Traditional classifications relied on morphology alone. The World Health Organisation Classification (2001) which includes immunohistochemistry and genetic data is now generally accepted. A simplified version follows:

NON-HODGKIN's LYMPHOMAS

B CELL (> 90%)

Small lymphocytic lymphoma
(equivalent to B cell, p.447).
Lymphoplasmacytic lymphoma.
Mantle cell lymphoma.
Follicular lymphoma.
Burkitt's lymphoma.
Diffuse large B cell lymphoma.
Extranodal marginal zone B-cell lymphoma
Myeloma/Plasmacytoma.

T CELL (< 10%)

T cell prolymphocytic leukaemia.
Peripheral T cell lymphoma.
Adult T cell leukaemia.
Angioimmunoblastic T cell lymphoma.
Anaplastic large cell lymphomas
  (some do not express T cell markers).
Enteropathy-type T cell lymphoma.
Mycosis fungoides (skin).

According to this classification each type is considered separately for treatment purposes.

The classification relies on cell surface markers which distinguish the B and T cells and their subsets. B and T cell monoclonality can be detected by gene rearrangements, and some types of lymphoma have characteristic translocations.

Subtyping of lymphoma

IMMUNOHISTOCHEMISTRY

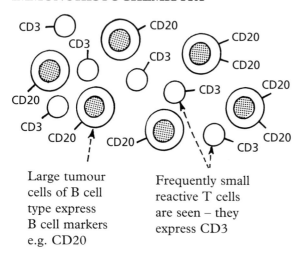

Large tumour cells of B cell type express B cell markers e.g. CD20

Frequently small reactive T cells are seen – they express CD3

MOLECULAR GENETIC ANALYSIS

In B cell differentiation different immunoglobulin genes are found by gene rearrangements, while in T cell differentiation a similar process occurs with T cell antigen receptors (p.92).

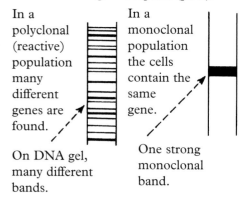

In a polyclonal (reactive) population many different genes are found.

On DNA gel, many different bands.

In a monoclonal population the cells contain the same gene.

One strong monoclonal band.

NON-HODGKIN'S LYMPHOMAS

FOLLICULAR LYMPHOMA

This is one of the commonest forms – a 'B' cell lymphoma.

The neoplastic follicles are the malignant equivalent of normal germinal centres.

The tumour cells express the anti-apoptosis gene bcl–2 which immortalises them. There is often a translocation t (14;18) which joins the bcl–2 gene to the immunoglobulin heavy chain gene.

The lymphoma is slowly progressive but often eventually fatal. Sometimes it transforms into a diffuse large 'B' cell lymphoma.

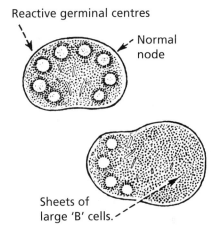

Reactive germinal centres

Normal node

Sheets of large 'B' cells.

BURKITT'S LYMPHOMA

This is a high grade lymphoma found mainly in Equatorial Africa, New Guinea and other malaria endemic areas. Similar tumours are seen in AIDS patients. The relationship with Epstein–Barr virus has already been discussed (p.81) – as has the translocation t (8;14) which activates the c-myc oncogene (p.152). The histological appearance is typical and striking.

Diffuse proliferation of lymphoblast-like B type cells

Cells medium-sized and uniform

Scattering of macrophages containing debris derived from very rapid cell turnover – contributing 'starry sky' appearance.

Mitoses frequent

Endemic (African type) Burkitt's lymphoma typically presents with lesions in the jaw, or in the abdomen, e.g. ovary, liver, gastrointestinal tract. The less common cases in the West typically involve lymph node, marrow and gut.
The disease may respond dramatically to aggressive treatment.

DIFFUSE LARGE B-CELL LYMPHOMA

This is the commonest type of lymphoma and may arise in nodes or extra-nodal sites. They rapidly disseminate. They are composed of sheets of large round cells. About 50% of patients survive.

PLASMA CELL TUMOURS

SOLITARY PLASMACYTOMA
A very small number of plasma cell tumours present as solitary growths, e.g. in a long bone, the nasopharynx, a lymph node, alimentary tract. In 50% of cases, multiple myeloma occurs within 10 years.

MULTIPLE MYELOMA (MYELOMATOSIS)
The great majority of plasma cell tumours present as widespread

deposits in the bone marrow. Classically the lesions are seen as punched out defects in the bones – the skull showing this appearance particularly well. These focal proliferations of plasma cells usually occur against a background of more diffuse infiltration throughout the marrow.

Binucleate cell –––

The disease has an incidence of 10/100 000 per annum with an age peak in the 7th decade.

The median survival, even with treatment, is 3 years.

Pathological effects are considered under two main headings:

1. Tumour growth and its effects

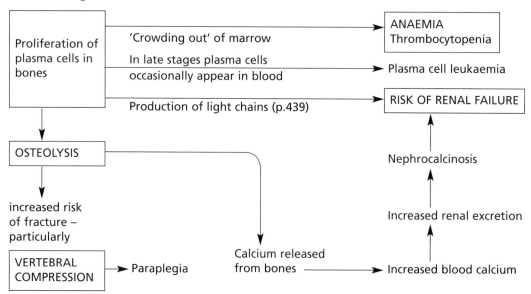

PLASMA CELL TUMOURS

Pathological effects (*continued*)

2. **Synthesis of immunoglobulin and its effects**

Myelomatosis, being a monoclonal tumour, will produce a single Ig, but the type of Ig varies from case to case, unlike Waldenström's macroglobulinaemia where the immunoglobulin is always IgM. The common heavy chains are G (60%) and A (20%). Light chains of κ type are encountered more frequently than λ reflecting the normal κ:λ ratio, i.e. 65:35. Thus myeloma of IgGκ is the most frequent.

The presence of a single type of Ig is reflected in the electrophoretic pattern

The other normal immunoglobulins are always decreased.

Spike of → 'M'yeloma protein

alb   α¹   α²   β   γ

In most cases high levels of 'M' protein cause:
1. High ESR
2. Marked rouleaux formation
3. Depending on type of Ig – increased blood viscosity.

Note: 'M' stands for myeloma and it does not signify IgM.

Release of light chains

In many myelomas, some of the Ig molecules are incompletely formed, and unattached light chains are released with important effects. Because of their low molecular weight the light chains:

(1) Pass through the glomerular filtrate,
(a) appearing in the *urine* as Bence Jones protein (precipitates during heating – redissolves between 90°–100°C).
(b) During passage through the tubules the protein precipitates as casts and also damages the epithelial cells.

Myeloma kidney

Note giant cells

(2) Pass through capillaries

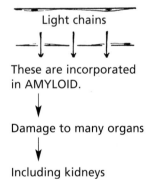

Light chains

These are incorporated in AMYLOID.

↓

Damage to many organs

↓

Including kidneys

Infections, often of opportunistic type, and particularly pneumonias are common because the immune response is deficient since the high levels of 'M' protein are non-functioning.

NON-HODGKIN'S LYMPHOMA – T CELL

MYCOSIS FUNGOIDES

This is a primary T cell (CD4) lymphoma of the skin occurring usually in middle aged men. It presents as a scaly, red macule progressing to skin plaques and then nodules.

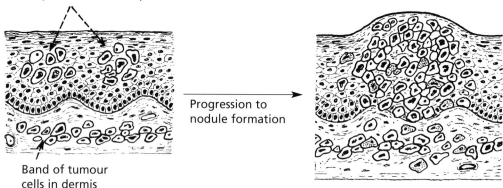

Foci of large neoplastic cells in epidermis (Pautrier abscesses)

Band of tumour cells in dermis

Progression to nodule formation

After many years the lymphoma may become generalised or exfoliate into the blood (Sézary syndrome).

ANAPLASTIC LARGE CELL LYMPHOMA

The large malignant T cells (usually expressing surface marker CD30) often spread within the sinuses of the node and, in the past, were mistaken for secondary carcinoma cells.

Some of the large tumour cells mimic the cells in Hodgkin's disease.

Although three-quarters of cases are of T cell type, the remainder are 'null' cell type, i.e. they express neither T nor B cell markers, causing further diagnostic difficulties.

The tumour shows 2 age peaks.

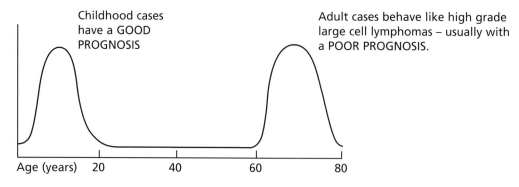

Childhood cases have a GOOD PROGNOSIS

Adult cases behave like high grade large cell lymphomas – usually with a POOR PROGNOSIS.

Age (years)   20   40   60   80

HODGKIN'S DISEASE

Incidence

This disease accounts for 20% of lymphomas. It may occur at any age but there are 2 peaks of incidence. The overall average incidence is 30 cases/million population but there are wide geographical variations.

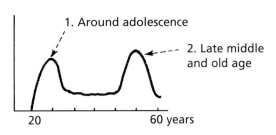

1. Around adolescence

2. Late middle and old age

20   60 years

Presentation

Most patients present with painless enlargement of one or more lymph node groups – cervical, axillary, mediastinal. One quarter complain of systemic 'B' symptoms (see Staging) – fever, night sweats, weight loss, itch. The risk of infections is increased by immunosuppression.

Spread and Staging

The disease spreads from one group to the next directly connected by lymphatics.

Normal nodes

Single node replaced by pale tumour tissue

Spread to adjacent nodes

Disease beginning in lymph node

Spreading to
1. Other lymphoid tissue
   (a) Nodes in central axis
   (b) Spleen
2. Other organs
   (a) Marrow
   (b) Liver
   (c) Miscellaneous, e.g. alimentary tract

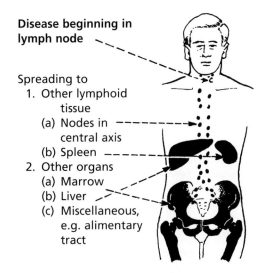

Staging (Ann Arbor system)

Stage I	Disease involving single node or group of nodes
Stage II	Disease in more than one site – all lesions either below or above the diaphragm
Stage III	Disease on both sides of diaphragm
Stage IV	Widespread involvement of extralymphoid sites ± lymph node involvement

The suffix (E) to the numeral indicates Extranodal disease, (A) denotes absence of systemic symptoms, (B) presence of these (see above).

441

HODGKIN'S DISEASE

Hodgkin's disease is diagnosed on the basis of distinctive large tumour cells known as Reed–Sternberg cells, which are now known to be 'B' cells of germinal centre origin.

Typical RS cell

30–60 μm diam.
Amphophilic cytoplasm

Peripheral clumping of nuclear chromatin

Mirror image nuclei

Large eosinophilic nucleoli

They express CD30 and CD15

Variants of RS cell

1. The lacunar cell

Shrinkage of cell cytoplasm towards cell wall and nucleus, leaving a clear space

2. Mononuclear Hodgkin's cell

Nuclear characteristic similar to RS cell but smaller

These cells are not specifically diagnostic of Hodgkin's disease.

There are two main types of Hodgkin's disease:

(a) Classical HD, probably caused by EBV. There are three main forms:

1. Nodular sclerosing (70%)

Thick bands of collagen separating Hodgkin's tissue

Lacunar cells often numerous

Often mediastinal presentation

2. Mixed cellularity (20%)

Plasma cells and eosinophils present in addition to RS cells and lymphocytes

3. Lymphocyte depleted (<2%)

Very numerous RS and mononuclear Hodgkin's cells – few lymphocytes ± diffuse fibrosis

(b) Nodular lymphocyte predominant Hodgkin's disease (6%) This form affects young males and has a good prognosis. The 'popcorn cells' express 'B' cell markers and not CD30 of classic Hodgkin's disease – it is an unusual 'B' cell lymphoma.

Sheets of small lymphocytes

Scattering of unusual Hodgkin's cells – 'popcorn' cells

LEUKAEMIAS

Leukaemias are primary malignant tumours of haemopoietic cells.

Neoplastic haemopoietic cells fill the marrow including long bones.

High marrow cellularity (no fat spaces)

(a) Spill over into blood

LEUKAEMIA

Increased WBC, e.g. 20 000 to 250 000/mm^3

(b) No spill over

ALEUKAEMIC LEUKAEMIA

WBC normal or low

Clinical Effects

The neoplastic cells replace the normal bone marrow

1. Deficiency of red cells ⟶ anaemia.
2. Deficiency of platelets ⟶ thrombocytopenia ⟶ bleeding.
3. Deficiency of white cells ⟶ infection.
4. Increased cell turnover ⟶ ↑DNA breakdown ⟶ ↑uric acid ⟶ gout.

Spread of leukaemia

Leukaemic cells circulate in blood and/or lymph and can therefore spread anywhere in the body. Nodular deposits are, however, uncommon.

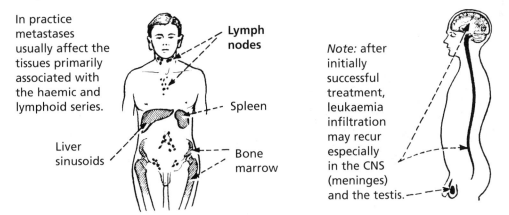

In practice metastases usually affect the tissues primarily associated with the haemic and lymphoid series.

Lymph nodes

Spleen

Liver sinusoids

Bone marrow

Note: after initially successful treatment, leukaemia infiltration may recur especially in the CNS (meninges) and the testis.

LEUKAEMIAS

Classification

Leukaemias are classified according to the rate of progression and the lineage of the tumour cells. The 4 main forms are:

	MYELOID (granulocyte: monocyte series)	LYMPHOID (B and T lymphocyte series)
ACUTE LEUKAEMIA – Rapid progression – Numerous primitive 'blast' cells.	(i) ACUTE MYELOBLASTIC LEUKAEMIA	(iii) ACUTE LYMPHOBLASTIC LEUKAEMIA
CHRONIC LEUKAEMIA – Slow progression – Cells almost mature.	(ii) CHRONIC MYELOID LEUKAEMIA	(iv) CHRONIC LYMPHOCYTIC LEUKAEMIA

Rare leukaemias affect red cells, megakaryocytes and plasma cells.

Aetiology

In most cases, the cause is unknown. Risk factors include:

1. Radiation e.g. post Hiroshima, Chernobyl, therapeutic X-ray.
2. Chemicals e.g. chemotherapy, benzene.
3. Genetic e.g. Down's syndrome.
4. Virus e.g. Human T-cell Leukaemia Virus-1.

CELL KINETICS

Even in acute leukaemias, increased cell longevity beyond the normal (due to failure of response to mechanisms controlling ageing and destruction) is as important as proliferative rates in increasing the marrow cell population.

ACUTE MYELOBLASTIC LEUKAEMIA

This is the commonest acute leukaemia of adults – 80% of patients are over 60 years old. Young adults and children may also be affected.

It may arise de novo or in association with chronic myeloid leukaemia, myeloproliferative disorders, myelodysplasia. The onset and progression to marrow failure is rapid, clinically presenting as anaemia, haemorrhage or serious infection.

The WHO classification describes four broad categories:

1. AML with recurrent genetic abnormalities. The differing genetic rearrangements have major implications for prognosis and treatment.

2. AML with multilineage dysplasia – usually following myelodysplastic syndrome.

3. AML, therapy related – usually after alkylating chemotherapy.

4. AML, not otherwise classified – a wide variety showing varying degrees of differentiation, e.g. acute monocytic, acute erythroblastic, acute myelomonocytic.

PATHOLOGY

The marrow

Over-run by blast cells

The blood

Decreased platelet count – **thrombocytopenia.**

2/3 cases: WBC 20 000–50 000 blast cells
1/3 cases: **aleukaemic**

Other organs may be involved: Splenomegaly, hepatomegaly and lymph node enlargement. More specific pathological clinical complications are seen in 2 subtypes.

Promyelocytic

Primitive cell with primary myeloid granules ---

A typical chromosomal translocation t(15:17) is found.

Patients often develop disseminated intravascular coagulation.

Myelomonocytic and Monocytic

Infiltration of the gums and central nervous sytem is often seen.

CHRONIC MYELOID LEUKAEMIA (CML)

This form of leukaemia arises from malignant transformation of a primitive stem cell – but with the production of differentiated cells – particularly neutrophils.

This is a disease of middle age. There are 3 phases:

1. **Chronic phase** – a period of slow evolution – 2–6 years is typical.
2. **Accelerated phase** – an increase in immature cells.
3. **Blast phase** – transformation to an acute leukaemia – myeloblastic or, very rarely, lymphoblastic.

Rarely patients develop myelofibrosis with marrow failure.

Marrow

Total cellularity: cells of granulocyte series – late forms numerous (including eosinophil and basophil types). Often increase in megakaryocytes; may be increased fibrosis. Increased pressure in bones may cause clinical tenderness and pain.

Blood
(a) WBC: 75 000–250 000/mm^3
Differential WBC
Blasts
Promyelocytes } <5%

Majority of cells are late myelocytes and mature granulocytes

(b) ANAEMIA

(c) THROMBOCYTOPENIA
(sometimes thrombocytosis)

Splenomegaly

Firm, may be massive, e.g. 3 kg

May be infarction

↓

Clinically painful

Lymphoid follicles inconspicuous

Red pulp with cells of granulocyte series ± megakaryocytes ± red cell precursors

Philadelphia (Ph) chromosome
In over 95% of cases of CML there is a specific cytogenetic change t(9;22)(q34;q11) with the formation of the 'Ph chromosome'.

The change involves a translocation of the c-abl gene (an oncogene) from chromosome 9 to chromosome 22 where hybridisation with the bcr gene occurs. A tyrosine kinase inhibitor (IMATINIB) which targets this pathway has been introduced.

CHRONIC LYMPHOCYTIC LEUKAEMIA

This is a common form of leukaemia (25% of all cases) and particularly affects middle aged and elderly patients. It is a monoclonal proliferation of small lymphocytes and is best regarded as the leukaemic form of lymphocytic lymphoma.

Most cases are of B cell type – less than 5% are of T cell lineage.

There is typically lymph node enlargement and splenomegaly.

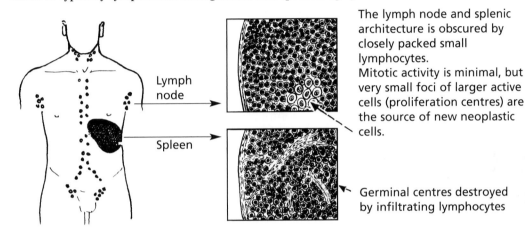

Lymph node

Spleen

The lymph node and splenic architecture is obscured by closely packed small lymphocytes.
Mitotic activity is minimal, but very small foci of larger active cells (proliferation centres) are the source of new neoplastic cells.

Germinal centres destroyed by infiltrating lymphocytes

In some cases the lymphoid enlargement precedes the leukaemic phase.

The marrow   *Early*   **The blood picture**

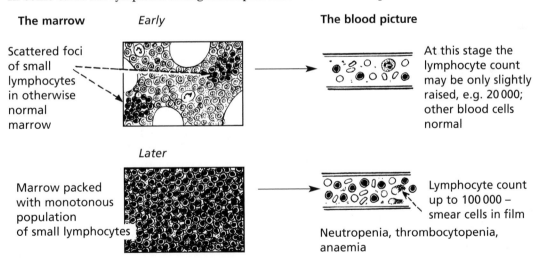

Scattered foci of small lymphocytes in otherwise normal marrow

At this stage the lymphocyte count may be only slightly raised, e.g. 20 000; other blood cells normal

Later

Marrow packed with monotonous population of small lymphocytes

Lymphocyte count up to 100 000 – smear cells in film

Neutropenia, thrombocytopenia, anaemia

In addition to anaemia these patients often suffer recurrent infections due to defective immunity.

In a minority of cases (approximately 5%) transformation to a high grade 'B' cell lymphoma results (Richter syndrome).

ACUTE LYMPHOBLASTIC LEUKAEMIA (ALL)

This term describes a group of leukaemias of lymphocytic precursors. ALL is the commonest form of childhood leukaemia but is also seen in adults.

Like AML, immunological and genotypic classification is increasingly important. Broadly, they are classified as follows:

- Precursor B cell > 80%
- Precursor T cell 15%
- Null cell.

ALL in Childhood

This is usually of Precursor B ALL type

The skin may show pallor or haemorrhage

Mediastinal mass is common in T-ALL

CNS involvement with increased intracranial pressure and nerve palsies in 5% of children. Without prophylactic intrathecal chemotherapy 75% relapse.

Lymphadenopathy

Mild hepatosplenomegaly is common.

Testicular involvement is common.

Bone and joint pain are common.

The marrow is packed with blast cells

Scanty cytoplasm
Small nucleoli

Most are small lymphoblasts

Blasts

Blood
WBC usually 5–25 × 10^{12}/l.

Childhood ALL is now potentially curable – 70% survive 5 years.

ALL in Adults
Adults have a worse prognosis and often require bone marrow transplantation as well as chemotherapy.

MYELOPROLIFERATIVE DISORDERS

In this group of diseases, neoplastic transformation of a haemopoietic precursor cell may lead to excess production of erythrocyte, leucocyte or white cell precursors. In many cases more than one element is affected. Transformation to acute leukaemia occurs in all forms. This can be summarised as follows:

In these conditions excess marrow proliferation may be seen in liver, spleen and other organs – EXTRAMEDULLARY HAEMOPOIESIS (EHM).

MYELOFIBROSIS

In this rare affection of the elderly, the haemopoietic cellular proliferation is overshadowed by progressive FIBROSIS of the marrow; SPLENOMEGALY (often of massive proportions) due to EXTRAMEDULLARY HAEMOPOIESIS is often found.

Marrow: ordinary marrow puncture usually results in a 'dry tap', therefore trephine or cutting needle biopsy is required

Total cellularity – all types of cell – very early reticulin increase.

Reticulin ++ – early fibrosis – cellularity decreasing.

Established fibrosis – only small foci of haemopoietic cells remaining.

At this stage bone changes may be seen on X-ray – OSTEOSCLEROSIS.

Blood findings

RBC low	WBC may be increased	Platelets may be increased

as marrow cells are replaced

↓

Progress to PANCYTOPENIA (this is exaggerated by enlarged spleen)

Film   *Leucoerythroblastic blood picture*

– – Nucleated reds
Poikilocytosis

– – 'Tear drop' cells

– – Abnormally large platelets

– – Myelocytes

2. MYELODYSPLASTIC SYNDROMES (MDS)

These are primary disorders of stem cells associated with several different chromosomal abnormalities. They lead to ineffective haemopoiesis of varying types, with the appearance in the peripheral blood of abnormal cells. A significant number progress to LEUKAEMIA.

449

CHAPTER 12

GENITOURINARY SYSTEM

KIDNEY – STRUCTURE AND FUNCTION

The kidney has several functions:

1. Eliminating waste products.
2. Controlling electrolyte and fluid balance.
3. Contributing to acid–base balance.

By filtering plasma and modifying the filtrate to produce urine.

It produces several hormones:

(i) *Renin*, which influences vascular tone and blood pressure.

(ii) *Erythropoietin*, which increases red blood cell production.

(iii) *1, 25 dihydroxy Vitamin D* – The active form is produced by 1α hydroxylation in the kidney. It promotes calcium absorption from the gut and is required for normal bone mineralisation.

Tests of renal function:

1. Blood analysis

Many substances will show altered values in renal failure, but the following are always elevated and are commonly used in estimating the progress of the disease.

(i) Urea – normal range 2.5–7.0 mmol/l.
(20–40 mg/100 ml)

(ii) Creatinine – 50–100 mmol/l.
(0.6–1.2 mg/100 ml)

2. Urine examination

(a) Tests for the presence of protein, red cells, haemoglobin and neutrophils in the urine. Estimation of specific gravity and measurement of urinary output.

(b) Urinary casts. These are composed of foreign elements of various types which are moulded into cylindrical form by passage along tubules and are seen on microscopy.

Protein casts (also called hyaline or colloid)

Red cell casts

Epithelial casts consisting of desquamated tubular epithelium

Granular casts; the remains of necrotic tubular cells

In jaundice, casts of bile-stained debris may be found and other solids may be seen floating freely.

(c) Other material seen on microscopy.

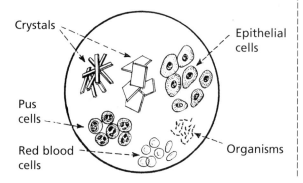

Crystals

Epithelial cells

Pus cells

Red blood cells

Organisms

3. **Clearance Tests** (typically creatinine clearance) give an indication of glomerular filtration rate: this is not absolute since some creatinine is secreted by renal tubules. The following formula is used to calculate the volume of blood cleared:

$$\text{Clearance} = \frac{UV}{P} \text{ where}$$

U = urinary concentration,
V = volume of urine per minute,
P = plasma concentration.

GLOMERULAR STRUCTURE AND FUNCTION

The glomerulus consists of an invagination of a capillary network, derived from the afferent arteriole, into Bowman's capsule – the beginning of the proximal tubule.

The glomerulus is an efficient filter with a large surface area – controlled by the structure of the glomerular capillaries.

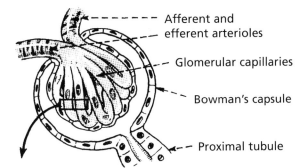

Afferent and efferent arterioles

Glomerular capillaries

Bowman's capsule

Proximal tubule

Ultrastructure

The barrier separating blood from the lumen of the nephron consists of 3 layers:

1. Endothelium (fenestrated)–
2. Basement membrane
3. Epithelium

Mesangial matrix

Capillary

Mesangial cell

Mesangial cells have three functions:
1. Contract and control blood flow
2. They are phagocytic cells and ingest proteins and immune complexes (p.101)
3. They form matrix and secrete inflammatory mediators.

These layers form a complicated sieve controlling glomerular permeability. Wide pores (70–100 nm) in the endothelium allow all components to reach the basement membrane.

The basement membrane has a strong anionic (negative) charge which repels major plasma proteins (also anionic). It has a central dense layer (lamina densa).

Foot processes

The epithelial cells are attached to the basement membrane by foot processes, separated by gaps 30–60 nm in diameter covered by a fine 'slit diaphragm'.

Filtration

The glomerular filtrate is virtually protein free plasma. Its rate of production is dependent upon:

Variation in any of these factors affects the output of urine. Diminished urinary output results from a reduction in renal blood flow as in shock, from an increase in osmotic pressure as in haemoconcentration, or from obstruction to the outflow of urine.

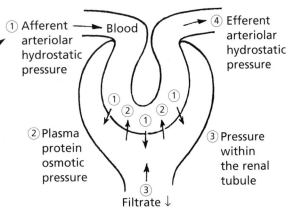

① Afferent arteriolar hydrostatic pressure

Blood

④ Efferent arteriolar hydrostatic pressure

② Plasma protein osmotic pressure

③ Pressure within the renal tubule

Filtrate ↓

GLOMERULAR DISEASES

Glomerular damage results in:
1. Reduction in urinary output.
2. Proteinuria.
3. Haematuria.

The mechanism underlying these changes is probably as follows:

Swelling of endothelium	Inflammation altering permeability of layers	Focal loss of epithelium and endothelium
↓		
Diminished blood flow		
↓	↓	↓
Reduction in urine	Proteinuria	Haematuria

These lead to 4 main clinical syndromes.

1. The NEPHRITIC SYNDROME – characterised by moderate proteinuria, haematuria, oedema, oliguria and often renal impairment. Hypertension is common.
2. The NEPHROTIC SYNDROME
   Heavy proteinuria (>3.5 g/day) ⟶ Hypoalbuminaemia ⟶ Oedema
3. RENAL FAILURE – chronic in type.
4. Asymptomatic haematuria or proteinuria

The main causes are:
(a) IMMUNE DAMAGE ⟶ GLOMERULONEPHRITIS
(b) DIABETES MELLITUS
(c) Vascular disease e.g. hypertension

The cause is best determined by renal biopsy.

The core of tissue obtained is examined by:

1. Light microscopy   **2. Immunofluorescence**   **3. Electron microscopy**

Shows   1. Increase in cells,
        2. Details of basement membrane and
        3. Mesangial matrix.

Immune complexes can be detected.
1. Linear
2. Granular

Detailed cellular and membrane damage can be seen.

The main forms of glomerular disease are described in the following pages.

ACUTE DIFFUSE PROLIFERATIVE GLOMERULONEPHRITIS

This disease classically follows 2–3 weeks after an infection – usually pharyngitis due to Group A haemolytic streptococci. It is commonest in children and young adults who develop the NEPHRITIC SYNDROME: oliguria, proteinuria, haematuria (urine is smoky and dark), moderate hypertension and facial (periorbital) oedema. This disease is now uncommon in fully developed countries.

The lesion is essentially acute inflammation of all glomeruli.

- Glomerulus large, fills capsular space: solid and cellular
- Projects into tubule

- Endothelial and mesangial cells swollen and more numerous
- Capillary lumen narrowed
- Neutrophils present

Necrosis of individual endothelial and epithelial cells occurs

Immune complexes are identified by:

1. Electron microscopy

Electron-dense granular deposits constantly seen in subepithelial position

Capillary lumen

and 2. Immunofluorescence

– demonstrates granular deposition of IgG and C3 (complement component 3)

The clinical findings can be correlated with pathology as follows:

Prognosis – The disease usually resolves in 1–2 weeks, particularly in children, but in adults complications are more common.

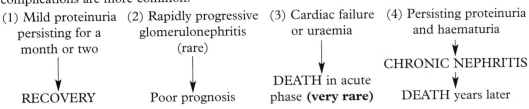

(1) Mild proteinuria persisting for a month or two → RECOVERY

(2) Rapidly progressive glomerulonephritis (rare) → Poor prognosis

(3) Cardiac failure or uraemia → DEATH in acute phase (**very rare**)

(4) Persisting proteinuria and haematuria → CHRONIC NEPHRITIS → DEATH years later

RAPIDLY PROGRESSIVE GLOMERULONEPHRITIS (RPGN)

As the name suggests, this disease progresses to end-stage renal failure in weeks or months. The histological hallmark is **crescent formation** in >50% of glomeruli. It is sometimes called 'crescentic glomerulonephritis'.

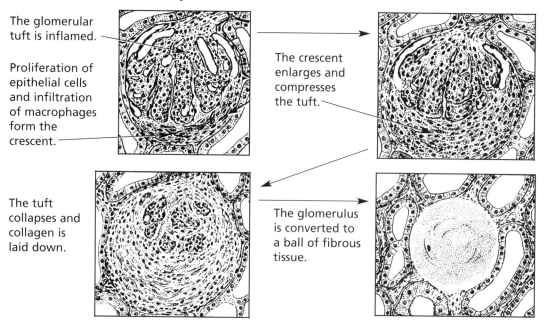

The glomerular tuft is inflamed.

Proliferation of epithelial cells and infiltration of macrophages form the crescent.

The crescent enlarges and compresses the tuft.

The tuft collapses and collagen is laid down.

The glomerulus is converted to a ball of fibrous tissue.

RPGN may complicate most types of glomerulonephritis. It occurs in several circumstances:

1. **Goodpasture's syndrome**
   In this serious disorder there is both renal and pulmonary damage. Immunofluorescence shows the cause – an antibody to type IV collagen in the glomerular basement membrane (anti-GBM) which also damages pulmonary alveolar membranes.

   IF shows linear deposits of IgG and C3 in the capillary basement membranes

Anti-GBM antibody ⟶ Renal damage (RPGN)
⟶ Lung damage (haemorrhage) } Renal and/or pulmonary failure

Note: In some cases the lungs are not affected.

RPGN may complicate:
2. **Vasculitis** – e.g. Wegener's granulomatosis, microscopic polyarteritis nodosa.
3. **Systemic Lupus Erythematosus.**
4. **Acute diffuse proliferative glomerulonephritis,** especially in adults.

Prognosis – Without treatment, most patients die within 6 months.
Immunosuppressive drugs (e.g. prednisolone, cyclophosphamide) and plasma exchange (to remove anti-GBM antibodies) improve the prognosis but many patients require dialysis or transplantation. Hypertension is a further serious complication.

MEMBRANOUS GLOMERULONEPHRITIS

This accounts for around 30% of cases of the nephrotic syndrome in adults; some patients present with asymptomatic proteinuria.

Aetiology
1. Around 85% of cases are IDIOPATHIC.
2. Drugs e.g. penicillamine and gold – in treatment of rheumatoid arthritis.
3. Tumours e.g. carcinoma of lung, melanoma.
4. Infections e.g. malaria, HIV, hepatitis B and C.

Pathology – There is generalised thickening of capillary basement membrane.

Tuft enlarges

Diffuse hyaline thickening of capillary

Glomeruli not hypercellular

Specific silver staining of the basement membrane shows a typical pattern.

Basement membrane material is increased and shows spikes

Immunofluorescence reveals deposition of IgG in the capillary walls.

Electron microscope findings explain this appearance.

Loss of foot processes

Basement membrane material between deposit ≡ spikes

Subepithelial deposits

Single layer of basement membrane

In the later stages there is a massive increase in basement membrane material.

Silver staining shows

A double-contoured basement membrane with joining spikes (rail track)

Electron microscope shows

Two layers of basement membrane

Deposits

Capillary lumen

Tubular changes – In the early stages, protein droplets and lipid globules appear in the tubular epithelium. If the disease progresses there is atrophy of the tubules and interstitial fibrosis.

Prognosis – In about 35% of patients the disease remits spontaneously, the remainder continuing to have proteinuria and in 40% chronic renal failure eventually supervenes.

MESANGIOCAPILLARY (MEMBRANOPROLIFERATIVE) GLOMERULONEPHRITIS

In this form of glomerulonephritis there is an increase both in **cells** and **mesangial matrix** within glomeruli.

Tufts are lobulated and hypercellular

Capillaries narrow

Increase of mesangium between capillaries; sometimes areas of hyalinosis

Epithelial cells swollen; occasionally crescents form

Silver staining of basement membrane

Duplication of basement membrane as in membranous glomerulonephritis, but without spikes.

These changes are due to **'mesangial interposition'**

Epithelial layer

Basement membrane

Mesangial cells growing between endothelial layer and basement membrane

A **new layer** of basement membrane is laid down

Endothelial layer

Using electron microscopy and immunofluorescence, 2 types are identified.

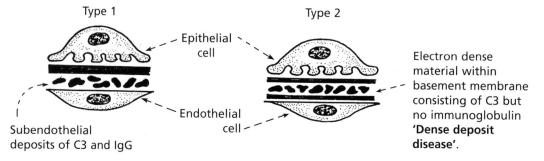

Type 1

Epithelial cell

Endothelial cell

Subendothelial deposits of C3 and IgG

Type 2

Electron dense material within basement membrane consisting of C3 but no immunoglobulin **'Dense deposit disease'**.

Aetiology
Complement activation is a feature of both forms. In Type 1 this is due to immune complexes by the classical pathway (p.99). In Type 2 there is activation by the alternative pathway by an autoantibody which stabilises C3 converting enzyme. Serum C3 is low in both forms.

Clinical features
Children and young adults are usually affected, they display the **nephrotic syndrome** or simple proteinuria or the nephritic syndrome.
In half of patients there is progression to renal failure (with hypertension) within a decade.

FOCAL GLOMERULONEPHRITIS

In contrast to the glomerular diseases discussed hitherto, focal glomerulonephritis affects only a proportion of glomeruli and only part of those glomeruli (segmental).

Major portion of glomerulus normal

Affected lobule hypercellular – mesangial proliferation

Thrombosis of capillary loops common

Adhesions to capsule develop

Red cells in capsular space

In *focal segmental* (necrotising) *glomerulonephritis*, part of the tuft becomes necrotic and there is related inflammation. Crescents are sometimes seen. This pattern is seen in:

- Systemic vasculitis, e.g. polyarteritis nodosa
- IgA nephropathy and Henoch–Schönlein purpura
- SLE (systemic lupus erythematosus)
- Some cases of Goodpasture's syndrome.

The pattern is associated with haematuria or nephrotic syndrome. Segmental lesions heal by fibrosis.

Focal Segmental Glomerulosclerosis (FSGS)

In this pattern of disease, a segment of glomerulus undergoes sclerosis without inflammation, but with an increase in mesangial matrix.

Sclerosis

Increase in mesangial matrix

Primary FSGS presents as nephrotic syndrome and despite treatment may progress to chronic renal failure: it may recur within a transplanted kidney.

Secondary FSGS may complicate a variety of preexisting conditions including those associated with focal segmental glomerulonephritis.

IgA NEPHROPATHY

This very common disease can present with microscopic haematuria, nephrotic syndrome and may lead to chronic renal failure. It typically affects young males, who often suffer recurrent episodes after upper respiratory infections.

The blood IgA level is raised and glomerular damage is due to IgA immune complexes. Sometimes crescentic glomerulonephritis is seen.

Mechanism

IgA immune ──▶ Glomeruli ──▶ **Often focal** ──▶ Activation of ──▶ **Often focal**
complexes in   **deposition**   complement (C3)   **damage**
blood

Immunofluorescence

Shows deposits of
IgA and C3 within
the mesangium: the
capillary loops are
not usually affected.

Note: The focal deposition is
dependent on the molecular
size of the complex and failure
of mesangial clearance.

Henoch–Schönlein purpura has similar renal changes but also skin rash and gastrointestinal symptoms.

MINIMAL CHANGE GLOMERULONEPHRITIS

This disorder affects any age but is the major cause of nephrotic syndrome in children. It typically responds to a short course of steroids.

Normal

Foot processes

The glomeruli are histologically normal, but electron microscopy reveals fusion of podocyte foot processes. This is a finding in many causes of proteinuria.

Minimal change

Fusion of foot
processes

CHRONIC GLOMERULONEPHRITIS (GN)

This is the end stage of many forms of glomerulonephritis.

Rapidly progressive GN   IgA nephropathy   Mesangiocapillary GN

CHRONIC GN

Membranous GN   Focal glomerulosclerosis

Pathology The kidneys are both small – granular contracted kidney.

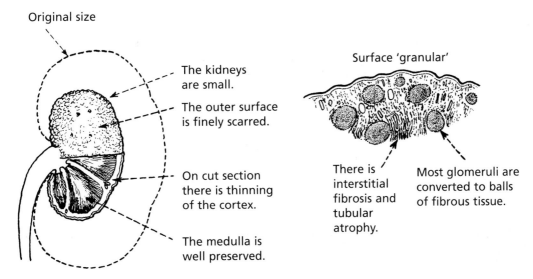

Original size

The kidneys are small.

The outer surface is finely scarred.

On cut section there is thinning of the cortex.

The medulla is well preserved.

Surface 'granular'

There is interstitial fibrosis and tubular atrophy.

Most glomeruli are converted to balls of fibrous tissue.

In chronic glomerulonephritis a vicious cycle is set up.

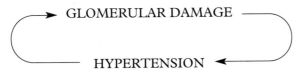

GLOMERULAR DAMAGE

HYPERTENSION

Patients may first present with chronic renal failure, or this may develop after years of glomerulonephritis.

GLOMERULONEPHRITIS – DISEASE MECHANISMS

The mechanism in most forms of GN is:

Immune complex formation → Activation of **complement** < **Cell damage** / **Neutrophil** activation → Glomerular injury

The glomerulus is central to immune complex deposition and formation due to its **fenestrated endothelium** and **high intraluminal pressure**.

Immune complexes can occur in glomeruli as follows:
1. Deposition of circulating complex.
2. In situ formation of complexes
   (a) Deposited antigens. (b) Glomerular antigens.

Localisation of complexes
This depends on the size of the complexes and their ability to penetrate the basement membrane.

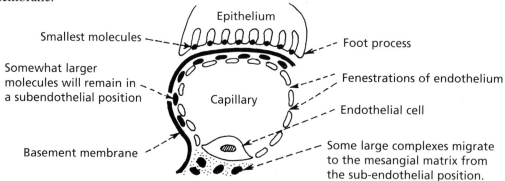

Other factors modifying the pathological changes are:
(i) Amount of antigen, (ii) Intensity of the immune reaction, (iii) Type of antibody (especially IgA), (iv) Availability of complement, (v) Degradation of complexes by macrophages and mesangial cells, (vi) Secondary tubular damage has important effects on renal function.

Note: In addition to its damaging consequences, complement activation does **solubilise complexes** allowing their disposal. Thus complement deficiency may predispose to immune complex disease e.g. in systemic lupus erythematosus (SLE).

GLOMERULAR DISEASE IN SYSTEMIC DISORDERS

SYSTEMIC LUPUS ERYTHEMATOSUS (SLE)
At least 50% of patients with SLE have clinical evidence of renal involvement, and almost all will have abnormalities on renal biopsy.

The main consequences are   (1) Proteinuria ⟶ nephrotic syndrome.
    (2) Microscopic haematuria.
    (3) Hypertension.
    (4) Progression to renal failure.

The renal changes form a spectrum.

Minimal
abnormalities

Diffuse proliferative
glomerulonephritis

Focal glomerulonephritis

MILD ⟶ **SEVERE**

On immunofluorescence, IgG, C3 are almost always present and IgA, IgM, Clq and C4 are often also seen.

AMYLOIDOSIS
The general features of amyloidosis have already been described (p.24). Amyloid is deposited around the capillary basement membranes of the glomeruli and in the renal vessels and interstitium.

Thickening of capillary basement membranes

Progressive obliteration of capillaries

Arteriolar lumen

Still patent

Severely narrowed

Gross proteinuria leading to a nephrotic syndrome is common. Interstitial fibrosis results from tubular degeneration and ischaemia due to glomerular and arteriolar lesions. Chronic renal failure results.

Parasitic glomerulopathies
The kidney and particularly the glomeruli are damaged in many parasitic infections in the tropics. **Malaria** and **schistosomiasis** are especially important.

Mechanism
Parasitic antigen + antibody (IgM in early stages; then IgG, IgE) (Immune complex)

glomerulus ⟶ membranous GN ⟶ progression to chronic GN.

Clinically
Progression from mild proteinuria ⟶ nephrotic syndrome ⎫
⟶ nephritic syndrome ⎭ ⟶ renal failure

463

THE KIDNEY and HYPERTENSION

There are two aspects to the relationship of the kidney and high blood pressure.
    (a) Many renal diseases lead to hypertension (p.197).
    (b) Hypertension leads to renal damage.

A vicious circle can be set up:

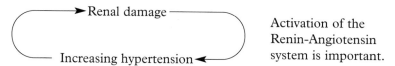

                  Renal damage   Activation of the
                                          Renin-Angiotensin
                    Increasing hypertension   system is important.

The renal consequences of benign and malignant hypertension differ, but in each, vascular changes are important.

BENIGN HYPERTENSION

Afferent arterioles   **Interlobular arteries**

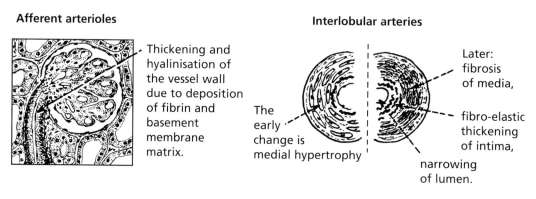

Thickening and hyalinisation of the vessel wall due to deposition of fibrin and basement membrane matrix.

The early change is medial hypertrophy

Later: fibrosis of media,

fibro-elastic thickening of intima,

narrowing of lumen.

These arteriolar changes lead to glomerular ischaemia.

Adhesions develop

Increasing fibrosis of capsule

Capillaries collapse and disappear

Late

Glomerulus completely sclerosed

The tubules atrophy and there is interstitial fibrosis.

These changes are patchy in distribution so that renal failure rarely occurs.

THE KIDNEY AND HYPERTENSION

BENIGN HYPERTENSION (*continued*)

Kidney may be slightly smaller

Surface granular with depressed dark red scars

Dilated tubules

Depressed scar

Sclerosed glomeruli

Hypertrophied glomerulus

Fibrous tissue infiltrated by lymphocytes and plasma cells

Tubules absent

It is now thought that small emboli from atheroma of the aorta are responsible for much of the scarring in benign hypertension.

MALIGNANT HYPERTENSION

In this form of hypertension, the blood pressure rises very rapidly and damages renal arteries, arterioles and glomeruli. Renal failure is common unless the disease is treated.

Afferent arterioles: the hallmark is **fibrinoid necrosis.**

Fibrinoid necrosis heals with the production of an 'onion-skin' lesion.

Escape of red cells into capsular space

Crescent formation stimulated by haemorrhage and fibrin formation

Fibrinoid necrosis of arteriole

Thrombosis extending into tuft

Interlobular arteries

Lumen reduced

Concentric fibrous layers (onion skin) in intima

Increase in medial layer

These changes account for the gross appearance.

Blotchy haemorrhages shine through capsule ('Flea bitten' kidney)

Surface smooth

Kidney normal size

Cortical haemorrhages

Occasional tiny infarct

465

CHRONIC RENAL FAILURE

Progressive renal damage in many kidney diseases eventually leads to chronic renal failure. The major causes include:

(a) Chronic glomerulonephritis.
(b) Chronic pyelonephritis and interstitial nephritis.
(c) Diabetic nephropathy.
(d) Obstructive uropathy.
(e) Polycystic kidneys.

In many cases the underlying cause cannot be determined.

The severity of renal failure is monitored by the serum urea, creatinine and by the glomerular filtration rate (GFR).

GFR (normal approximately 100 ml/min)

50 –
30 – } Mild renal failure – usually asymptomatic, hypertension may develop.
10 – } Moderate – anaemia, fatigue and hypertension.
5 – } Severe – marked fluid retention, anorexia, vomiting.
0 – } End stage – pulmonary oedema, coma, death

The rate of decline depends on the underlying cause

Compensatory mechanisms:

As nephrons are lost, the surviving nephrons show (1) COMPENSATORY HYPERTROPHY and are (2) CONTINUALLY ACTIVE with no 'down time'. (In the normal kidney, the nephrons do not all function simultaneously.)

Normal glomerulus

Afferent vessel — Efferent vessel

Filtration pressure

Compensatory hypertrophy

Dilatation

Constriction

Glomerulus is subjected to increased 'wear and tear'

Increased filtration pressure

Sclerosis

Effects of chronic renal failure:

1. WATER and ELECTROLYTE BALANCE

Loss of tubular resorptive power

↓ Glomerular filtration rate
↓
Retention of Na+ ——→ Retention of water
↓
Hypertension

↓ Excretion of K+
↓
Hyperkalaemia
↓
Cardiac arrhythmias

Urine concentration is lost – with production of urine of fixed specific gravity – 1010.

CHRONIC RENAL FAILURE

Effects of Chronic Renal Failure (*continued*)

2. DISTURBANCE OF ACID–BASE BALANCE

Reduced tubular production of ammonia \ / Reduced bicarbonate reabsorption

ACIDOSIS

Reduced excretion of H^+ ions

3. URAEMIA

The kidney also fails to excrete nitrogenous waste products, which accumulate. Although urea concentrations rise and are used to monitor renal function, retention of urea is not in itself harmful.

In uraemia, patients are lethargic. Anorexia, nausea and vomiting are common, with confusion, convulsions and death.

4. HORMONAL ABNORMALITIES

Three main hormones are involved: Erythropoietin, parathormone and vitamin D.

(i) Reduced renal mass

Reduced **erythropoietin**

ANAEMIA
(usually normochromic, normocytic)

(ii) Retention of phosphate

Hypocalcaemia

Secondary
hyperparathyroidism

(iii) Reduction of renal mass

Reduced 1α hydroxylase

Reduced vitamin D

RENAL OSTEODYSTROPHY

5. HYPERTENSION – This is almost inevitable and several consequences are possible.

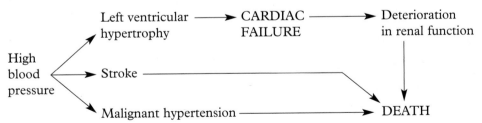

High blood pressure

Left ventricular hypertrophy ⟶ CARDIAC FAILURE ⟶ Deterioration in renal function

Stroke

Malignant hypertension ⟶ DEATH

6. **Fibrinous exudates**, e.g. **fibrinous pericarditis, 'uraemic pneumonitis' with pleural exudate, uraemic colitis.**

7. **Haemorrhagic ulcers** of the gastro-intestinal tract.

8. **Depression of immunological reaction.** Infections are common and will in turn affect renal function.

467

INFECTIONS OF THE KIDNEY

The kidney can become infected through 2 main routes.

(1) **Ascending infection** usually associated with **lower urinary tract infection** (obstruction and/or vesico-ureteric reflux are often present). This is by far the commoner route and gives rise to PYELONEPHRITIS.

(2) Blood borne (haematogenous) infection by pyogenic organisms (e.g. from septicaemia) or in tuberculosis (the latter now uncommon).

ACUTE PYELONEPHRITIS

This is an acute ascending pyogenic infection and the patient exhibits the usual general features of pyrexia, nausea, vomiting, headaches, rigors, etc., plus localising signs, e.g. frequency, dysuria, loin pain and sometimes haematuria.

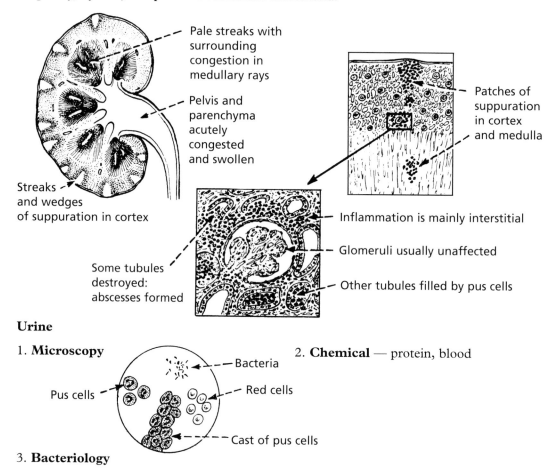

Pale streaks with surrounding congestion in medullary rays

Pelvis and parenchyma acutely congested and swollen

Streaks and wedges of suppuration in cortex

Patches of suppuration in cortex and medulla

Inflammation is mainly interstitial

Glomeruli usually unaffected

Other tubules filled by pus cells

Some tubules destroyed: abscesses formed

Urine

1. **Microscopy**

Bacteria

Pus cells

Red cells

Cast of pus cells

2. **Chemical** — protein, blood

3. **Bacteriology**

Large numbers of bacteria are found in the urine, several hundred thousand per ml in the acute phase.

The commonest infecting organism is *Escherichia coli*, but other faecal bacteria may also be found, e.g. proteus, *Streptococcus faecalis*.

ACUTE PYELONEPHRITIS

Causes

In women, cystitis is common, particularly in the sexually active. Ascending infection is often provoked by vesico-ureteric reflux during micturition. Pyelonephritis is common in pregnancy.

In men, urinary tract obstruction is usually found, typically due to prostatic enlargement. A number of causes of obstruction are seen in both sexes e.g. calculi or tumours in renal pelvis, tumours pressing on ureter, calculi in ureters and tumours of bladder.

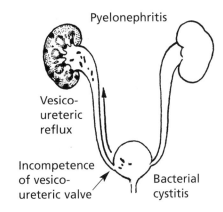

Influence of urinary tract obstruction

Obstruction of the urinary tract acts in 3 ways to promote infection:

1. The urine tends to stagnate and encourages growth of bacteria.
2. A tendency to vesico-ureteric reflux during micturition develops especially when cystitis occurs.
3. Catheterisation is commonly carried out in these cases and can introduce infection. In this case the infection is likely to be mixed.

Progress The possibilities are as follows:

Perinephric abscess and papillary necrosis are now rare due to specific antibiotic therapy.

Papillary necrosis (maximal at the kidney poles) is most apt to occur in cases associated with urinary obstruction, diabetes, analgesic nephropathy (e.g. aspirin and phenacetin), sickle cell anaemia and severe hypotension.

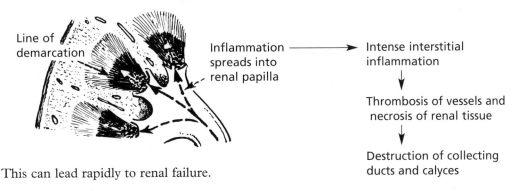

This can lead rapidly to renal failure.

CHRONIC PYELONEPHRITIS

Chronic pyelonephritis is essentially the result of repeated attacks of inflammation and healing. Vesico-ureteric reflux in early life, often associated with congenital anomalies of the urinary tract, is now regarded as important. The process can be visualised as follows:

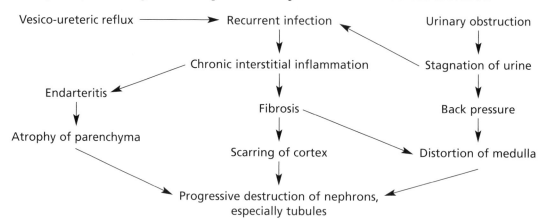

Kidney structure and function may be further prejudiced by the onset of hypertension. In cases with urinary obstruction, the external size of the kidney may remain normal or even be increased. Those with no underlying abnormality, commoner in the female, show progressive contraction of the kidney which becomes greyish white. The majority of cases are of this type.

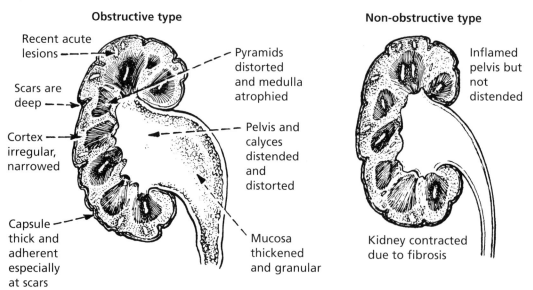

Depending on the cause, only one or both kidneys may be affected to variable degrees (c.f. chronic glomerulonephritis).

CHRONIC PYELONEPHRITIS

Microscopically, 3 types of lesion are seen in most cases:

1. Extensive interstitial fibrosis, inflammation and parenchymal loss.

2. Occasionally acute suppurative lesions due to recent infection.

Periglomerular fibrosis

Heavy chronic infiltration
Absence of tubules

Endarteritis obliterans

3. Foci of dilated tubules in the cortex. This is due to destruction of the collecting tubules so that they end blindly. Upper tubules dilate, develop colloid casts and come to resemble thyroid tissue.
The patchy inflammation results in fibrosis and atrophy irregularly distributed throughout the cortex and medulla.

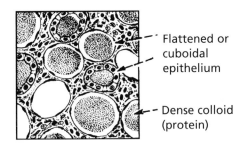

Flattened or cuboidal epithelium

Dense colloid (protein)

Clinical effects

These are due to destruction of tubules and distortion of the anatomy of the renal medulla.

1. There is a progressive loss of the renal concentrating power.

2. The sodium pump effect of the counter-current mechanism is upset (see p.475); base is lost thus causing acidosis.

Renal failure with uraemia develops, although the patient may still be passing relatively large quantitites of dilute urine. Chronic pyelonephritis is an important cause of end stage renal failure. Where unilateral obstruction is the cause only one kidney is affected and uraemia is not a feature.

3. Hypertension is common. Ninety per cent of patients are hypertensive when renal failure occurs. Malignant hypertension develops in some cases of severe chronic pyelonephritis. Where the inflammation is confined to one kidney, its removal relieves the hypertension in some cases.

TUBERCULOSIS OF THE KIDNEY

This is now uncommon in many Western countries, due to BCG vaccination for tuberculosis and the effect of specific treatment. It is due to **blood spread of infection** from another site, e.g. the lungs. Alternatively, but much less commonly, there may be an ascending infection from some other part of the genitourinary system, e.g. epididymis.

As usual, the tuberculous process develops slowly and lesions in the lungs which are the source of infection may have healed and disappeared by the time kidney damage is clinically apparent. The disease is commonly unilateral.

Stages

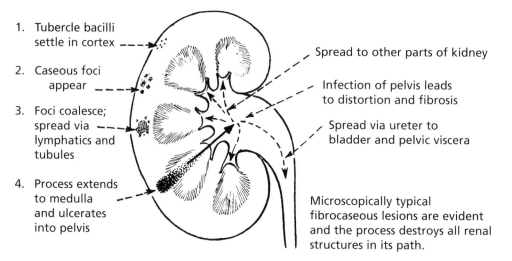

1. Tubercle bacilli settle in cortex

2. Caseous foci appear

3. Foci coalesce; spread via lymphatics and tubules

4. Process extends to medulla and ulcerates into pelvis

Spread to other parts of kidney

Infection of pelvis leads to distortion and fibrosis

Spread via ureter to bladder and pelvic viscera

Microscopically typical fibrocaseous lesions are evident and the process destroys all renal structures in its path.

Clinical features

There may be no localising features, the patient merely showing the general features of tuberculous infection – fever, night sweats and loss of weight. Lumbar discomfort or pain, dysuria and haematuria can develop. Secondary pyogenic infection is common leading to pyuria. Tubercle bacilli can usually be demonstrated in the urine either on direct microscopic examination or by culture. If, however, the ureter is blocked by caseous material, the urine, now coming solely from the uninfected kidney, may be sterile.

The danger is that infection may spread to the unaffected kidney and lead to renal failure.

INTERCURRENT RENAL CONDITIONS

DIABETES

Renal complications are common in diabetes. Up to 30% of diabetics develop proteinuria, usually after many years and may go on to chronic renal failure.

The renal lesion is essentially a special form of the 'small vessel disease' seen systemically in insulin dependent diabetes e.g. diabetic retinopathy. Rarely similar changes can be seen in non diabetics.

Diabetic glomerulosclerosis. This takes one of two forms:

Diffuse

Capsular hyaline deposits

Capsule thickened

Capillary basement membranes thickened

PAS-positive hyaline material is deposited in the mesangium in a diffuse or nodular manner

Afferent and efferent arterioles both show hyaline thickening

Nodular

Tubular atrophy

The basement membrane thickening is due to deposition of abnormally glycosylated proteins. The nodular form is often termed the Kimmelstiel–Wilson lesion. Progressive closure of capillaries can occur together with fibrous obliteration of the capsular space and the whole glomerulus. Haemodynamic changes, especially hyperfiltration, lead to sclerosis. Secondary tubular atrophy follows.

Clinical effects

Screening for microalbuminuria is important to detect early disease. Proteinuria may result in the nephrotic syndrome. Hypertension leads to further renal damage: control of blood pressure, and of diabetes itself, is important to delay the onset of renal failure.

Pyelonephritis

This is common in diabetes and may be complicated by papillary necrosis.

Atheroma

This disease is common in the renal arteries and their branches in diabetes. It increases the renal ischaemia.

INTERCURRENT RENAL CONDITIONS

RENAL FUNCTION AND PREGNANCY

Four conditions affecting renal function may arise in pregnancy.

1. **Acute pyelonephritis** is relatively common, possibly due to (a) the effects of uterine pressure on the ureters and (b) relaxation of smooth muscle allowing ureteric dilatation and reflux.

2. **Pre-eclampsia and eclampsia.** This is a syndrome characterised by hypertension, increasing unselective proteinuria and oedema. Placental ischaemia with stimulation of vasoconstriction leads to disseminated intravascular coagulation (DIC). The essential kidney lesion is glomerular; tubular changes are secondary.

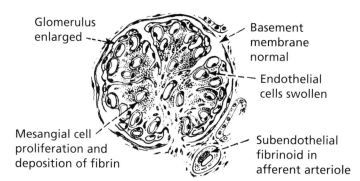

Glomerulus enlarged

Basement membrane normal

Endothelial cells swollen

Mesangial cell proliferation and deposition of fibrin

Subendothelial fibrinoid in afferent arteriole

EM examination shows mesangial deposits of fibrin, fibrinogen, IgM and complement.

The lesion appears to resolve rapidly after parturition. So far as kidney function is concerned, the danger of eclampsia lies in the occasional development of acute renal failure from (3) and (4) below.

In addition there is often severe liver damage and cerebral injury indicated first by convulsions.

3. **Acute tubular necrosis.** This is associated with complications of pregnancy causing SHOCK e.g. septic abortion, retroplacental haemorrhage and postpartum haemorrhage.

4. In more severe cases **bilateral cortical necrosis** may occur especially if disseminated intravascular coagulation (DIC) is superadded.

RENAL TUBULE – STRUCTURE AND FUNCTION

The renal tubules modify the glomerular filtrate. Initially isotonic and neutral, it becomes hypertonic and quite strongly acid. Within 24 hours, 180 litres of filtrate are reduced to 1.5 litres of urine. The main functions of this process are:
- (a) to get rid of waste products, particularly those of protein metabolism.
- (b) to aid in maintaining the normal acid–base balance.
- (c) to conserve fluid, electrolytes and other essential substances.

Three mechanisms are involved:
1. Active absorption of substances from the filtrate by the tubular epithelium.
2. Passive interchange between the filtrate and the interstitial tissues to maintain osmotic equilibrium.
3. Secretion by the tubular epithelium.

Note: 1. Active reabsorption requires energy, and there is a limit to the capacity of the process – maximal tubular capacity (Tm). When this is exceeded, the particular substance involved will appear in the urine. Glucose is an example. In diabetes, the amount of glucose in the filtrate far exceeds the absorptive capacity, and glycosuria results.

    2. **Urinary acidification**

        H ions, excreted by distal tubule, take part in 3 reactions:

        1. $H + HCO_3 = H_2 CO_3$
        2. $H + NH_3 Cl = NH_4 Cl$ ⎫ Urinary excretory products
        3. $H + HPO_4 + Na = NaH_2 PO_4$ ⎭

Effects of tubular damage

Damage to the tubules results in gross biochemical changes.
1. Loss of mechanisms controlling balance of electrolytes, water and urea.
2. Upset in acid–base balance.
3. Loss of substances in urine normally completely or almost completely reabsorbed – glucose, potassium, amino acids.

Glomerular lesions and pathological changes in the renal pelvis also upset tubular function by interfering with blood supply.

ACUTE TUBULAR NECROSIS

This arises in 2 circumstances:

1. During a state of shock, e.g. due to haemorrhage, burns, trauma, acute intestinal obstruction, incompatible transfusion and acute pancreatitis.
2. Following administration of toxic substances, e.g. carbon tetrachloride, cis-platinum, lithium, mercury, and various drugs e.g. antibiotics.

The gross appearance of the kidneys is the same in both groups, although the type and distribution of the lesions are different.

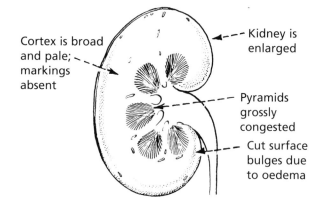

Cortex is broad and pale; markings absent

Kidney is enlarged

Pyramids grossly congested

Cut surface bulges due to oedema

Shock cases

The lesions are the result of ischaemia, and this determines the part of the kidney affected and the portion of the tubule damaged.

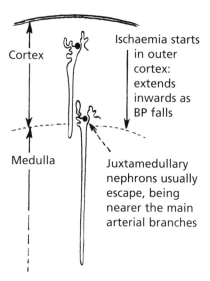

Cortex

Ischaemia starts in outer cortex: extends inwards as BP falls

Medulla

Juxtamedullary nephrons usually escape, being nearer the main arterial branches

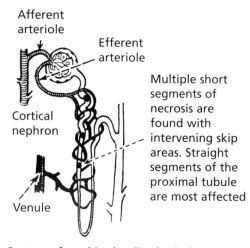

Afferent arteriole

Efferent arteriole

Cortical nephron

Multiple short segments of necrosis are found with intervening skip areas. Straight segments of the proximal tubule are most affected

Venule

Casts are found in the distal tubules, protein, haemoglobin or myoglobin according to the cause.

ACUTE TUBULAR NECROSIS

Toxic cases

The lesions are evenly distributed, affecting all nephrons. They are maximal in the proximal tubules and are the direct result of the poison, the action of which is intensified by the concentrating activity of the tubule.

Degenerate proximal tubules containing debris

Normal distal tubule

Clinical effects

There are two clinical phases:

1. *Oliguria*

The glomerular filtration rate is greatly reduced due to reduced renal blood flow. Unselective reabsorption of the filtrate occurs through the damaged tubule. The effects are:

Reduced GFR   Tubular damage

Retention of non-protein nitrogen

Retention of fluid

Upset in electrolyte balance

Acidosis due to inability to control hydrogen ion concentration of urine

Uraemia

Danger of pulmonary oedema

Hyperkalaemia

Possible cardiac arrest

2. *Diuresis*

This occurs following healing of the lesions. The damaged tubular epithelium is replaced by a simple type which has not yet developed selective activities. Large volumes of dilute urine are passed. The clinical results are:

Absence of concentration

Continued retention of non-protein nitrogen

Loss of electrolytes including K^+

Loss of fluid

Upset in acid–base balance

Possible cardiac irregularity

Dehydration

Provided the patient can be maintained by countering the various biochemical upsets, the prognosis is good. The tubular epithelium has a great capacity for regeneration and ultimately regains its selective powers.

TUBULO-INTERSTITIAL DISEASES

In this group of disorders there is damage to the renal tubules and to the interstitial tissues. The main forms are:

    (a) Acute tubular necrosis
    (b) Infection – Pyelonephritis   } Pages 469, 476, 477
    (c) Interstitial nephritis.
    (d) Metabolic conditions – e.g. gout, nephrocalcinosis, hypokalaemia.
    (e) Myeloma cast nephropathy.
    (f) Renal tubular abnormalities.

TUBULO-INTERSTITIAL NEPHRITIS

This occurs in 2 forms – acute and chronic, both typically associated with an immunological reaction to drugs.

ACUTE: Symptoms develop 10–14 days after exposure to drugs e.g. methicillin and NSAIDs e.g. mefenamic acid. Patients are febrile, there is haematuria, proteinuria. Arthralgia is common. Renal impairment varies in severity – may cause ACUTE RENAL FAILURE.

Pathology

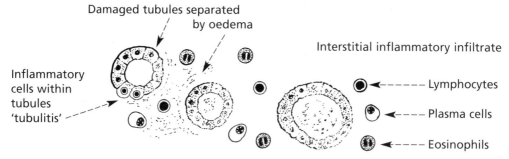

Prognosis   (i)   Complete remission may follow withdrawal of drug and/or treatment with steroids.
        (ii)   Continuing exposure ⟶ chronic renal impairment.

CHRONIC: Long-standing interstitial nephritis leads to interstitial fibrosis, inflammation and continuing tubular damage with tubular loss and atrophy. Many patients present with chronic renal failure. In many cases no definite underlying cause can be found. One such example is 'Balkan nephropathy' found in the river Danube valley perhaps due to ingestion of fungal toxins.

ANALGESIC NEPHROPATHY

This is a distinctive disorder caused by long term exposure to analgesics e.g. phenacetin (historically) and NSAIDs.
Interstitial inflammation and tubular damage may proceed rapidly to papillary necrosis (p.469).
There is an associated increased risk of transitional cell carcinoma of the kidney and ureter (p.487).

TUBULAR LESIONS OF METABOLIC ORIGIN

This type of lesion is brought about by a metabolic defect which may arise outside the kidney (primary) or be the result of renal dysfunction (secondary).

The basic pathological mechanism is very similar in many of the conditions:

High plasma concentration of metabolite → Appearance in glomerular filtrate → Concentration and precipitation

Necrosis of tubules → Interstitial fibrosis

Formation of calculi → Secondary inflammation and other complications

Progressive renal damage and failure

The following are some examples:

(a) **Hypercalcaemic nephritis**

Calcium is deposited in tubular epithelial cells with subsequent fibrosis and calcification – **nephrocalcinosis.**

The usual causes of hypercalcaemia are malignant tumours, primary hyperparathyroidism, hypervitaminosis D and sarcoidosis.

(b) **Urate nephropathy** occurs in patients with long standing **gout**.

Increased primary secretion of uric acid leads to uric acid crystal formation in the acid environment of the distal tubule.

The tubular wall is destroyed

Interstitial giant cell reaction and fibrosis Nephron loss

(c) **Myeloma cast nephropathy**

This is dealt with on pages 438 and 439.

RENAL TUBULAR ACIDOSIS

The tubules, either due to an inherited defect or to damage secondary to other renal diseases, are unable to produce an acid urine.

There are 2 main forms:
1. In Type I the defect is in the distal tubule.
2. In Type II the function of the proximal tubule is abnormal and there are usually other abnormalities in addition to acidosis e.g. in the Fanconi syndrome there is aminoaciduria, glycosuria and hypophosphataemia.

HAEMOLYTIC URAEMIC SYNDROME

This is a rare complication of many apparently dissimilar conditions. The mechanism appears to be as follows:

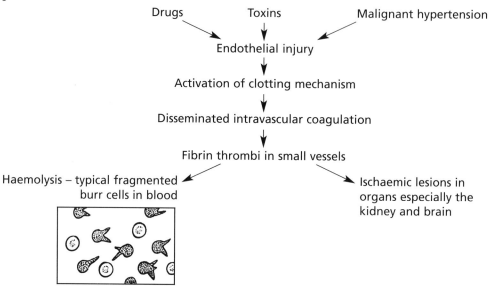

The renal lesions are similar to those seen in malignant hypertension. There is fibrinoid necrosis of the afferent arterioles and capillaries of the glomeruli, and resulting areas of tubular necrosis. In the most extreme cases, bilateral cortical necrosis of the kidneys may occur. The underlying pathology is sometimes termed thrombotic microangiopathy. Clinical manifestations are varied. Renal failure, haemolytic anaemia, hypertension, and sometimes purpura with thrombocytopenia are the main features, but lesions in other organs and the symptoms of the initiating disease produce a complicated picture.

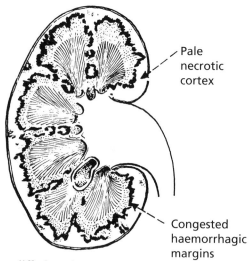

Aetiology

Activation of the clotting system can occur in many differing circumstances:

1. In children there is a close association with alimentary infections: particularly by *E. coli* 0157 which produces a verocytotoxin.

2. Shock conditions, e.g. following abruptio placentae in pregnancy, endotoxic shock.

3. Malignant hypertension. This can be a sequel to the syndrome and equally can predispose the patient to it.

4. Drugs e.g. contraceptive pill, immunosuppressive drugs.

PATHOLOGICAL COMPLICATIONS OF END-STAGE THERAPIES

The prognosis of end-stage renal failure has been greatly improved by (1) Dialysis and
(2) Renal Transplantation. The following possible pathological complications are important:

1. Dialysis

(a) *Haemodialysis*

    (i) **Local** – infection and thrombosis at site of vessel access.

    (ii) **Systemic** – aluminium toxicity: historically, severe dementia or severe osteomalacia
was caused by using water containing excess aluminium. Aluminium and other
impurities are now removed.
In some cases of long-standing dialysis, small amounts of absorbed aluminium may
be associated with mild mental deterioration.
Amyloidosis affecting synovial tissues (e.g. carpal tunnel syndrome: joint stiffness)
due to raised circulating β_2 microglobulin.

(b) **Continuous Ambulatory Peritoneal Dialysis (CAPD)** – peritonitis: especially due to
Staphylococci, Gram –ve organisms and fungi.

2. Renal transplantation

Rejection is the main complication, depending on the extent of HLA matching between
donor and recipient. The Banff classification is used to type rejection. There are four forms
of rejection:

(a) *Hyperacute rejection* – within minutes or hours
Pre-existing antibodies ⟶ Binding to ⟶ Thrombosis
against donor HLA or ABO   endothelial cells   and necrosis

(b) *Acute cellular rejection* – within days to months (Banff type I)
Cell mediated response ⟶ Interstitial lymphocytic ⟶ Tubular
against donor cells   infiltrate and 'tubulitis'   destruction

(c) *Acute vascular rejection* – days to months (Banff types II and III)
Cell mediated immune ⟶ Infiltration of vessel wall by ⟶ Thrombosis
response to epithelial cells   lymphocytes 'endotheliitis'   and necrosis

(d) *Chronic rejection* – months to years
Continuation of ⟶ Vascular occlusion, ⟶ Ischaemia and
immune attack   glomerular sclerosis   renal failure

Other complications

1. Cyclosporin toxicity
2. Opportunistic infections   } Associated with therapeutic immuno-suppression.
3. Increased incidence of
tumours, particularly
LYMPHOMAS

Note: Many lymphoproliferative disorders are due to
Epstein–Barr virus infection and some respond to
reduction in immuno-suppressive therapy.

4. Recurrence of original renal disease e.g. IgA nephritis in transplanted kidney.

Note: Similar complications occur in other transplant situations.

CONGENITAL DISORDERS

Malpositions and malformations of the kidney are relatively common and the variations are numerous. Some of the commoner are:

1. Ectopic kidney (pelvic kidney)

One or both kidneys fail to reach the normal adult position. The condition causes difficulty:

(a) During parturition
(b) In differential diagnosis of pelvic neoplasms and infections
(c) When the renal artery originates at the normal level and the long vessel creates problems in arterial supply.

2. Fusion of kidneys

This is usually partial, producing the so-called 'horse-shoe' kidney. The ureters may be partially obstructed leading to hydronephrosis, infection and calculus formation. Frequently the kidneys are also ectopic, adding another hazard.

3. Single kidney

This may be a form of fusion and there may be two ureters. In other cases, there is absence (agenesis) of one kidney, usually the left. There is no interference with renal function unless, of course, the single kidney becomes diseased.

4. Bilateral agenesis (Potter's syndrome)

This is incompatible with life. The affected infants have a distinctive appearance, with low set ears, receding chin, parrot beak nose and wide set eyes.

POLYCYSTIC KIDNEY DISEASE

This occurs in two main forms:

1. Adult polycystic disease (APKD)

This is relatively common, and varying degrees of the change may be seen from single cysts up to the classical type where the kidneys are converted into a mass of cysts.
It is an inherited autosomal dominant trait due to two genes, PKD-1 (85% of cases) which encodes a protein polycystin-1, and PKD-2 (15%) associated with milder disease.

Kidney greatly enlarged:
(often exceeds 1 kg)

Cysts vary in size
(largest 5 or 6 cm)

Many are brownish
(fluid serous or mucoid)

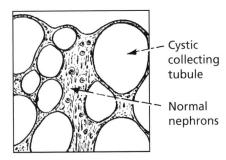

Cystic collecting tubule

Normal nephrons

The precise defect is unclear, with cyst formation in some of the collecting tubules, causing a mixture of normal and abnormal nephrons. Cystic change develops after birth and is progressive, resulting in atrophy of normal nephrons by pressure.

Intrahepatic cysts are often present but rarely numerous. Death from cerebral haemorrhage is more frequent than expected, partly due to the hypertension secondary to the kidney disorder and in some cases to aneurysms of cerebral arteries.

Clinical Findings
(a) Usually discovered during 3rd and 4th decades, rarely in childhood.
(b) Atrophy of the normal nephrons leads to chronic renal failure, and hypertension.
    Progress varies with the number of normal nephrons.

2. Infantile polycystic disease (Polycystic kidney of the newborn)

This is a rare condition.

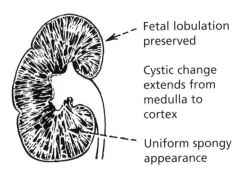

Fetal lobulation
preserved

Cystic change
extends from
medulla to
cortex

Uniform spongy
appearance

The nephrons are said to be normal in number and formation. Cystic dilatation is situated in the terminal branches of the collecting tubules. The disease, if severe, is incompatible with life, and death occurs shortly after birth. It is due to an autosomal recessive trait. Congenital hepatic fibrosis often coexists.

RENAL CALCULI

Three basic types of renal calculi are recognised.

 ← Surface is rough; colour brown, probably due to old blood pigment

← Smooth light brown colour

←-- Flaking surface, greyish white

(1) **Calcium oxalate** (80%)

(2) **Uric acid and urates** (5%)

(3) **Triple phosphates** (magnesium, ammonium and calcium) (15%)

Commonly the stones are mixed.

Sites of formation:
Precipitates form in the collecting tubules and pass into the renal pelvis where they enlarge.

Mode of formation. This is complex, but the the following theory is likely:

Excess excretion of stone substance (e.g. oxalate) + Calcium

↓

Supersaturated solution of salt

Bacteria e.g. nanobacteria

↓

Initiating nidus of calcium

← Lack of substances keeping calcium salts in solution (magnesium, phosphates, etc.)

← Lack of inhibitors of crystal formation

Precipitation and stone formation

Predisposing factors

1. **Urinary pH**. Urate and oxalate stones form in an acid urine; phosphate stones in alkaline urine.
2. **Dehydration** – causing increased urinary concentration.
3. **Stasis.** Obstruction to urine flow encourages salt precipitation.
4. **Renal disease.** The pH of the urine is frequently disturbed, and the composition of the urine is always altered.

Renal infection is one of the most important factors. In many cases of renal sepsis, the urine becomes alkaline, favouring phosphate precipitation. Ischaemia causing degeneration and necrosis induces calcification in many chronic renal diseases, and this may lead to stone formation.

RENAL CALCULI

Predisposing factors (*continued*)

5. **Metabolic factors.** These can operate by altering the pH of the urine and especially by increasing the output of substances e.g.
    (a) Hypercalcuria and hyperphosphaturia. These may be caused by:
    Hyperparathyroidism, primary or secondary to renal failure
    Vitamin D overdosage
    Diet, e.g. excessive milk and alkalis over years in peptic ulcer cases
    Immobilisation leading to loss of calcium from bones.
    (b) Oxaluria. Due to:
    Congenital metabolic defect
    Poisoning by ethylene glycol.
    (c) Urate excess
    (d) Rare stones, e.g. cystine, xanthine, are related to inborn metabolic defects.

Effects and complications

These are related to passage of the stone and develop in two situations.

(1) Passage of small stone → Injury to ureter
↓ ↓
Colic Stricture
↓
Subsequent impaction of stone

(2) Passage of larger stone → Impaction (at upper and lower ends of ureter, or at brim of pelvis)
↓
Stasis
↙ ↘
Hydronephrosis Infection

With the development of stasis and infection, further stone formation is encourgaged. This can lead to some peculiar results, e.g.:

Staghorn calculus

This large single stone is associated with suppuration and ulceration of the pelvis and calyces. It is composed mainly of phosphates.

Stones and infection in the pelvis can lead to squamous metaplasia of the epithelium. In a few instances this may develop into squamous carcinoma.

BLADDER CALCULI

These may have passed down the ureter. In the bladder they can increase greatly in size. Cystitis is common and the enlargement is due to deposit of phosphates. Stones may actually form in the bladder when there is urethral obstruction and chronic cystitis.

TUMOURS OF THE KIDNEY

MALIGNANT TUMOURS

Three are of importance: renal cell carcinoma, transitional cell carcinoma and nephroblastoma.

Renal cell carcinoma

This is the commonest primary malignant renal tumour. It usually has a typical appearance.

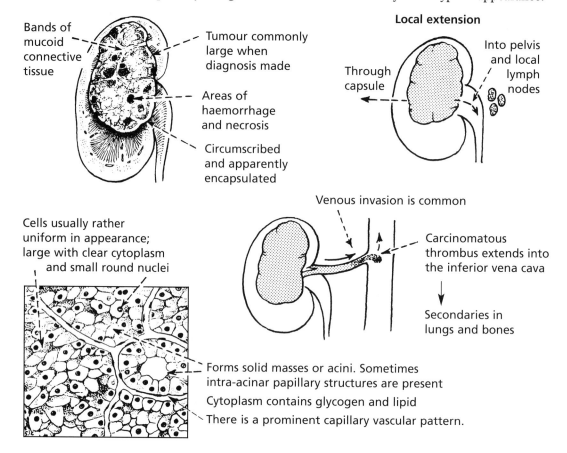

Local extension

Bands of mucoid connective tissue

Tumour commonly large when diagnosis made

Through capsule

Into pelvis and local lymph nodes

Areas of haemorrhage and necrosis

Circumscribed and apparently encapsulated

Venous invasion is common

Cells usually rather uniform in appearance; large with clear cytoplasm and small round nuclei

Carcinomatous thrombus extends into the inferior vena cava

Secondaries in lungs and bones

Forms solid masses or acini. Sometimes intra-acinar papillary structures are present

Cytoplasm contains glycogen and lipid

There is a prominent capillary vascular pattern.

Aetiology: Renal cell carcinoma is associated with:
(a) Cigarette smoking,
(b) Obesity,
(c) Cystic change in patients on haemodialysis,
(d) Genetic predisposition e.g. the von Hippel–Lindau syndrome (renal cysts, cerebellar haemangioblastoma) – associated with a gene on chromosome 3.

Systemic effects

Rarely, patients with renal carcinoma show:
  (i) Hypercalcaemia – parathyroid related hormone peptide production (PTHrP).
 (ii) Hypertension – increased renin production by tumour or in adjacent kidney.
(iii) Polycythaemia – increased erythropoietin.

TUMOURS OF THE KIDNEY

Malignant tumours (*continued*)

Transitional cell carcinoma
This tumour arises from the epithelium of the renal pelvis and is similar to the commoner transitional cell carcinoma of the bladder, with which it shares aetiological factors.

Patients usually present with haematuria.

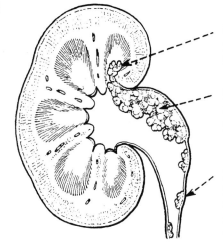

Invasion into renal parenchyma is often seen.

Papillary tumour arising in renal pelvis.

Multiple tumours may be seen in the ureter – representing a field change.
At surgery the entire ureter is usually resected.

Nephroblastoma (Wilms' tumour)
This is one of the commonest malignant tumours of childhood. It is an embryonic type of tumour derived from kidney rudiments, and forms a large well-circumscribed growth which rapidly invades blood vessels, giving rise to pulmonary secondaries. With modern therapy 90% long-term survival rates are achieved.

There may be skeletal muscle differentiation.

Much of the tumour consists of spindle cells resembling sarcoma

This merges with tubules and acini

Occasionally there are primitive glomerular structures

Mutation of a gene (WT-1) on chromosome 11 appears to be responsible for the development of this tumour.

BENIGN TUMOURS
1. **Fibroma.** This is the commonest simple tumour arising from interstitial cells. It is found incidentally at autopsy in the medulla as a tiny round white nodule, usually less than 1 cm in diameter.
2. **Adenoma.** This is a small nodular proliferation of tubular type epithelium. Histologically they are similar to renal cell carcinomas. It is arbitrarily stated that a tumour smaller than 2 cm in diameter is benign: larger than 3 cm may behave as a metastasising carcinoma.

DISEASES OF THE URINARY TRACT

The urinary tract is essentially a collecting and discharge system. There are 4 main pathological processes affecting its function: (1) obstruction, (2) infection, (3) calculus formation and (4) neoplastic disease.

Congenital anomalies, which are relatively rare, produce their effects by one or other of these processes.

Obstruction

Acute obstruction, if complete, causes rapid cessation of urine production. If both kidneys are involved, renal failure quickly follows. Chronic obstruction is more common and leads to anatomical changes, with sequels.

Hydronephrosis

This is a dilatation of the renal pelvis and calyces, due to chronic incomplete or intermittent obstruction.

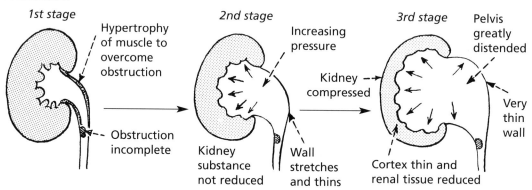

1st stage — Hypertrophy of muscle to overcome obstruction — Obstruction incomplete

2nd stage — Increasing pressure — Kidney substance not reduced — Wall stretches and thins

3rd stage — Kidney compressed — Pelvis greatly distended — Very thin wall — Cortex thin and renal tissue reduced

Microscopically, there is tubular atrophy and glomerular scarring. Superimposed infection is common and aggravates the renal damage.

Aetiology

The condition may affect one or both kidneys. This is related to the site of obstruction.

Unilateral obstruction: above the bladder

Common sites:
1. Pelvi-ureteric junction.
2. At pelvic brim.
3. At entrance to bladder.

Causes:
1. Calculus.
2. Tumour growth.
3. Inflammatory stricture.
4. Congenital abnormality.

Gross hydronephrosis is more commonly unilateral.

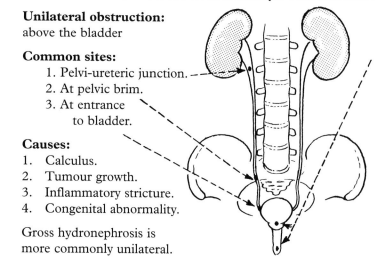

Bilateral obstruction: in or around bladder or urethra. The ureters are also affected and become dilated and tortuous.

Causes:
1. Prostatic enlargement.
2. Tumour of bladder.
3. Urethral stricture.
4. Pelvic neoplasm.
5: Retroperitoneal fibrosis.

URINARY TRACT INFECTION

Pyelonephritis has already been considered. Inflammation of the ureters is due to extension upwards from an infection of the bladder and urethra.

Acute cystitis

The bladder shows the usual signs of inflammation. Small haemorrhages are common in the oedematous mucosa. The following points are important:

1. It is common in females, especially frequent in pregnancy: and also associated with sexual intercourse.
2. In males it is usually secondary to obstruction, e.g. due to enlarged prostate or a urethral stricture.
3. Obstruction encourages infection, enhances its effects and prolongs the inflammatory process.
4. In non-obstructive cases, infection is usually due to *E. coli*. Mixed infections, proteus and staphylococcus, are common in obstructive cases.
5. Vesicoureteric reflux is very important allowing retrograde spread of infection to the kidneys. It occurs as a congenital defect in children but also may be secondary to cystitis.

Chronic cystitis

This is the result of repeated attacks of acute cystitis, but it is usually associated with obstruction of the urethra causing stasis of urine.

Mixed infection including *B. proteus* is common and, together with urea-splitting organisms forming ammonia, result in an alkaline urine. Phosphates precipitate and can form crumbling whitish calculi.

Tuberculous cystitis

This is always secondary to a tuberculous infection elsewhere, usually in the kidney. Less commonly, the epididymis is the source of infection. Small tubercles form in the submucous layer, usually at the bladder base. These ulcerate and secondary infection is common.

Urethritis

Acute inflammation of the urethra is commonly due to the gonococcus, but another form is now more common in Western countries: so-called non-specific urethritis is often due to chlamydia infection.

In Reiter's syndrome, in addition to urethritis, there is arthritis and conjunctivitis.

Schistosomiasis

Infection of the bladder with *Schistosoma haematobium* results in chronic granulomatous inflammation with urinary obstruction and haematuria. There is a strong association with the development of squamous cell carcinoma of the bladder.

TUMOURS OF THE URINARY TRACT

Transitional cell carcinomas occur in the bladder, ureters and renal pelvis. They arise from the stratified transitional epithelium lining the tract and are all considered to be CARCINOMAS but show a wide spectrum of malignant potential. They are graded I to III as follows, according to the World Health Organisation (WHO) classification.

GRADE I – These are **Papillary Tumours.** Tumours at the benign end of the spectrum have a uniform, well-differentiated epithelial covering showing no mitotic activity. They have a slender stalk and delicate branching fronds. With this structure, and their fine vascular connective tissue, haemorrhage is common.

GRADE II – These also are **Papillary.** The stalk of the tumour is broader and the epithelial cells show mitoses and variability. Early stromal invasion may be present.

The adjacent epithelium may show dysplasia

GRADE III are solid sessile tumours: They are distinguished by the degree of cellular anaplasia, mitotic activity and aggressive growth. Infection with ulceration and necrosis is common: local penetration into the bladder muscle and lymphatic invasion are usual. Squamous carcinoma and adenocarcinoma are rare tumours. Rhabdomyosarcoma may occur in the bladder in children.

Aetiology
Bladder tumours are an industrial hazard:
(a) in aniline dye manufacture due to beta-naphthylamine
(b) in the rubber industry
(c) in manufacturing processes involving benzene.

SMOKING and CHRONIC ANALGESIC ABUSE are important associations. In the MIDDLE EAST chronic infestation by **Schistosoma haematobium** is an important association, particularly with squamous carcinoma.

Mechanism

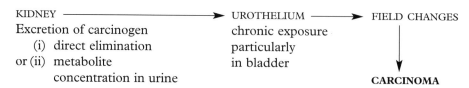

Note: (i) Urothelial tumours are often multiple and recurrence is common: long term surveillance is important.
(ii) Progression from a low grade to higher grades is frequent.

FEMALE GENITAL TRACT – ANATOMY AND PHYSIOLOGY

The ovaries, fallopian tubes, uterus, vagina and vulva form an integrated system which is unique in that full function is limited to a period of roughly 40 years from puberty to menopause. A two-tier system of hormonal control operates. Secretion of steroids by the ovary prepares the uterus for pregnancy, and the ovarian secretion is controlled by the anterior pituitary and hypothalamus.

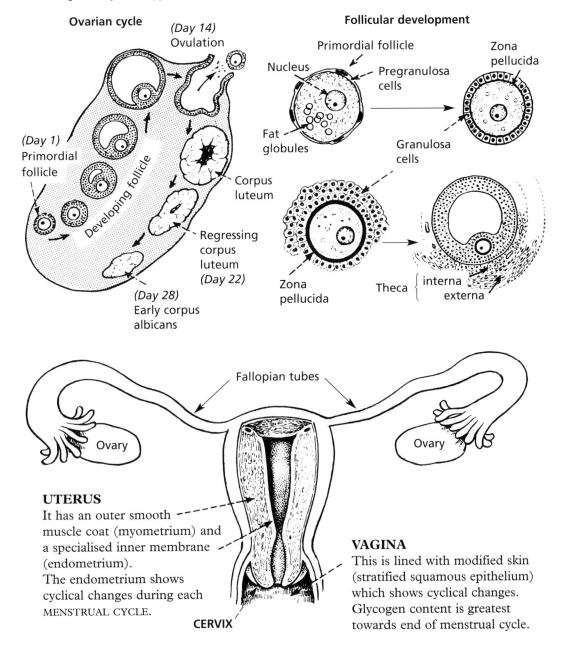

Ovarian cycle

(Day 14) Ovulation

(Day 1) Primordial follicle

Developing follicle

Corpus luteum

Regressing corpus luteum (Day 22)

(Day 28) Early corpus albicans

Follicular development

Primordial follicle

Nucleus

Pregranulosa cells

Zona pellucida

Fat globules

Granulosa cells

Zona pellucida

Theca { interna externa

Fallopian tubes

Ovary

Ovary

UTERUS
It has an outer smooth muscle coat (myometrium) and a specialised inner membrane (endometrium).
The endometrium shows cyclical changes during each MENSTRUAL CYCLE.

CERVIX

VAGINA
This is lined with modified skin (stratified squamous epithelium) which shows cyclical changes. Glycogen content is greatest towards end of menstrual cycle.

CYCLICAL ENDOMETRIAL CHANGES

Menstruation

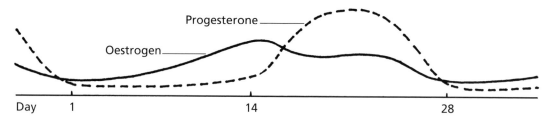

Proliferation   Secretion   Regression

Day   0   1   3   4   14   23   28

ASSOCIATED OVARIAN STEROID SECRETION

Progesterone

Oestrogen

Day   1   14   28

Proliferative phase
This is induced by oestrogen produced by developing ovarian follicles, stimulated by FSH from the pituitary.

Stromal cells, narrow spindles to begin with, become plump

Epithelium is cuboidal, growing taller as ovulation is approached

Glands are simple, narrow tubes dilating prior to ovulation. (Triggered by a surge of FSH and LH)

Secretory phase
Progesterone produced by the corpus luteum stimulates secretion by the glands. Oestrogen is also produced. The stromal cells enlarge (pseudo-decidual change), oedema is present and vascularity greatly increased.

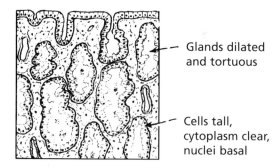

Glands dilated and tortuous

Cells tall, cytoplasm clear, nuclei basal

Premenstrual regressive phase
Endometrial growth ceases 5–6 days before menstruation. Prior to menstruation, it shrinks due to decreased blood flow and discharge of secretion. This increases the tortuosity of glands and blood vessels.

DISEASES OF THE ENDOMETRIUM

Endometritis is now an unusual condition.

Acute infection is almost confined to infection associated with parturition and abortion – often related to retention of products of conception. Historically, criminal abortion in non-sterile conditions led to severe infection. Gonococcal infection does not commonly extend beyond the cervix but can lead to acute endometritis. Chlamydia may cause acute or chronic endometritis.

Chronic endometritis
This is a rare lesion as a primary condition. It can follow an acute endometritis which may be mild. The uterine changes occur in 2 phases:

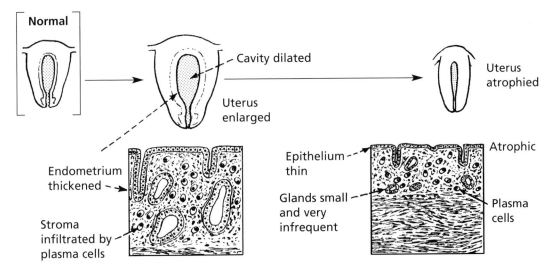

The normal cyclical changes may fail to take place.

Tuberculous endometritis
This is now uncommon in the British Isles. It is the result of infection spreading from the fallopian tubes. If the patient is still menstruating, the tubercles are shed each month: diagnostic curettage should be done as late in the cycle as possible to allow new tubercles to develop. In some cases, menstruation ceases and caseation occurs.

Intrauterine anti-fertility devices
A mild chronic inflammation may be associated with the use of these devices. There may be focal atrophy with mild plasma cell infiltration. Irregular bleeding may result.

Oral contraceptives
These are commonly a combination of an oestrogen with a progestogen. They tend to induce atrophy of the endometrium, the glands becoming small, inactive and infrequent. The stroma appears relatively abundant and progestogen-containing devices cause stromal decidualisation.

DISEASES OF THE ENDOMETRIUM

ENDOMETRIOSIS
This consists of deposits of endometrium outside the uterine cavity.

In most cases, the disease is confined to the pelvis and the genital tract.

Sites:
Fallopian tube
Ovary
Broad ligament
Surface of uterus

Other sites: Caecum and appendix, bladder, rectum, umbilicus, laparotomy scar.

These deposits react to the stimulus of ovarian steroids and show cyclical changes. The result is haemorrhage into the local tissues at the time of menstruation. Adhesions develop, often leading to infertility. Malignant change to endometrioid adenocarcinoma occurs uncommonly.

Aetiology
In some instances deposits are formed in laparotomy scars after uterine operations, but in most cases there has been no surgical interference. Three theories have been proposed.

1. Retrograde spill of menstrual debris – perhaps the most favoured.
2. Metaplasia of tissues into Müllerian duct elements.
3. Lymphatic and blood borne emboli of endometrial tissue.

ADENOMYOSIS
This is a condition of ectopic endometrial deposits in the myometrium. There is an accompanying overgrowth of muscle and connective tissue. Two macroscopic forms occur:

1. **Diffuse**
   Deposits are confined to inner part of myometrium. Foci of endometrium often brownish in colour

2. **Localised**
   Resembling fibroid but with brownish foci

The endometrial deposits communicate with the uterine cavity, but despite this they often contain altered blood in the glands which become cystic. The diffuse type is commoner. Adenomyosis is not related to endometriosis.

ENDOMETRIAL HYPERPLASIA

Endometrial hyperplasia occurs in 3 forms: Simple hyperplasia, complex hyperplasia and atypical hyperplasia. Of these, atypical hyperplasia is most important as it is associated with an increased risk of malignancy.

SIMPLE HYPERPLASIA

This tends to occur in the peri-menopausal period. It is due to excess oestrogen stimulation – particularly associated with **anovulatory** cycles, but rarely with oestrogen therapy or oestrogen-secreting tumours.

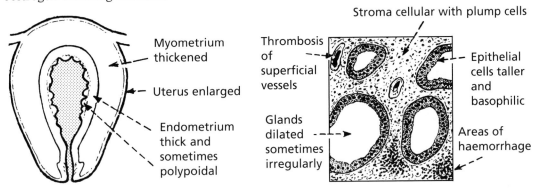

Myometrium thickened

Uterus enlarged

Endometrium thick and sometimes polypoidal

Thrombosis of superficial vessels

Glands dilated sometimes irregularly

Stroma cellular with plump cells

Epithelial cells taller and basophilic

Areas of haemorrhage

Clinically, there is irregular, frequent and heavy bleeding.

COMPLEX HYPERPLASIA

In this form, hyperplasia is often focal and glands but not stroma are affected. Thus the glands appear crowded, but show no atypia. There is no increased risk of malignancy.

ATYPICAL HYPERPLASIA

In this condition the hyperplasia is focal and cytological atypia with mitotic figures is common. Intervening endometrium may show simple hyperplasia. The importance of atypical hyperplasia is its relationship to the development of adenocarcinoma i.e. it is considered to be pre-cancerous, with a risk of around 20%.

Epithelium tall, sometimes stratified

Normal endometrium

Stroma reduced in adenomatous areas. Cellular atypia and mitoses. Variation in size of glands.

ENDOMETRIAL POLYP

This is a localised proliferation of endometrial glands which becomes pedunculated.

Sometimes polyps are associated with general endometrial hyperplasia. Progressive elongation of the pedicle jeopardises the blood supply. Compression by the uterine muscle results in venous congestion at the tip leading to bleeding and necrosis.

495

ENDOMETRIAL CARCINOMA

This common gynaecological cancer particularly affects postmenopausal patients, who typically present with vaginal bleeding.

CARCINOMA
This growth may form a *localised* plaque or polyp.

In some cases, however, it appears as a *diffuse* change involving much of the endometrium. It grows initially within the endometrial layer, bulging into the uterine cavity. Surface necrosis occurs at an early date.

Most growths are well-differentiated adenocarcinomas

but anaplastic growths are not uncommon →

Areas of squamous metaplasia are relatively common (adeno-acanthoma); they have no prognostic implication

In some cases with a particularly poor prognosis malignant squamous epithelium is admixed with the adenocarcinoma – so-called ADENOSQUAMOUS carcinoma.

The endometrium possesses no lymphatics and invasion of the myometrium takes place slowly.

Local extension: this may take place in several directions.

Spread towards tube

Penetration of uterus and growth in the parametrium

Spread to cervix and vagina

Direct invasion of the bladder

Metastases

1. Via lymphatics

Para-aortic nodes

Internal iliac nodes

By local lymphatic channels to vagina

2. Via blood vessels
Secondary deposits in the vagina and ovaries may be due to this mode of spread

3. Via fallopian tube

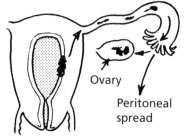

Ovary

Peritoneal spread

4. Distant metastases. At a late date, secondaries may appear in the liver, lungs and bones. These may be the result of lymphatic or blood spread.

ENDOMETRIAL CARCINOMA

Prognosis

Post-menopausal bleeding may give early warning of the disease. Lack of lymphatics in the endometrium limits extension for some time. The most important prognostic factor is the **stage** of the tumour, usually expressed in the FIGO (International Federation of Gynaecology and Obstetrics) system. The histological grade and subtype are also important. Overall a 60% 5 year survival is seen.

Aetiology

Endometrial carcinoma is uncommon before the 5th decade. The most important factor is prolonged OESTROGENIC stimulation due to:

(a) endogenous overproduction e.g. in cases of oestrogen-secreting ovarian tumours.

(b) exogenous oestrogen therapy.

(c) in OBESITY: increased conversion of androstenedione (from adrenals) to oestrone.

(d) ATYPICAL HYPERPLASIA is an important precancerous stage.

Other endometrial malignancies:

ENDOMETRIAL STROMAL SARCOMAS

These rare tumours may be of low grade or high grade.

Low grade tumours – infiltrate extensively through the lymphatics of the myometrium. The cells are cytologically bland and mitoses are few. About one fifth of patients eventually die from the disease.

High grade stromal sarcomas – are highly malignant spindle celled tumours, with poor prognosis. It may be difficult to separate these from uterine leiomyosarcomas.

MIXED MESODERMAL TUMOURS (CARCINO-SARCOMA)

These uncommon tumours can differentiate both into endometrial carcinoma and stromal sarcoma. They often present as soft fleshy masses protruding from the cervix into the vagina.

The tumour contains carcinoma and stromal elements.

If these resemble endometrial stroma, the tumour is described as

HOMOLOGOUS

Sometimes stromal elements include malignant cartilage; sometimes striated muscle.

The tumour is then described as

HETEROLOGOUS

DISEASES OF THE MYOMETRIUM

MYOMETRIUM
Tumours of the myometrium are extremely common.

LEIOMYOMA (fibroid)
This is a circumscribed growth derived from uterine muscle.

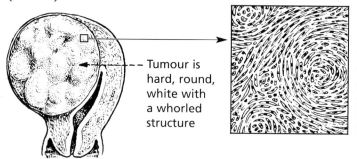

Tumour is hard, round, white with a whorled structure

The cells are typical long spindle muscle cells, arranged in interlacing bundles

They vary in size from tiny (mm) growths to several cm in diameter and are frequently multiple. Apparent encapsulation is due to compression by adjacent muscle. Fibroids may be found in any part of the uterus.

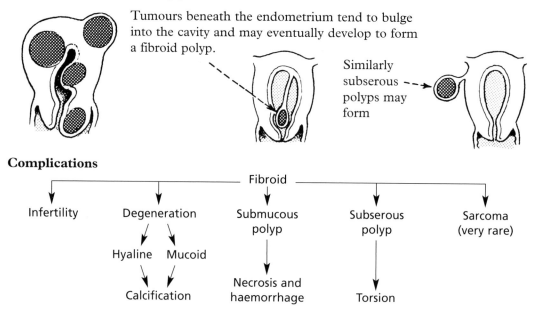

Tumours beneath the endometrium tend to bulge into the cavity and may eventually develop to form a fibroid polyp.

Similarly subserous polyps may form

Complications

Fibroid

Infertility	Degeneration	Submucous polyp	Subserous polyp	Sarcoma (very rare)
	Hyaline Mucoid			
	Calcification	Necrosis and haemorrhage	Torsion	

Leiomyoma is one of the commonest tumours, occurring in 15–20% of women over the age of 35. Growth ceases at the menopause.

LEIOMYOSARCOMA
This is a rare tumour which may arise from a preceding leiomyoma, but usually does not. Some tumours are highly malignant but in others with few mitotic figures it is difficult to predict the outcome – these are known as Smooth Muscle Tumours of Unknown Malignant Potential (STUMP).

DISEASES OF THE CERVIX

The cervix constitutes the lower one third of the uterine body.

It is in two parts: endocervical and vaginal or ectocervical. The dividing line is quite sharp and is determined by the character of the lining epithelium.

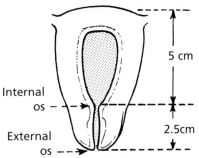

Internal os —

External os — —

5 cm

2.5cm

The remainder of the cervical wall consists of circular smooth muscle lying in abundant fibroelastic tissue.

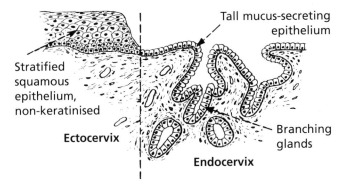

Tall mucus-secreting epithelium

Stratified squamous epithelium, non-keratinised

Ectocervix

Branching glands

Endocervix

At the internal os, the structure gradually merges with that of the uterus proper, the branching glands giving place to the simple tubules of the endometrium, and the proportion of muscle increases greatly.

CERVICITIS
Inflammation of the cervix may be acute or chronic. Acute cervicitis may be due to gonorrhoea or follow cervical laceration at childbirth.

Chronic cervicitis is commoner. Candida, trichomonas (p.503) and chlamydia may be responsible. The last is associated with reactive lymphoid follicles (follicular cervicitis).

Viral infections of the cervix include Herpes Simplex Virus (Type II) and human papilloma viruses (HPV). The latter can cause simple viral warts or be associated with cervical intraepithelial dysplasia and neoplasia (CIN) and invasive carcinoma (p.501).

CERVICAL POLYP
This is a local proliferation of endocervical mucosa which becomes pedunculated and may protrude through the cervix.

Cystic glands are common due to obstruction by chronic inflammation

CERVICAL INTRAEPITHELIAL NEOPLASIA (CIN)

The transformation zone

From puberty onwards and particularly in pregnancy the squamo-columnar junction presents on the vaginal surface of the external os. This is the area where **squamous metaplasia** occurs. It is important because cervical squamous carcinoma and its precursor **cervical intraepithelial neoplasia** (CIN) begin there. Within this metaplastic epithelium, **dysplastic** changes may develop. They are graded as CIN I, II and III. Later, in some cases, invasive squamous carcinoma develops.

CIN I = Mild dysplasia.

Upper $^{2}/_{3}$: → Stratified.

Basal $^{1}/_{3}$: High nucleo-cytoplasmic ratio; pleomorphic nuclei

CIN II = Moderate dysp.

Superficial stratification

Cellular abnormalities extending up into middle one third

CIN III = Severe dysp. and Carcinoma in situ.

May be 1 or 2 layers of stratified epithelium on surface.

Remainder: Immature; large nuclei; mitoses.

Koilocytes (cells with a wrinkled pyknotic nucleus and perinuclear cytoplasmic clearing) are often seen in the suprabasal layers indicating HPV infection.

CYTOLOGY and CIN

The cervical screening programme aims to detect CIN and thus prevent the development of invasive carcinoma. Smears from the squamo-columnar junction obtained by a wooden spatula are stained by Papanicolaou's method. The cells can be examined for dysplasia – so-called dyskaryosis. Inflammatory changes e.g. due to candida infection may be seen. Liquid based cytology is increasingly replacing conventional smears.

Normal smear

Abundant cytoplasm

Small pyknotic nucleus

Large squame

Dyskaryosis

High nucleus: cytoplasmic ratio

Nuclei hyperchromatic

The cytology is a SCREENING TEST. Patients with abnormalities are referred for colposcopy where abnormal epithelium turns white on exposure to acetic acid (acetowhite). Punch biopsy to assess dysplasia is often followed by laser ablation. New techniques to identify proliferating and malignant cells are being rapidly developed.

CARCINOMA OF CERVIX

CARCINOMA

This is the most common malignant tumour of the female genital tract, even where there is a vigorous campaign for early diagnosis and eradication of carcinoma in situ. The growth is a squamous carcinoma in 90% of cases, and an adenocarcinoma in 10%. Most squamous carcinomas arise at the squamo-columnar junction: a minority and most adenocarcinomas arise within the endocervical canal.

The cervix becomes very indurated; necrosis and ulceration commonly follow quickly.

Later, a large fungating mass is produced. Sloughing may leave an excavated crater.

Microinvasive carcinoma is the earliest stage of invasive cancer – where spread is less than 5 mm in depth. This is associated with an excellent prognosis.

Spread

Until a very late stage, the disease is confined to the pelvic cavity. The patient commonly dies before distant metastases appear.

Local spread takes place in several directions:

1. **Downward extension.**

2. **Lateral extension.** The anatomy of this region is important.

Uterus

Trigone of bladder

The ureters come very close to the cervix in their travel to the bladder, and are apt to be involved in extension of the growth to the parametrium. The ureters may be obstructed by pressure or invasion. Renal infection and failure follow.

(a) The growth encircles the external os. In some cases it causes obstruction of the cervical canal and pyometra may develop.

(b) Extension to the vagina takes place in direct continuity.

CARCINOMA OF CERVIX

Spread of carcinoma (*continued*)

3. **Anterior and posterior extension**

Direct invasion of the bladder or rectum results in fistulous communications. Spread along the uterosacral ligaments involves the sacral nerves, causing intractable pain.

4. **Lymphatic spread**
This occurs early and involves the chains of lymph nodes in the pelvis.

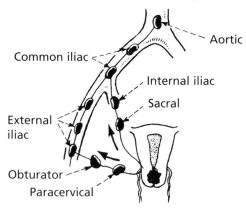

Prognosis

With modern treatment there is an 80% 5-year cure rate when the disease is diagnosed early i.e. confined to the cervix: it falls significantly if spread to the pelvis has occurred.

Previously death was commonly due to a combination of renal failure and sepsis: fatal haemorrhage from eroded vessels also occurred. With better local control death is usually due to metastases.

Aetiology

1. ***Epidemiological facts***
   (a) The disease is rare in virgins (in a community of nuns, no cases were seen) and the incidence is highest in prostitutes. The disease is rare in strictly orthodox Jewish women and significantly increased in less strict Jewish communities.
   (b) Historically the disease was seen most commonly in the 4th and 5th decades. Nowadays, in Western Societies, dysplasia and carcinoma are seen in younger women (3rd decade) and the prevalence has greatly increased. These changes are statistically related to sexual promiscuity and early age of first coitus.
   (c) The use of barrier methods of contraception is associated with a decreased incidence.

2. ***Virus Infection***
   In the great majority of cases HUMAN PAPILLOMA VIRUS (HPV) is associated with cervical carcinoma and is the postulated carcinogenic agent with male to female transmission.

Associations

HPV types 6, 11, 42	CIN I and condylomata
HPV types 16 or 18	CIN III and invasive carcinoma

3. Of other possible co-factors or mutagens ***Tobacco*** heads the list.

4. It seems likely that in many cases initiation of the progression to cancer begins at an early age before the cervical muco-squamous junction has stabilised.

DISEASES OF VAGINA AND VULVA

Trichomonas vaginalis

Vaginal discharge is a common complaint especially in parous women. In many cases it is related to chronic cervicitis. There are however a number of inflammatory conditions which arise primarily in the vagina.

Gonococcal infection may produce an acute inflammation with purulent discharge but it is often asymptomatic.

Purulent discharge is also associated with infection by a protozoon, *Trichomonas vaginalis*. The discharge tends to be frothy. It is commonly transmitted during sexual intercourse. The male can also be infected.

Candida albicans infection is common in pregnancy and in patients undergoing antibiotic or immunosuppressive therapy.

PRIMARY TUMOURS of the VAGINA are rare. Squamous carcinoma occurs in the upper vagina of women and may lead to fistula formation between the vagina and the bladder or rectum. Vaginal intraepithelial neoplasia (VAIN) may be associated with CIN and VIN. Historically, clear cell carcinoma was sometimes found in adolescent girls, due to the effect on the fetus of administration of diethylstilbestrol to the patient's mother during early pregnancy. It arose in a background of vaginal adenosis – a proliferation of glands within the vaginal wall.

VULVAL INFLAMMATION is common in post-menopausal women. It is related to atrophy of the skin, which has very thin epithelial covering at this phase of life and is easily abraded. Inflammation at other periods of life frequently involves Bartholin's gland.

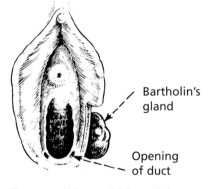

Bartholin's gland

Opening of duct

The duct which opens into the vagina in front of the hymen is apt to become blocked. If the inflammation subsides a simple cyst of the duct arises but an abscess may form.

Two conditions which mainly occur in the tropics and are seen only very occasionally in temperate countries are:

1. **Lymphogranuloma venereum.** This is a chlamydial infection which starts as an ulcer on the vulva or in the vagina. It heals in a short time, only to be followed by a chronic suppurative reaction in the inguinal and sometimes pelvic lymph nodes. This leads to extensive scarring and sometimes fistulous openings in the pelvic viscera.
2. **Granuloma inguinale.** This begins as a papule on the vulva, perineum or vagina. It ulcerates and can spread widely, causing extensive destruction of tissue. Histologically, it is a granuloma and the infecting organism (*Calymmatobacterium granulomatis*) can be seen in macrophages.

DISEASES OF VAGINA AND VULVA

LEUKOPLAKIA AND PREMALIGNANCY

Leukoplakia is a descriptive term meaning white patches. These are common on the vulval and perineal regions in almost any chronic inflammatory skin condition due to the local moist conditions, e.g. chronic dermatitis (lichen simplex), fungal infection and lichen sclerosis.

There is however one type of lesion appearing as white patches in this region which shows epithelial dysplasia and is premalignant.

Hyperkeratosis and Parakeratosis
Epithelial hyperplasia with mitotic activity and abnormal cells

Chronic inflammatory reaction

Hyalinisation of superficial dermis

The degree of dysplasia varies, amounting to carcinoma in situ in some cases.

These changes are now numerically graded VIN I, II and III, i.e. Vulvar Intraepithelial Neoplasia (analogous to CIN).

TUMOURS OF THE VULVA

Simple tumours are common. CONDYLOMATA ACUMINATA are papillary proliferations due to infection by Human Papilloma Virus (HPV) types 6 or 11. Koilocytosis (see p.500) in the superficial keratinocytes is the histological marker.

Sweat gland tumours (hidradenomas) may also occur.

Carcinoma of vulva

This is a rare condition found usually in women in the 6th and 7th decades of life.

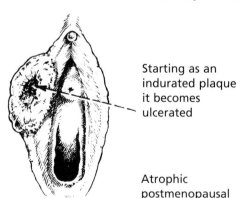

Starting as an indurated plaque it becomes ulcerated

The inguinal glands on both sides are invaded at an early date. The growth is usually a squamous carcinoma.

Atrophic postmenopausal vulva

DISEASES OF THE FALLOPIAN TUBE

Acute Salpingitis

The inflammation is the result of ascending infection from the endometrium: some cases follow abortion and puerperal infection. In addition to the infecting organisms causing acute endometritis (see p.493) Chlamydia is a cause of acute salpingitis.

The inflammation is usually bilateral and primarily involves the tubal plicae which are congested and oedematous: there is a purulent exudate.

If resolution of the acute inflammation does not occur (antibiotic therapy is important) chronic salpingitis and its possible complications are established. The term 'pelvic inflammatory disease' is used.

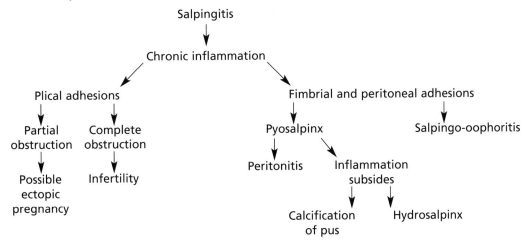

Tuberculous salpingitis

Tuberculous infection of the female genital tract, for some unexplained reason, almost always starts in the fallopian tube. It is usually due to blood spread from some other site: only very occasionally it is secondary to tuberculous peritonitis.

The complications are those expected of a chronic salpingitis with the added element of caseation.

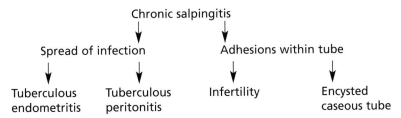

Tumours of the fallopian tube

Benign tumours such as fibroma and myoma occasionally occur. Small cysts of congenital origin are common around the fimbrial ends of the tubes.

Carcinoma, usually a papillary adenocarcinoma, is extremely rare. There may be a profuse watery secretion which appears as a vaginal discharge.

DISEASES OF THE OVARIES

Oophoritis

Inflammation of the ovaries is always secondary to disease of the fallopian tubes or peritoneum. In the case of the tube, the inflamed fimbrial end becomes adherent to the ovary and direct spread of infection occurs. Tubo-ovarian inflammation is also associated with the presence of an intra-uterine contraceptive device (see p.493). Important local complications may follow.

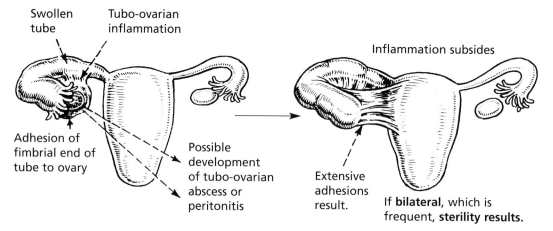

Swollen tube · Tubo-ovarian inflammation · Inflammation subsides · Adhesion of fimbrial end of tube to ovary · Possible development of tubo-ovarian abscess or peritonitis · Extensive adhesions result. · If **bilateral**, which is frequent, **sterility results**.

The ovary may be similarly involved in tuberculous salpingitis, and caseating lesions can occur.

Ovarian changes of functional origin

The control mechanisms of ovarian function frequently develop faults resulting in abnormalities of structure:

Follicular cysts

These may be single or multiple. The maximum diameter of a normal Graafian follicle is 1.5–2 cm. Single follicular cysts may be several centimetres in diameter. Amenorrhoea is common in such instances. Multiple follicular cysts, usually small, are associated with endometrial hyperplasia.

Granulosa cells lining cyst

Theca lutein cysts

These are cysts from which the granulosa cells have disappeared, leaving cysts surrounded by luteinised thecal tissue. Bilateral, multiple small cysts of this nature occur in polycystic ovarian disease and are associated with obesity, hirsutism and oligomenorrhoea (Stein–Leventhal syndrome).

DISEASES OF THE OVARIES

A multiplicity of types of ovarian tumours exists. Various classifications have been suggested; none is completely satisfactory. The following is a simple working classification:

1. Epithelial tumours (derived from surface epithelium).
2. Sex cord/stromal tumours.
3. Germ cell tumours.
4. Secondary (metastatic) tumours.

COMMON EPITHELIAL TUMOURS

These comprise 60% of all ovarian tumours and 90% of malignant tumours and are found in adult life, very rarely in children.

Histogenesis: The ovarian surface epithelium and the various mature Müllerian structures have a common origin in EMBRYONAL COELOMIC epithelium. The ovarian surface epithelial stem cells retain the ability to differentiate along different pathways: this explains the histological appearance of these tumours.

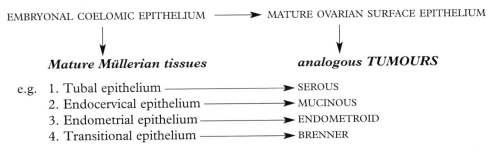

EMBRYONAL COELOMIC EPITHELIUM ⟶ MATURE OVARIAN SURFACE EPITHELIUM

Mature Müllerian tissues   *analogous* **TUMOURS**

e.g.
1. Tubal epithelium ⟶ SEROUS
2. Endocervical epithelium ⟶ MUCINOUS
3. Endometrial epithelium ⟶ ENDOMETROID
4. Transitional epithelium ⟶ BRENNER

The histological features relate to a spectrum of behaviour:

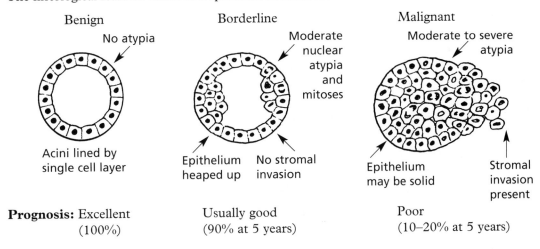

Benign — No atypia — Acini lined by single cell layer
Prognosis: Excellent (100%)

Borderline — Moderate nuclear atypia and mitoses — Epithelium heaped up — No stromal invasion
Usually good (90% at 5 years)

Malignant — Moderate to severe atypia — Epithelium may be solid — Stromal invasion present
Poor (10–20% at 5 years)

507

COMMON EPITHELIAL OVARIAN TUMOURS

Serous cystadenoma

Twenty-five per cent of all ovarian tumours are of this variety. In a third of cases they are bilateral, but they almost never reach the large size of the mucinous growths.

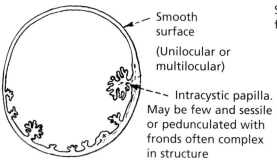

Smooth surface

(Unilocular or multilocular)

Intracystic papilla. May be few and sessile or pedunculated with fronds often complex in structure

Some tumours have small loculi with papillary formations making them appear solid.

Epithelium cuboidal with central nuclei. Fluid is watery.

Psammoma bodies with concentric layers of calcification are commonly seen.

Complications

1. Torsion may occur
2. Malignant transformation is common and 30% of malignant tumours are bilateral.

Mucinous cystadenoma

This accounts for 20% of all ovarian tumours. It can reach a very large size and is typically multilocular. 25% are bilateral.

Slightly nodular due to loculi

The cut surface shows the multilocular mosaic pattern

Mucin secretion

Nuclei basal

Tall columnar epithelium (septa from the capsule support cyst)

Smooth peritoneal covering

The tumour is usually unilateral

Complications

1. **Torsion of the pedicle.** This is not uncommon with a large ovarian tumour of any type.
2. **Rupture.** This may lead to seeding of the mucin-secreting epithelium on the peritoneum. It continues to secrete, leading to the condition 'pseudomyxoma peritonei', with a peritoneal cavity filled with mucin. Many of these tumours appear to have originated in the appendix.
3. **Malignant transformation** including borderline tumours. Cells are large, with large irregular nuclei. Mitoses are common; slight secretion present (see over).

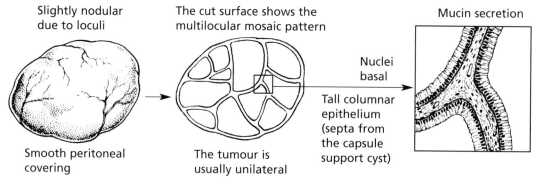

Congestion, often infarction due to interruption of blood flow

Brenner tumours

These are essentially benign and show islands of transitional epithelium in a fibrous stroma.

CARCINOMA OF THE OVARY

Mucinous cystadenocarcinoma

This accounts for 20% of all cases of primary carcinoma of the ovary. It almost always arises as a malignant transformation of a benign cystadenoma.

Areas of solid growth appear in the cyst wall.

Frequently in the malignant areas, florid papillary structures are formed and where the change is widespread it may be difficult to differentiate it from the malignant form of papillary cystadenoma.

Papillary (serous) cystadenocarcinoma

This is the commonest malignant tumour of the ovary – responsible for 40% of the total. Usually it takes the form of exuberant papillomatous growths extending over the surface and obliterating the ovarian structure. It is often bilateral.

Mitotic figures common

Invasion of capsular tissues

Endometrioid carcinoma

In a considerable number of cases, ovarian carcinoma has a solid or semi-solid appearance and as such starts off as a growth smaller than either of the cystic tumours.

Microscopically, they are frequently anaplastic, but sometimes they show differentiation towards an endometrial pattern and are termed 'endometrioid'. There is no 'benign' equivalent, but some cases arise in endometriosis.

Progress in ovarian carcinoma

Spread of ovarian cancer in the early stages is by direct extension to the pelvic peritoneum. The papillary serous cancer seeds widely in the peritoneal cavity and only later are lymphatics invaded and metastases appear.

The mucinous variety rarely spreads by lymphatics.

The overall 5-year survival rate for ovarian cancer is only 30% and death often takes place within 2–3 years due to cachexia and interference with intestinal and renal function.

Aetiology

Most cases are sporadic. Nulliparous women with a late menopause have an increased risk. There is a family tendency – especially in women with mutation of the BRCA-1 gene.

Tumour marker

CA125 is a glycoprotein: serum levels are raised in about 50% of patients with ovarian carcinoma.

TUMOURS OF THE OVARY – MISCELLANEOUS

SEX CORD and STROMAL TUMOURS

These may be divided into two broad groups:

1. Those tending to produce excess oestrogen: granulosa cell tumours and thecomas.
2. Those producing androgens and virilisation: Sertoli–Leydig cell tumours, hilus cell tumours and lipid cell tumours.

Granulosa cell tumour

This is composed of cells resembling the granulosa cells lining Graafian follicles. They vary in size from a few mm to large cystic structures. Commonly, the smaller varieties are found deep in the ovarian substance. This tumour may be found at any age: 5% occur in children; 50% in the child-bearing years; 40% postmenopausally.

Rosettes of cells with nuclei radially arranged are common (Call–Exner bodies)

All granulosa cell tumours are potentially malignant – they may recur, sometimes many years after removal.

Measurement of serum **inhibin** (a glycoprotein produced by granulosa cells) is useful in following progress.

Thecoma

This is a growth consisting of spindle cells. They are found mainly during the 3rd, 4th and 5th decades of life. They are benign and rarely recur.

Function of these tumours varies widely. Oestrogenic manifestations consist of:
1. Precocious puberty in children.
2. Hyperplasia of endometrium. This may be atypical and carcinoma is said to develop occasionally.
3. Enlargement of breasts.

Fibromas are histologically similar but do not produce hormones. They may be associated with pleural effusion (Meig's syndrome).

Sertoli–Leydig cell tumours (androblastoma)

Tubules lined by SERTOLI cells, sometimes pyramidal with clear cytoplasm.

LEYDIG cells occasionally with Reinke crystalloids in their cytoplasm

This typifies the virilising tumour group. It is a rare tumour. The degree of virilisation varies. Usually a small yellow tumour within the ovarian substance, it has a characteristic microscopic structure.

Some of these tumours are malignant and consist of poorly differentiated spindle cells with occasional tubule formations.

The androgens, if secreted, result in:
1. Atrophy of breasts and external genitalia
2. Deepening of voice, temporal recession of hair
3. Growth of facial and body hair
4. Enlargement of clitoris.

TUMOURS OF THE OVARY – MISCELLANEOUS

GERM CELL TUMOURS

These arise from primitive germ cells capable of differentiating in many ways. The following diagram indicates the main varieties of tumour produced.

Primitive germ cells: Embryonic differentiation: Extra-embryonic differentiation

No differentiation   Mature teratoma   Immature teratoma   Yolk sac tumours   Choriocarcinoma

Dysgerminoma

Dysgerminoma

This is a solid tumour of characteristic appearance. It is usually ovoid with a smooth capsule, greyish colour and rubbery consistency. Like all germ cell tumours it is commoner in younger age groups and is often bilateral. Some cases are found in association with intersex.

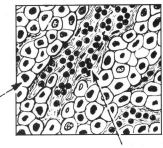

Lymphocytes

Microscopically, it consists of large clear round cells with large nuclei resembling germ cells. These are arranged in alveoli separated by fine connective tissue infiltrated by lymphocytes. These histological appearances are identical to those of seminoma of the testis.

Dysgerminomas are malignant tumours spreading to para-aortic lymph nodes. They are radio-sensitive and also respond to chemotherapy.

Teratomas

These are of two main varieties: (1) Mature and (2) Immature.

Mature cystic teratoma (dermoid cyst)

Hairs

Tooth

Eminence

This is one of the commonest ovarian tumours and it occurs at all ages.

It is unilocular with an eminence on one aspect from which hairs grow. Teeth may be present on this eminence. The cyst is lined by stratified squamous epithelium. Sebaceous glands, nervous tissue, respiratory, intestinal epithelium and thyroid tissue may also be present.

Very occasionally the squamous epithelium may undergo malignant change.

Hairs

Sebaceous glands

511

TUMOURS OF THE OVARY – MISCELLANEOUS

Teratomas (*continued*)

Immature teratoma

The tumours are predominantly solid and are malignant. They contain immature tissues, typically of primitive nerve tissue and mesenchymal tissue. They may metastasise to the peritoneum where the nerve tissue may differentiate (gliomatosis peritonei).

Chemotherapy has greatly improved the prognosis in these cases.

Solid tumours are occasionally seen consisting only of thyroid tissue (struma ovarii) or carcinoid tumour cells.

Extra-embryonic tumours (yolk sac tumours, choriocarcinoma).

These are very rare. The main feature in all of them is their extreme malignancy, but modern chemotherapy has revolutionised the outlook.

SECONDARY TUMOURS

The ovaries are often the site of metastatic growths from the breast, lung, intestinal system, etc. They are commonest during the child-bearing years.

Krukenberg tumour

This is a very characteristic secondary tumour due to metastatic deposits from an undiscovered stomach carcinoma in a pre-menopausal woman. Both ovaries are involved. They are firm and fibrous, of equal size, smooth and slightly lobulated. No adhesions are present.

Histologically they may be mistaken for a spindle cell sarcoma, but among the undifferentiated cells are large cells with eccentric nuclei and clear cytoplasm containing mucin (signet ring cells).

ECTOPIC PREGNANCY

This means implantation of the fertilised ovum outside the uterine cavity.

Sites of implantation

Ampullary implantation
This is the commonest.

Interstitial implantation (rare)

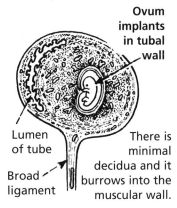

Ovum implants in tubal wall

Lumen of tube

Broad ligament

There is minimal decidua and it burrows into the muscular wall.

Uterine changes

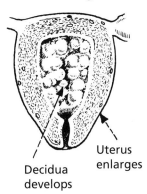

Decidua develops

Uterus enlarges

Erosion of the tubal tissues by the ovum results in **rupture**.

This is the commonest finding.
The direction of rupture varies:

(1)

Rupture into the lumen of the tube and leakage into peritoneal cavity.

(2)

Rupture directly into the peritoneal cavity. If the implantation is interstitial, there may be a further complication – damage to the uterine arteries with **arterial bleeding.**

Exceedingly rarely the whole pregnancy – ovum and placental tissue – aborts into the peritoneal cavity where it reimplants. Usually development is limited and the fetus dies, but continuation of the pregnancy almost to term has been reported.

Aetiology. Most commonly the tube has been previously damaged by salpingitis, leading to partial blockage of the tube. There has been an increased incidence of ectopic pregnancy in women fitted with intrauterine contraceptive devices.

(3)

Rupture into the broad ligament

Extraperitoneal haematoma

TROPHOBLAST DISEASE

HYDATIDIFORM MOLE
This occurs in two forms:

1. **Complete.** This is a pregnancy lacking a fetus. The mole starts early in pregnancy and the uterus is filled by cysts of varying size.

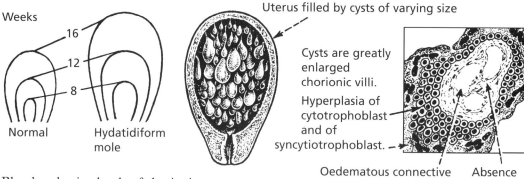

Weeks

Normal   Hydatidiform mole

Uterus filled by cysts of varying size

Cysts are greatly enlarged chorionic villi.

Hyperplasia of cytotrophoblast and of syncytiotrophoblast.

Oedematous connective tissue containing cisterns   Absence of vessels

Blood and urine levels of chorionic gonadotrophin are high.

1a. **Invasive mole.** Villi may penetrate the myometrium and invade blood vessels with pulmonary 'metastases'. There is usually complete regression after hysterectomy however.

Prevalence: Uncommon in the West (1 in 1500 pregnancies) but common in the East (1 in 120 pregnancies).

Genetics: The genetic sex of the complete form is XX, but both chromosomes are paternal. It is thought that a single sperm penetrates a dead or dying ovum.

Progress: Abortion is the usual outcome: there is a 2–3% risk of CHORIOCARCINOMA developing.

2. **Partial mole.** Sometimes only part of the placenta shows hydatid change and a fetus, usually malformed, may be present. Genetic analysis shows a typical triploid karyotype i.e. 69 chromosomes. While trophoblast may persist there is no risk of choriocarcinoma.

CHORIOCARCINOMA
This is the malignant tumour of the trophoblast and is by definition of fetal origin. It usually follows hydatidiform mole. Pleomorphic cytotrophoblast and syncytiotrophoblast, showing numerous mitoses, invade blood vessels causing haemorrhage and early lung metastases

Clot

either as a single large 'cannon-ball' haemorrhagic mass or multiple small emboli ('snow-storm' lung). The high blood and urine concentrations of chorionic gonadotrophin are used to monitor progress and treatment which is now usually successful.

The myometrium is infiltrated by masses of malignant trophoblast and blood venous sinuses are eroded.

BENIGN DISEASES OF THE BREAST

Acute inflammation is an occasional complication of **lactation**.

Fissures or abrasions of the nipple predispose to the condition. Infection is transmitted by the suckling neonate who is carrying hospital staphylococci. Abscesses may form in the lobules of the breast leading to scarring during healing.

Chronic infection e.g. tuberculosis is very uncommon.

Duct ectasia (plasma cell mastitis)
This chronic inflammatory reaction is associated with ectasia of the ducts (cystic dilatation).

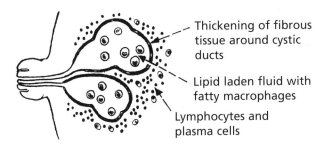

Thickening of fibrous tissue around cystic ducts

Lipid laden fluid with fatty macrophages

Lymphocytes and plasma cells

Infection of the dilated ducts allows escape of contents into the tissues resulting in *granulomatous* reaction. Clinically it may raise suspicion of duct carcinoma.

Traumatic Fat Necrosis occurs in obese pendulous breasts and results in an irregular granulomatous fibrous reaction which may mimic carcinoma.

In some cases of **Silicone Implant**, continuing granulomatous inflammation with fibrosis occurs in the 'capsule' due to leakage of silicone.

Fibrocystic change
In this condition there are four characteristic features, and the form which the disease takes varies according to the relative proportions of these features:

1. **Fibrosis**. There is progressive hyalinisation of the stroma.

2. **Cyst formation.** Obstruction of ducts leads to dilatation of the ducts and acini. The lining epithelium may show apocrine metaplasia.

3. (a) **Adenosis**. This is an increase in the number of lobules and in the size of existing lobules.

Hyperplastic lobules

Normal lobule

(b) **Sclerosing adenosis**
This is a localised condition which may simulate carcinoma. There is proliferation of acini and stroma, and mitotic activity can be marked but there is no danger of malignancy.

BENIGN DISEASES OF THE BREAST

Fibrocystic change (*continued*)

4. **Epithelial hyperplasia** is the most important component because it forms a link between simple proliferation and malignant change.

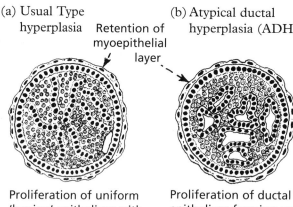

(a) Usual Type hyperplasia

Retention of myoepithelial layer

(b) Atypical ductal hyperplasia (ADH)

(c) Atypical lobular hyperplasia (ALH)

Proliferation of uniform 'benign' epithelium with 'streaming' pattern.

Proliferation of ductal epithelium forming an irregular network: epithelial cells showing mild atypia.

Uniform proliferation of acinar epithelium without acinar expansion.

Fibrocystic change is very common, and the various changes are ascribed to abnormal and exaggerated responses of the breast tissues to the cyclical physiological menstrual hormonal stimuli; they are essentially benign, but a link with carcinoma has been established when there is hyperplasia with cytological atypia (i.e. ADH, ALH). In these circumstances, particularly if the changes are widespread, the risks of carcinoma are increased.

Lesions related to Fibrocystic change

1. **Fibroadenoma**

    This is a benign nodular proliferation, now considered to be a component of fibrocystic change and not a true neoplasm. It is usually single, occurring in young women. It presents clinically as a small, firm, mobile lump.

Microscopic appearance

Gross appearance
Well circumscribed, rounded and elastic in consistency: glistening, greyish cut surface 1–3 cm diam.)

Small acinar and duct structures resembling normal breast

Fibrous tissue arranged around acini

Epithelium forms clefts: these are due to pressure from the projecting fibrous tissue

2. **Radial scar**

    This small (up to 1 cm diam.), firm lesion shows a central dense fibrous core with radiating fingers of fibrosis entrapping and distorting glandular elements. It is benign but can be confused with carcinoma even on histological examination.

    Similar but larger lesions, also detected by mammography, are known as **complex sclerosing lesions**.

BENIGN BREAST TUMOURS AND IN SITU CARCINOMA

Duct papilloma
This tumour may develop in any part of the duct system of the breast, but is most common in the lacteal sinuses at the nipple. Two forms exist:

1. **Solitary papilloma.** These are almost always near the nipple.

Complex branching pedunculated tumour filling lacteal sinus

Columnar epithelium with underlying myoepithelium

Connective tissue core

Prominent myoepithelium gives a double layer of cells covering the fronds.

2. **Multiple papillomata**
These may be distributed throughout the duct system. In this form, multicentric carcinoma occasionally develops.

In both forms, there may be discharge from the nipple which may be haemorrhagic. Examination of the discharge will reveal the tumour epithelial cells which are benign. Other benign breast tumours are rare.

Ductal carcinoma in-situ (DCIS)
This is a non-invasive carcinoma of the ducts. It may be visible as greyish-white material filling the dilated ducts, and central necrotic debris may be squeezed out of the ducts (comedocarcinoma).

Solid or cribriform cylinders of cells show the usual features of malignancy – variation in size and shape of both cell and nucleus, relatively greater size of nuclei, mitotic figures, etc. The condition has to be differentiated from atypical ductal hyperplasia.

Solid proliferation of pleomorphic cancer cells

Necrotic debris

No myoepithelium

Thinning of duct wall

Cribriform pattern with rigid 'Roman bridges'

DCIS is graded into high and low grade, the former having a higher risk of invasive malignancy.

Lobular carcinoma in situ. This lesion is usually multifocal and bilateral. The breast acini of affected lobules are distended by fairly uniform carcinoma cells which grow into the duct system or break through basement membrane to become infiltrative carcinoma, either of lobular or ductal type.

517

CARCINOMA OF THE BREAST

This is the commonest form of malignancy in the female. It may be found in any part of the breast but most frequently it is in the upper outer quadrant.

INFILTRATING DUCTAL CARCINOMA

This, the commonest form, presents as a firm to hard lump. The following illustrations show a large carcinoma with significant local spread. It is emphasised that modern screening methods aim to detect the disease at a much earlier stage.

Gross appearance

Surface shows a coarse texture (peau d'orange)

Nipple often retracted in late stages

Strands of fibrous tissue extend in all directions

Localised, hard, craggy mass greyish-white in colour with yellow flecks ('unripe pear' appearance)

Often fixed to underlying muscle

Microscopic appearance

On section the growth has a crab-like shape – due to lines of infiltration.

Cords of spheroidal cells

Dense collagenous stroma

Occasional acinar formation

INFILTRATING LOBULAR CARCINOMA

Ten per cent of breast cancers are of this type. Based on distribution of the 'in situ' precursor, this tumour may be multicentric within the breast and there is a 30% chance of a similar tumour arising in the contralateral breast. Microscopically the tumour infiltrates the tissues as single files of malignant cells.

Infiltrating lobular carcinoma

Medullary carcinoma

Large spheroidal cells

Fine stroma often heavily infiltrated by lymphocytes

More rare forms of breast cancer are TUBULAR CARCINOMA – showing well differentiated cells often with intra-tubular calcification: MEDULLARY CARCINOMA – a highly cellular tumour with a florid lymphocytic infiltrate, and MUCOID CARCINOMA where the malignant cells lie in pools of mucin.

CARCINOMA OF THE BREAST

Local Spread: Breast cancers are usually slow growing: tumour size is proportional to duration. In late stages local infiltration causes skin ulceration and there may be direct penetration of the chest wall. In addition, intra-epithelial spread occurs. The classical example is **PAGET'S DISEASE OF THE NIPPLE** – which may complicate intra-duct carcinoma. (Occasionally an infiltrating component is absent.)

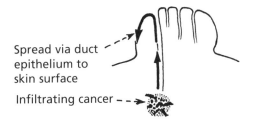

Spread via duct epithelium to skin surface

Infiltrating cancer

Nipple is red, swollen and inflamed with crusts on the surface.

Fluid exudes from surface

Microscopic examination reveals:

Packets of pale cells in the epithelium

Marked inflammatory reaction in dermis with plasma cells.

Paget cells (nuclei large with prominent nucleoli: cytoplasm clear)

Occasional mitosis

Metastatic Spread: This is by lymphatic and blood streams.

Early (When the tumour is still small) 	*via LYMPHATICS* 1. To axillary nodes from all sites of breast. 2. Through internal mammary lymphatics to thorax (esp. in cancers sited medially).	*via BLOOD STREAM* ? to bone marrow where cells can lie dormant for long periods.
Late	Local spread via skin lymphatics causing: (a) Widespread lesion – skin becomes stiff and board-like: 'cancer-en-cuirasse'. (b) Blockage of dermal lymphatics: oedema of skin except at anchorage points, giving a fine mamillated appearance: 'peau d'orange' (see p.240).	Secondaries appear in many viscera, particularly liver, lung and bone (spine, long bones)

519

CARCINOMA OF THE BREAST

Prognosis

The most important factors determining prognosis are:

1. Size – lesions under 1 cm rarely metastasise.
2. Number of lymph nodes involved – divided into three groups
   (a) no nodes involved
   (b) 1–3 nodes
   (c) ≥ 4 nodes.

3. Histological grade (graded 1,2,3) on the basis of
   (a) extent of tubule formation
   (b) nuclear pleomorphism
   (c) mitotic activity
4. Hormone receptor status – oestrogen receptor positive tumours respond better to tamoxifen and other anti-oestrogen drugs. Progesterone receptors are also detected. Demonstration of overexpression of the oncogene C-erb B-2 allows treatment by monoclonal antibodies (herceptin) directed against the protein.

These factors are summarised in prognostic indices such as the Nottingham Prognostic Index, based on size, lymph node status and grade.

Aetiology

Breast cancer is uncommon below the age of 30 years. The risk increases with age, the maximal incidence being in the later decades.
The important risk factors are:

1. Genetic:

There is a strong familial association. Mutation of genes, BRCA1 on chromosome 17 and BRCA2 on chromosome 11, are responsible for many cases of breast cancer in young women with a positive family history. Deletion of tumour suppressor genes has been identified (mutation of suppressor gene p53 is common) – Li–Fraumeni syndrome.

2. Sex hormone associations: (a) Commoner in nulliparous women.
(b) Early menarche and late menopause increase risk – ? prolonged cyclical exposure to sex hormones.
(c) Breast feeding reduces risk.

Screening for Breast cancer

The aim of screening is to detect either pre-malignant conditions or cancer at an early stage and is very important where there is a family history of cancer. Mammography is capable of detecting intra-duct carcinoma and pre-cancerous lesions. Focal calcification is an important indicator but is not diagnostic of malignancy because it also occurs in benign lesions. Whatever method of screening is used the diagnosis must be established on morphological evidence using fine needle aspiration, needle biopsy and, sometimes, open biopsy.

Other rare tumours of the breast include PHYLLODES TUMOUR – large and usually benign, affecting elderly women: occasionally sarcoma of the stroma is present. Soft tissue sarcomas and primary lymphoma are rare.

THE MALE BREAST

The breast is seldom the seat of disease in males. Abnormal enlargement – gynaecomastia – may occur in a temporary form at puberty or as a permanent feature in Klinefelter's syndrome (XXY). Oestrogen metabolic upsets (e.g. in liver disease) or excess intake (e.g. treatment of prostatic cancer) are other causes. All tumours are rare.

THE PROSTATE

The prostate surrounds the bladder neck and urethra. Although traditionally divided into five lobes, it is now regarded as having four major zones, which tend to be affected by different disorders.

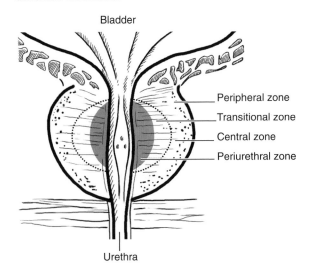

Its internal structure is a series of branching glands in a fibromuscular stroma.

There are three main disorders of the prostate:

1. Prostatitis
2. Benign prostatic hyperplasia
3. Prostatic carcinoma.

Prostatitis

There are three forms:

1. *Acute bacterial prostatitis* – associated with urinary tract infections – usually by Gram negative bacilli such as *E. coli*. Instrumentation, e.g. catheterisation may provoke the episode.
2. *Chronic bacterial prostatitis* – due to repeated urinary tract infections, usually by the same group of organisms.
3. *Chronic abacterial prostatitis* – the cause of this is unknown. The patient complains of urinary symptoms such as dysuria and frequency, low back pain and perineal discomfort.

DISEASES OF THE PROSTATE

Benign prostatic hyperplasia

This is an extremely common finding in over 70% of men over 60 years. The prostate is enlarged often over 100 g (normal prostate 20 g). The transitional and periurethral zones are most affected.

Normal

Urethra is compressed

Periurethral glands are hypertrophic

Peripheral main glands are compressed and atrophic

Glandular papillary projections

Cystic spaces common

Aetiology

It is clear that androgens are responsible for prostatic proliferation with conversion of testosterone to dihydrotestosterone by the enzyme 5α-reductase, found mainly in prostatic stromal cells. Use of 5α-reductase inhibitors is effective treatment in many cases; often combined with α adrenergic blockers.

Complications

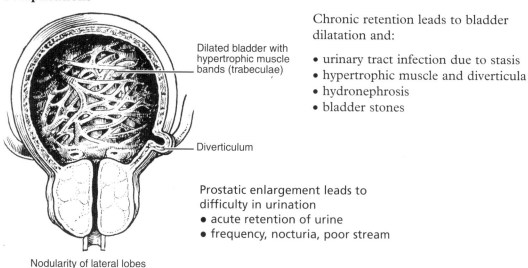

Dilated bladder with hypertrophic muscle bands (trabeculae)

Diverticulum

Nodularity of lateral lobes with compression of urethra

Chronic retention leads to bladder dilatation and:

• urinary tract infection due to stasis
• hypertrophic muscle and diverticula
• hydronephrosis
• bladder stones

Prostatic enlargement leads to difficulty in urination
• acute retention of urine
• frequency, nocturia, poor stream

DISEASES OF THE PROSTATE

CARCINOMA OF THE PROSTATE

This is the second commonest cancer in men in the UK and a major cause of cancer death. It is rare below the age of 40 and rises to very high prevalence in men over 80.

It takes origin from the peripheral zone, or in the transition zone. Often the prostate also shows benign hyperplasia, but this is coincidental and not causally related. It is almost always an adenocarcinoma.

Closely set small irregular acini lined by a single layer of epithelium

Histological grading:

The GLEASON system (Grades 2 through 10) indicates the degree of differentiation from (2) very well differentiated to (10) aggressive anaplastic tumours. Grading correlates well with prognosis.

Spread

1. Direct spread occurs throughout the prostate and outwards to the pelviprostatic tissue.
2. Lymphatic spread is the main mode of extension. There is a rich lymphatic plexus and the perineural lymphatics are particularly affected. The pelvic nodes are invaded and subsequently the abdominal chain.
3. Bone metastases tend to be common, especially in the vertebrae. This is due to retrograde spread from the prostatic venous plexus to the vertebral veins. These secondaries are often characterised by the formation of new dense bone around them (osteosclerosis).

Biochemical tests

1. Prostatic specific antigen (PSA) measured in the blood using an immuno-histochemical technique is a useful diagnostic marker.
2. These tumours produce prostatic acid phosphatase and, when metastases are present, an increased level may be found in the blood. When bones are invaded, blood alkaline phosphatase may also rise due to osteoblastic activity.

So-called latent carcinoma

Small subcapsular foci with the histological features of very well differentiated carcinoma may be found in a prostate showing benign hyperplasia. They are discovered incidentally at autopsy in patients dying from causes unconnected with prostate disease. The incidence increases with age and reaches 80% at age 80.

Prostatic intraepithelial neoplasia (PIN), analogous to CIN (p.500), has been recognised as a pre-invasive stage of the disease. Low grade PIN starts in early middle age and high grade PIN is strongly associated with development of invasive cancer.

DISEASES OF THE PENIS

TUMOURS of the PENIS

Papillomatous proliferations (condylomata acuminata), sometimes sessile but often florid, usually arise in the coronal sulcus or glans. They are due to sexually transmitted infection by Human Papilloma Virus (HPV) Types 6 and 11, and are analogous to similar lesions in the female genitalia

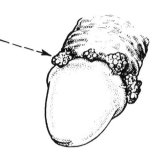

Peyronie's disease is a cellular fibromatosis related to Dupuytren's contracture.

Precancerous lesions

So-called leukoplakia and Bowen's disease are occasionally found on the penis. Another condition involving epithelial hyperplasia is Queyrat's erythroplasia. The histological appearances vary in these lesions, but all show epithelial dysplasia and usually amount to carcinoma-in-situ.

Carcinoma of the Penis

Accounts for less than 1% of all male malignancy and affects middle-aged and elderly men. The site of growth is usually in the preputial area, often in the coronal sulcus, but it extends to involve the glans penis. Two forms of growth occur:

Ulcer with sloughing base and hard rolled edges; usually it is adherent to the underlying tissues

Soft cauliflower growth

The growth spreads by the lymphatics to the regional (inguinal) nodes. Distant metastases occur late. The prognosis is reasonably good, 5-year survival rate being greater than 50%.

Aetiology

1. Early circumcision virtually confers immunity against carcinoma; the risk is greatly increased in the presence of poor penile hygiene.
2. Human Papilloma Virus (HPV) Types 16 and 18 are the initiating carcinogens. Inspissated smegma trapped behind the foreskin may be an important promoter (cofactor).

Inflammation

A wide variety of infections affect the penis, and are usually sexually transmitted. They include bacteria, e.g. syphilis and gonorrhoea, and viruses, e.g. genital herpes.

CANCER of the SCROTUM

This is a lesion which is rarely seen nowadays. Previously it was an occupational disease due to exposure to carcinogenic agents, e.g. soot, industrial oils, arsenic, etc.

DISEASES OF THE TESTIS

EPIDIDYMITIS AND ORCHITIS

Acute inflammation due to bacteria is uncommon in these organs, but spread of urinary infection via the vas deferens does occasionally take place and may result in destructive suppuration. Gonorrhoea and chlamydia are seen in young men.

In 20% of adult cases of mumps, the epididymis and testis become acutely inflamed. The condition is usually unilateral, but if bilateral there is a distinct danger of subsequent infertility.

Acute inflammation of the testis may be confused with **torsion**. Torsion generally occurs within the tunica vaginalis and leads to obstruction of the testicular vessels. Infarction results, with destruction of the tissue. Recurrent minor degrees of torsion can cause atrophy. Since the torsion may be bilateral, prophylactic surgery may reduce the risk of a second event.

Chronic inflammations are important, although rare, in this region.

Chronic granulomatous orchitis

This is a condition of unknown origin. The testis is infiltrated by macrophages, plasma cells and lymphocytes. Atrophy of the germinal epithelium occurs and the testis becomes fibrotic.

Tuberculosis

The epididymis is affected first; spread may have come from the prostate or vas deferens.

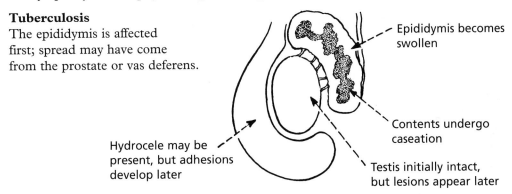

Epididymis becomes swollen

Contents undergo caseation

Testis initially intact, but lesions appear later

Hydrocele may be present, but adhesions develop later

Syphilis

Apart from the primary sore on the penis, the only other genital site involved is the testis. These are common in the tertiary stage. Two types of lesion are seen.

1. **Gumma**

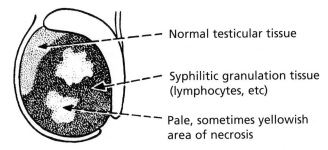

Normal testicular tissue

Syphilitic granulation tissue (lymphocytes, etc)

Pale, sometimes yellowish area of necrosis

2. **Granulomatous lesion** leading to scar formation with destruction of seminiferous tubules.

TUMOURS OF THE TESTIS

GERM CELL TUMOURS of the TESTIS

These tumours make up 2% of cancers in men and the incidence is rising steeply in Western countries. They are the commonest form of malignancy in young men. Tumours are more common in cases of undescended testicles.

The 2 main tumour types are SEMINOMA and TERATOMA.

Seminoma This corresponds to the dysgerminoma in the female. It is rare before puberty and has its peak incidence in adults in their 30s. It accounts for 50% of all testicular tumours.

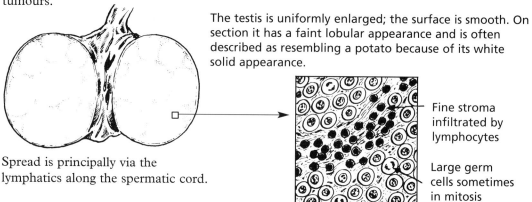

The testis is uniformly enlarged; the surface is smooth. On section it has a faint lobular appearance and is often described as resembling a potato because of its white solid appearance.

Spread is principally via the lymphatics along the spermatic cord.

Fine stroma infiltrated by lymphocytes

Large germ cells sometimes in mitosis

The growth is extremely radiosensitive and chemosensitive. Orchidectomy and adjuvant therapy give a >95% cure rate. In older men 'spermatocytic seminoma' is a rare variant but has an excellent prognosis.

Malignant teratoma (non-seminomatous germ cell tumour)

This type represents 35% of malignant testicular growths. It takes origin from totipotent germ cells capable of differentiating into derivatives of ectoderm, endoderm and mesoderm. It is customary to classify them according to the degree and type of differentiation exhibited. The lack of differentiation indicates the malignancy of the tumour.

The tumours form a spectrum of well differentiated to anaplastic highly malignant growths and are classified in various ways. The following is often used:

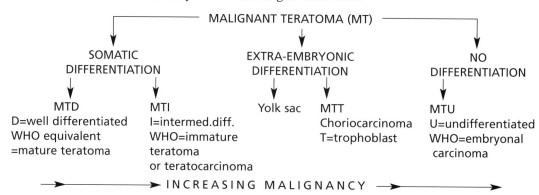

MALIGNANT TERATOMA (MT)

| SOMATIC DIFFERENTIATION | | EXTRA-EMBRYONIC DIFFERENTIATION | | NO DIFFERENTIATION |

MTD
D=well differentiated
WHO equivalent
=mature teratoma

MTI
I=intermed.diff.
WHO=immature
teratoma
or teratocarcinoma

Yolk sac

MTT
Choriocarcinoma
T=trophoblast

MTU
U=undifferentiated
WHO=embryonal
carcinoma

INCREASING MALIGNANCY

TUMOURS OF THE TESTIS

Malignant teratoma (*continued*)

These tumours, unlike seminoma, are usually irregular in shape and show focal haemorrhage and necrosis: in the better differentiated tumours small cysts are common.

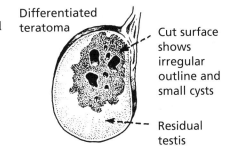

Differentiated teratoma

Cut surface shows irregular outline and small cysts

Residual testis

1. **MTD** – In this tumour organoid differentiation is easily recognisable (e.g. formation of intestinal glands, squamous epithelium, cartilage etc.): it is unlike its ovarian counter-part in important respects, however (a) it is very rare and (b) although apparently histologically benign, metastases may occur.
2. **MTI** – In addition to mature organised tissue this tumour contains varying amounts of clearly malignant tissue (e.g. adenocarcinoma)
3. **MTU** – These tumours are almost completely anaplastic showing only focal areas of poor attempts at differentiation.
4. **Yolk sac and Trophoblastic elements** occur commonly in malignant teratomas: pure forms are rare. α-Fetoprotein (from yolk sac elements) and chorionic gonadotrophin (from trophoblastic elements) are used in diagnosis and monitoring progress.
5. **Combined Germ-Cell Tumours** – Between 10 and 15% of germ-cell tumours consist of a mixture of seminomatous and teratomatous elements.

Spread
Lymphatic spread to paraortic lymph nodes is the usual mode of spread: vascular invasion with lung metastases also occurs.

Prognosis
Modern therapy has greatly improved the overall prognosis.

Large cells resembling those of seminoma

Intratubular germ cell neoplasia
There is an 'in situ' form of germ cell tumour, often found in association with the malignant tumours described above and thought to represent a precursor form.

Tubular basement membrane intact

MISCELLANEOUS TUMOURS
The following tumours are rare: Sertoli tumours,
Leydig cell tumours,
Lymphoma.

It should be remembered that leukaemia often involves the testes (p.443).

INFERTILITY

There are numerous causes which affect females or males. The causes are classified as follows:

1. **Pregonadal** – usually endocrine disorders of pituitary or adrenal origin.

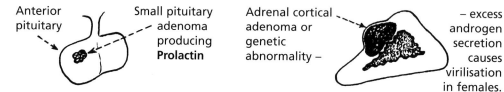

2. **Gonadal** — failure of production of gametes.

	Male	Female
(i) *Chromosomal defects*	**Klinefelter's syndrome**	**Turner's syndrome**
	XXY	XO
(ii) *Germ cell aplasia*	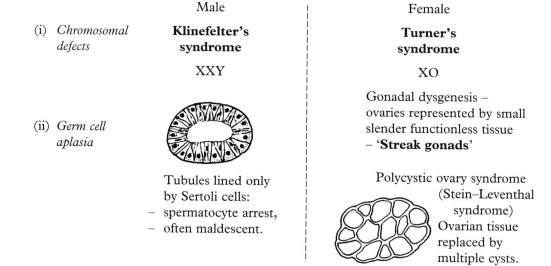 Tubules lined only by Sertoli cells: – spermatocyte arrest, – often maldescent.	Gonadal dysgenesis – ovaries represented by small slender functionless tissue – '**Streak gonads**' Polycystic ovary syndrome (Stein–Leventhal syndrome) Ovarian tissue replaced by multiple cysts.

(iii) *Iatrogenic causes:* **Irradiation, chemotherapy,** hormones e.g. the 'pill' and oestrogens in treatment of prostatic carcinoma.

3. **Postgonadal** – obstruction of passage of gametes.

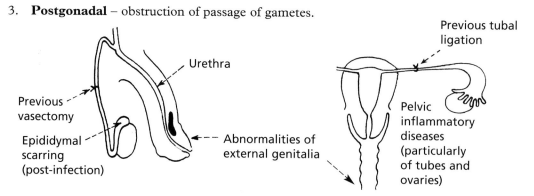

Note: In some cases of infertility no cause can be detected.

CHAPTER 13

NERVOUS SYSTEM

NERVOUS SYSTEM – ANATOMY AND PHYSIOLOGY

Considerations of anatomy and physiology have important applications to diseases of the central nervous system (CNS), particularly their effects and spread.

The anatomy of the various coverings is important.

The skull and vertebrae form a rigid compartment protecting the delicate CNS tissues.

This rigidity has serious disadvantages when pressure inside the skull increases, e.g. an expanding lesion soon takes up the small reserves of space available and the delicate brain tissues are progressively compressed, with very serious results.

Meninges and cerebrospinal fluid (CSF)

The CSF circulating freely in the subarachnoid space over the whole CNS surface and in the ventricular system acts as a protective water bath.

Diseases (particularly infections) at this site are usually *widespread* over the whole brain and cord surfaces, e.g. meningitis. Impediment to the flow of CSF causes serious effects – hydrocephalus.

The detailed arrangement of the meninges is important.

The thick **dura**, closely applied to the skull, acts as the periosteum – its rigid reflections (falx cerebri and tentorium cerebelli) complicate the effects of increased intracranial pressure.

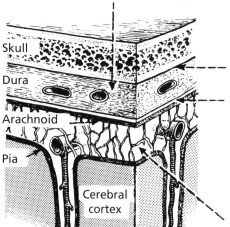

Skull
Dura
Arachnoid
Pia
Cerebral cortex

Extradural lesions tend to be localised; they have to strip the dura from the bone.
Subdural lesions remain local but can spread more widely since the arachnoid and dura are loosely attached.

The **arachnoid**, a delicate membrane, is loosely attached to the dura and sends trabeculae across the subarachnoid space which contains the cerebral blood vessels and the CSF.

Disease in the **subarachnoid** space can spread widely over the whole surface of the brain and spinal cord but is prevented from penetrating into the brain tissue by the **pia**.

NERVOUS SYSTEM – ANATOMY AND PHYSIOLOGY

The **pia** is invaginated into the brain substance along with the small penetrating vessels.

The dura, arachnoid and pia act as barriers which selectively separate the CSF and the blood from the CNS tissues.

It is important to understand that, although the CSF is very similar in composition to the extracellular fluid of the brain, changes in the CSF only very indirectly reflect changes in the CNS in disease.

The pia's barrier function is reinforced by the membrane formed by the foot processes of astrocytes:

1. on the brain surface
2. around the penetrating vessels. The potential space between the vessel wall and the pia is called the Virchow–Robin space.

3. at capillary level the pia is not present, but the foot processes along with the capillary endothelium and basement membrane form a specialised and selective 'blood-brain barrier'.

Thus the pia and the membrane formed by the foot processes of the astrocytes separate types of tissue derived from two embryological layers.

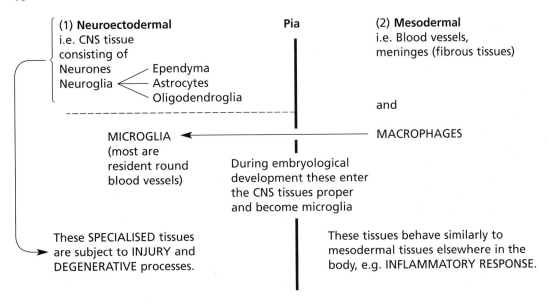

(1) Neuroectodermal
i.e. CNS tissue consisting of
Neurones
Neuroglia ⟨ Ependyma
Astrocytes
Oligodendroglia

Pia

(2) Mesodermal
i.e. Blood vessels, meninges (fibrous tissues)

MICROGLIA
(most are resident round blood vessels)

During embryological development these enter the CNS tissues proper and become microglia

and

MACROPHAGES

These SPECIALISED tissues are subject to INJURY and DEGENERATIVE processes.

These tissues behave similarly to mesodermal tissues elsewhere in the body, e.g. INFLAMMATORY RESPONSE.

NEURONAL DAMAGE

NEURONES are sensitive to damage by a wide variety of agents including anoxia, hypoglycaemia, virus infections and intracellular metabolic disturbances (e.g. associated with vitamin B deficiencies).

There are two main types, depending on the rapidity of the changes.

1. *Rapid NECROSIS* – associated with acute failure of function.

Healthy cell → Damaging agent e.g. hypoxia → Nuclear pyknosis, cytoplasmic shrinkage → Dissolution of cell with phagocytosis of debris

2. *Slow ATROPHIC CHANGES* – associated with gradual loss of function.

Healthy cell → Damaging agent → Cells usually smaller – but may be distended with abnormal metabolites → Eventual dissolution

The process of ageing involves cumulative atrophy and disappearance of neurones; in some individuals the process is speeded up resulting in ***presenile dementia***.
Note: There is no regeneration of destroyed neurones.
A large group of disorders of cerebral function seen in psychiatric practice have (as yet) no morphological evidence of nerve cell damage. They are caused by disturbances of poorly understood biochemical control mechanisms within the brain.
In addition to the PRIMARY degenerations described above, neurones are subject to SECONDARY degeneration in certain circumstances.

1. ***Retrograde degeneration*** – when the main axon is damaged there is degeneration of the neurone as well as the classical distal degeneration of the axon.

Normal — Damage here

Retrograde degeneration of neurone — Wallerian degeneration distally with loss of myelin sheath

Cell swollen; pale staining; loss of Nissl substance (chromatolysis) → Proceeds to eventual disappearance of cell

2. ***Trans-synaptic degeneration*** – in closely integrated neurone systems, neurone loss may be followed by degeneration of associated neurones across synapses.

Degeneration — Damage — Degeneration

GLIAL REACTIONS

The glial cells react vigorously in many diseases of the CNS.

1. The **NEUROGLIAL** cells have supportive and nutritive functions.

(a) The **astrocytes** with their numerous fibrillary processes give structural support. They are less susceptible to damage than neurones.

Normal — Damage not sufficient to kill the cell — Cells multiply, and enlarge / Increase in fibril production — Later, cells atrophy leaving dense meshwork of fibres

This process is called GLIOSIS. It is a feature of many diseases and is analogous to scar tissue. These cells and fibres contain Glial Fibrillary Acidic Protein (GFAP), recognition of which, using antibodies, is useful in histological sections.

Note: Collagenous scar tissue is only formed in the CNS when mesodermal structures such as large blood vessels are damaged.

(b) The **oligodendrocytes** – small cells with short processes – have a nutritive function in respect of neurones and especially myelin. This reaction is best seen when neurones are damaged.

Neurone / **Normal** / Oligodendrocytes — Swollen neurone showing chromatolysis — Increased numbers of larger oligodendrocytes — this process is called **SATELLITOSIS**.

2. The **MICROGLIAL** cells are members of the mononuclear-phagocytic system. Reaction is best seen when there is necrosis of tissues.

Normal — Necrosis

Microglial cells resident near blood vessels

Activated microglia phagocytose degradation products, e.g. lipids, haemosiderin. Blood monocytes augment resident cells.

Microglial cells are well seen in and around infarcts; the activated cells which have ingested lipids are strikingly different from the small inactive microglia.

Eccentric nucleus / Foamy cytoplasm

These cells have been given a variety of names: e.g. 'gitter' cells, or lipophages (lipid phagocytes).

INCREASED INTRACRANIAL PRESSURE

INCREASED INTRACRANIAL PRESSURE (ICP) occurs in two main circumstances:

1. Due to the presence of an EXPANDING LESION
2. Due to obstruction of the free flow of the CSF – this causes hydrocephalus and is dealt with on page 574.

INTRACRANIAL EXPANDING LESIONS

These lesions may occur within the brain substance or in the meninges. Important examples are:

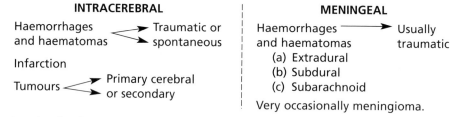

INTRACEREBRAL

Haemorrhages and haematomas → Traumatic or spontaneous

Infarction

Tumours → Primary cerebral or secondary

MENINGEAL

Haemorrhages → Usually traumatic
and haematomas
(a) Extradural
(b) Subdural
(c) Subarachnoid
Very occasionally meningioma.

The situation is often aggravated by cerebral OEDEMA.

The severity of the effects is modified by two important factors:
(1) the size of the lesion and (2) the rapidity of expansion.

There are three stages in the progress of increased intracranial pressure (ICP).

(1) The stage of **Compensation**

Expanding lesion
↓
Potential ICP ↑

↑CSF absorption
↓CSF formation

Vasoconstriction

↓CSF VOLUME

↓Intracranial BLOOD VOLUME

Allows brain to expand without serious effects

(2) The stage of **Decompensation**

At this stage there are herniations and distortions of the brain with their associated complications including:
- reduction in level of consciousness
- dilatation of pupil ipsilateral to mass lesion and papilloedema
- bradycardia with raised blood pressure ('Cushing' effect)
- Cheyne–Stokes' respiration

(3) A vicious circle is established leading to the stage of **vasomotor paralysis**.

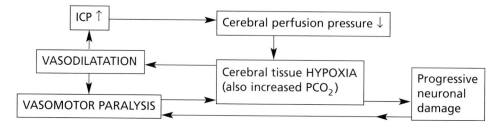

ICP ↑ → Cerebral perfusion pressure ↓

VASODILATATION

VASOMOTOR PARALYSIS

Cerebral tissue HYPOXIA (also increased PCO_2)

Progressive neuronal damage

INCREASED INTRACRANIAL PRESSURE

Effects

DISTORTIONS and DISLOCATIONS of the brain substance

These are to some extent dependent on the site of the initiating lesion; the effects of a unilateral expanding lesion are illustrated.

(1) Flattened cerebral convolutions (diminished subarachnoid space)

(2) Herniation of cingulate gyrus under the falx (supracallosal hernia)

(3) Movement of interventricular septum across the mid-line with distortion of ventricles

(4) Herniation of parahippocampal gyrus past the free edge of the tentorium cerebelli (tentorial hernia)

(5) Midbrain pushed against tentorium of opposite side (Kernohan notch); may give rise to paradoxical signs

(6) Cerebellar tonsils and medulla pushed down into foramen magnum

Falx

Skull

Dura

Expanding lesion (extradural haemorrhage)

Tentorium cerebelli

Foramen magnum

Note: The sudden removal of even small amounts of CSF by **LUMBAR PUNCTURE** may precipitate medullary 'coning' with fatal results due to damage to the 'vital centres'.

CEREBRAL OEDEMA

Swelling of the brain, of which oedema is the major component, is an important complication of many brain diseases because the enlargement either initiates or aggravates increased intracranial pressure.

The process may be localised or generalised depending on the type of initiating disorder.

Localised conditions

Examples:

    Infarcts, and local ischaemia

    Haematomas (due to vessel
       rupture and injury)

    Tumours

Generalised conditions

    Examples: Intoxications

    Metabolic disturbances, e.g. hypoglycaemia

    Generalised hypoxia

    Severe head trauma

    Malignant hypertension

The pathological mechanism is as follows:

Notes

(a) Components (1) and (2) overlap.

(b) The oedema fluid tends to spread in the white matter.

(c) The severity of oedema formation is very variable and unpredictable clinically.

(d) In clinical practice, therapy has two aspects:

    1. Treatment of the initiating disorder by any appropriate means.

    2. Minimising the formation of oedema by the use of

        (i) osmotic agents, e.g. urea or mannitol

        (ii) steroids.

INCREASED INTRACRANIAL PRESSURE

SECONDARY COMPLICATIONS

1. Vascular damage

(a) Compression of the central retinal vein causes PAPILLOEDEMA, an important clinical sign of raised ICP. *Note:* Axonal flow in the optic nerve is reduced, contributing to swelling of the optic disc.

Oedema of optic disc

Swelling and blurring of disc margin

(b) Stretching and compression of blood vessels may cause haemorrhage and infarction quite remote from the initiating lesion – secondary midbrain and calcarine infarction and haemorrhage are common.

2. Intracranial nerve damage

Oculomotor (III) and abducens (VI) nerves are particularly prone to damage, giving rise to paralysis of ocular movements in varying combinations.

The VIth nerve is specially vulnerable due to its long subarachnoid course. It is often the nerve on the side opposite the lesion which is stretched giving rise to paradoxical signs.

III

Vessels compressed

3. Obstruction of flow of CSF

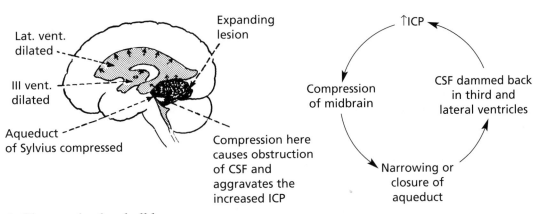

Lat. vent. dilated

III vent. dilated

Aqueduct of Sylvius compressed

Expanding lesion

Compression here causes obstruction of CSF and aggravates the increased ICP

↑ICP

CSF dammed back in third and lateral ventricles

Narrowing or closure of aqueduct

Compression of midbrain

4. Changes in the skull bones

Long continued ICP causes bone erosion and thinning visible on X-ray.
(a) Erosion of posterior clinoid processes of sphenoid bone.
(b) In children, before the skull is fully ossified, the inner table is thinned at the sites of convolutional pressure giving a striking X-ray appearance.

CIRCULATORY DISTURBANCES

(1) Hypoxia and ischaemia and (2) intracranial haemorrhage are the important and common mechanisms causing brain damage.

ACUTE HYPOXIC DISORDERS

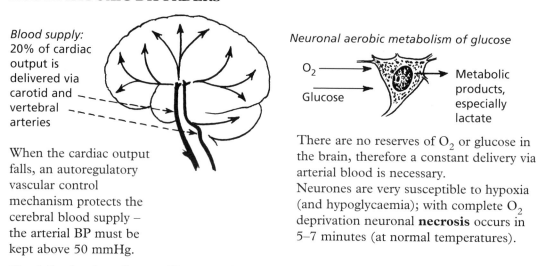

Blood supply: 20% of cardiac output is delivered via carotid and vertebral arteries

Neuronal aerobic metabolism of glucose

When the cardiac output falls, an autoregulatory vascular control mechanism protects the cerebral blood supply – the arterial BP must be kept above 50 mmHg.

There are no reserves of O_2 or glucose in the brain, therefore a constant delivery via arterial blood is necessary.

Neurones are very susceptible to hypoxia (and hypoglycaemia); with complete O_2 deprivation neuronal **necrosis** occurs in 5–7 minutes (at normal temperatures).

The following flow diagram illustrates the factors which influence availability of O_2 and the conditions giving rise to hypoxia.

These conditions, singly or together, can be responsible for cerebral hypoxia.

CEREBRAL INFARCTION

This condition, the commoner of the two main types of stroke (the other is spontaneous intracerebral haemorrhage), is caused by failure of the supply of oxygen (and glucose) to maintain the viability of the tissues in the territory of a cerebral arterial branch. This is not always due to simple local arterial occlusion, and very often a component of central circulatory deficiency is contributory. The lesion is essentially necrosis of all the tissues in the affected territory.

Mechanism

Precipitating condition ——➤ Perfusion failure ——➤ INFARCTION (ischaemic necrosis)

LOCAL ARTERIAL DISEASE (particularly ATHEROMA) and its complications, are the most common.

1. Arterial occlusions

(a)
THROMBOSIS on atheromatous plaque in

Intracerebral artery

Internal carotid artery

(b)
EMBOLISM commonly derived from heart
  (i) atrial fibrillation;
  (ii) endocarditis;
  (iii) mural thrombus complicating myocardial infarction.

Emboli derived from ulcerated atheroma in carotid artery are an important cause of infarcts

2. Arterial stenosis

ATHEROMA – the widespread loss of arterial lumen potentiates cerebral perfusion deficiency in two ways: (1) by distributing the normal arterial flow and (2) by prejudicing anastomotic communications.

Atheromatous stenosis alone is not usually a cause of infarction, but when central circulatory deficiency is added, infarction is common, e.g. this may vary from the slight fall in BP during sleep to the severe hypotension of shock or myocardial infarction.

Other rarer causes of arterial stenosis are dissecting aneurysm and arteritis. Arterial spasm is even rarer.

CEREBRAL INFARCTION

SITES

While infarcts may occur anywhere in the brain, depending on the vagaries of the precipitating arterial lesions, certain sites are more commonly affected.

1. In cases of local arterial occlusion, **internal structures supplied by 'end' arterial branches** are particularly vulnerable. The cortex is often protected in variable degree by anastomoses of other cerebral arteries. This is illustrated in the territory of the middle cerebral artery.

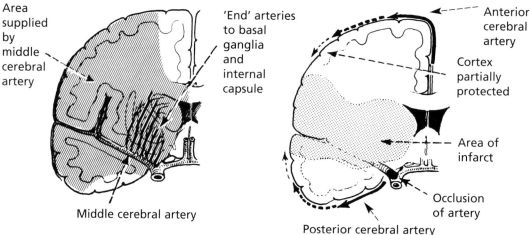

Area supplied by middle cerebral artery

'End' arteries to basal ganglia and internal capsule

Middle cerebral artery

Anterior cerebral artery

Cortex partially protected

Area of infarct

Occlusion of artery

Posterior cerebral artery

2. **Boundary zones** (see p.176)

    The cortex in particular is damaged in boundary zone infarction. In these cases, central circulatory deficiency is an important component, e.g. hypotension.

BRAIN DAMAGE DUE TO CARDIAC ARREST

This is characterised by widely distributed selective neuronal necrosis – the neurones are more susceptible to hypoxia than the supporting cells.

Affected areas – total cortical necrosis
or
most sensitive zones – hippocampus
– layers III, V, VI of cortex
– within sulci
– Purkinje cells of cerebellum.

Note: (a) These changes do not become apparent unless the patient survives at least 12 hours after the arrest.

(b) Similar types of neuronal damage can be seen in severe acute hypoglycaemia, carbon monoxide or barbiturate poisoning.

540

CEREBRAL INFARCTION

The diagram below illustrates the evolution of an infarct, e.g. in the territory of the middle cerebral artery. Up to 24 hours there is virtually no visible change.

18–24 hr	After 24 hours	After a few days	After weeks/months
Gross appearances			
	Less difficult to see	Line of demarcation seen	Demolition + scarring
Very difficult to see			
	Slight swelling / Blurring of white/grey junction	Necrotic tissue. Soft to touch; usually pale but may be congested if blood has permeated in (haemorrhagic infarct)	Cyst with pale or yellowish fluid / Shrinkage of scarred area: compensatory dilatation of ventricle
Microscopic appearances			
Early neuronal damage	Early neuronal damage ↓ Necrosis of neurones	Organisation of infarct begins Macrophages appear; capillary sprouting; oedema diminishing	Organisation well established; neurones disappear; numerous macrophages; gliosis
Clinical associations			

FUNCTIONAL LOSS

Effects are maximal in the early stages when oedema and circulatory disturbance in the adjacent tissues augment the functional loss caused by infarct. Larger infarcts may be associated with loss of consciousness.

The prognostic assessment of final functional loss cannot be made until the changes have subsided and any possible functional compensations have been established. This takes many weeks. Complete clinical recovery may follow small infarcts. Prompt thrombolytic therapy with tissue plasminogen activator can limit the degree of permanent disability.

CEREBRAL HAEMORRHAGE

Spontaneous intracranial bleeding is the second main type of stroke. In the great majority of cases there is localised arterial disease aggravated by hypertension. A small number are associated with cerebral tumours, systemic bleeding diathesis or arteriovenous malformations.

In most hypertensives over middle age, **microaneurysms** are found in the very small cerebral arteries. It is believed that rupture of one of these aneurysms is the immediate cause of intracerebral haemorrhage.

Rupture

Haematoma forms. Commonest site is branches of middle cerebral artery to basal ganglia and internal capsule; also occurs in pons and cerebellum.

Thin-walled microaneurysm

Progress
The onset is usually sudden with headache and, because of the high blood pressure, progress is rapid and the haemorrhage large.

↓

Associated raised ICP effects

↓

Death in many cases

When the bleeding is limited, there is survival with varying residual paralysis.

Final outcome
Cystic space containing yellow-brown fluid walled off by gliosis.

Apoplectic cyst

Note: Intracerebral bleeding may track irregularly and often reaches the subarachnoid space and ventricles.

SUBARACHNOID HAEMORRHAGE

This is commonly but not exclusively the result of rupture of a 'berry' aneurysm at or near the circle of Willis. The basic abnormality is a congenital weakness of the elastic tissues in the arterial wall; only rarely is an aneurysm present at birth, and while subarachnoid haemorrhage does occur in young people, the incidence increases with age. Hypertension is an important contributing factor.

Sites Often multiple, near arterial junctions.

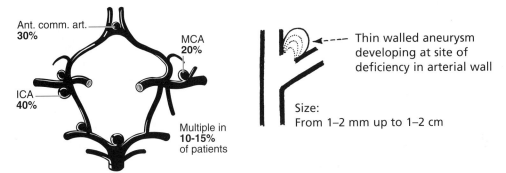

Not all aneurysms rupture; they are found incidentally at autopsy.
Massive haemorrhage may be preceded by one or more small leaks – marked by headache without functional loss.

Progress

Haemorrhage spreading throughout subarachnoid space – generalised ICP increased; blood-stained CSF.

Local infarction may be a complication

Irritant effect of haemorrhage causes local arterial spasm

Note: The aneurysm may rupture directly into the brain and mimic an intracerebral haemorrhage.

CSF findings

1–24 hours – blood stained; blood content constant in sequential samples (distinguishes blood derived from a traumatic tap)
– centrifuge supernatant – may be pink due to haemolysis.

24 hours onwards – supernatant shows xanthochromia (yellow colour due to presence of blood degradation products).

Other causes of cerebral haemorrhage of either type are vascular malformations and coagulation disorders.

HEAD INJURY

Head injuries of varying severity are common nowadays, particularly as a consequence of road traffic accidents. Immediate damage is caused by two main mechanisms which overcome the protection of the vulnerable cerebral tissues provided by the skull and the CSF 'water cushion'.

1. **Direct blows to the head** (e.g. **missile head injury**)

usually cause injury to the soft tissues of the scalp and often fracture of the skull with contusion or laceration of the underlying brain.

Scalp – laceration ± haematoma

Skull – fracture often comminuted ± depressed fragments

Brain – contusion, laceration or haematoma

2. **Non-missile head injury**

Since the head is usually freely moveable on the neck, the sudden application of forces derived from **acceleration, deceleration** and, particularly, **rotation** of the head often causes serious brain injury.

(a) **Skull fractures**

(i) *Skull damage*

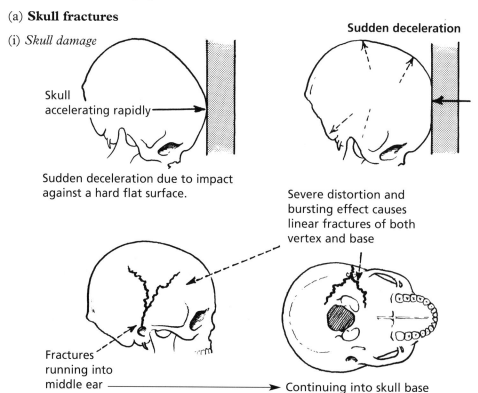

Skull accelerating rapidly

Sudden deceleration due to impact against a hard flat surface.

Sudden deceleration

Severe distortion and bursting effect causes linear fractures of both vertex and base

Fractures running into middle ear ⟶ Continuing into skull base

HEAD INJURY

Acceleration/deceleration injury

(ii) *Brain damage*

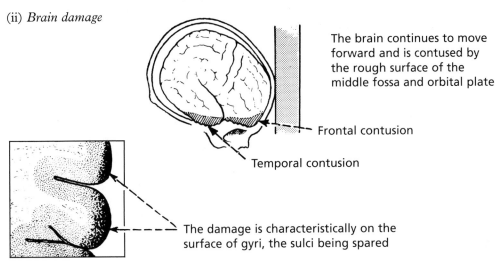

The brain continues to move forward and is contused by the rough surface of the middle fossa and orbital plate

Frontal contusion

Temporal contusion

The damage is characteristically on the surface of gyri, the sulci being spared

(b) **Rotation**

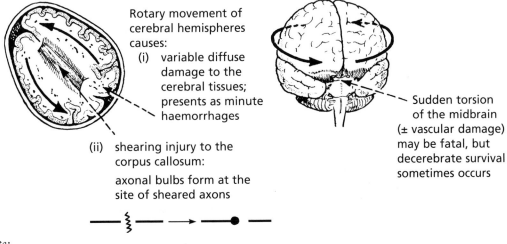

Rotary movement of cerebral hemispheres causes:
(i) variable diffuse damage to the cerebral tissues; presents as minute haemorrhages

(ii) shearing injury to the corpus callosum:

axonal bulbs form at the site of sheared axons

Sudden torsion of the midbrain (± vascular damage) may be fatal, but decerebrate survival sometimes occurs

Note:
It will be appreciated that more serious cerebral damage is the result of interaction of complex physical forces and anatomical features. An understanding of these mechanisms explains why serious cerebral injury is not uncommon in the absence of damage to the scalp or fracture of the skull, and also why brain damage may be remote from the site of impact: so-called 'contre-coup' injury is sustained when the brain tissue opposite the site of impact is contused.

HEAD INJURY

DELAYED COMPLICATIONS

In addition to damage sustained immediately at the time of impact, certain serious complications may supervene over the next hours or few days.

1. Haemorrhages

(a) **Extradural haematoma**

This type of haemorrhage classically occurs as a complication of linear fracture of the skull vault when the middle meningeal artery is torn.

Artery torn at site of fracture   Haemorrhage gradually strips dura from bone   A large, saucer-shaped haematoma forms

The classic clinical association is a direct blow to the head from which recovery is rapid. After a lucid interval of varying duration up to several hours, signs of increased intracranial pressure supervene. This chain of events is explained by the time taken for the haemorrhage to accumulate by stripping the dura from the skull.

(b) **Subdural haematoma**. This may occur at any site and is often extensive because of the loose attachment of the dura and arachnoid membranes. It is usually due to rupture of small bridging veins.

Skull ----

Bridging vein

Venous sinus in dura

Rupture of vein at entry into dura;

Dura

Blood spreads in subdural space

These acute subdural haematomas are often associated with subarachnoid haemorrhage and cerebral contusions.

(c) **Intracerebral haematomas** occur in association with cortical contusions particularly in the temporal and frontal lobes (burst lobe); but also at random deep within the hemispheres due to shearing at the time of impact. Large haematomas are uncommon.

HEAD INJURY

Delayed complications (*continued*)

2. **Cerebral oedema** is an important complication.

   Increased intracranial pressure ——► Cerebral hypoxia.

3. **External leakage of CSF** (and blood) from the ear and nose may complicate fractures of the skull base. This complication may be of long duration and is always a potential entry for infection.

4. **Local infection** may complicate compound fractures and progress to meningitis.

LATE COMPLICATIONS

1. **Epilepsy**

   Head injury is an important cause of epilepsy. The risk is highest in severe missile head injury and may be related to ischaemic brain damage.

2. **Chronic subdural haematoma**

   A thick layer of fluid and partially clotted blood gradually accumulates between the dura and arachnoid membranes which show considerable reactive thickening.

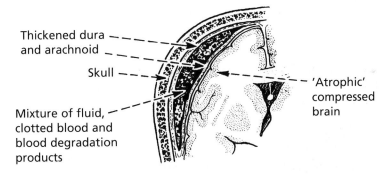

The precise cause is not known; most cases occur in alcoholics or in elderly people already suffering from cerebral atrophy, and it is possible that the small bridging veins are unduly stretched and become more susceptible to damage.

The clinical signs are usually insidious in onset and progressive, and in many cases there is a history of either no or only very trivial injury.

AGEING and DEMENTIA

Normal Brain Ageing

With normal ageing the brain becomes atrophic, but the morphological changes described below are not necessarily accompanied by loss of intellect.

Changes in old age

Gross as seen naked-eye at autopsy

Normal (3rd decade)

Mean weight
♂ – 1450 g
♀ – 1350 g

Granulations

Small

Thin arachnoid
Gyri – slightly rounded
Sulci – narrow

Aged brain
looks smaller

Sulci appear prominent due to cortical shrinkage

Mean loss 100 g – often much more

Large and numerous

Thick arachnoid

Gyri – narrow

Sulci – broad

There is compensatory enlargement of the lateral ventricles.

Dementia

Dementia is defined as 'an acquired progressive global impairment of intellect, memory and personality, without impairment of consciousness'. Around 5% of the population over 65 years are affected and the proportion rises to over 20% of these over 80 years.

Main causes are:
1. Alzheimer's diseases 70%
2. Multi-infarct dementia 10–15%
3. Lewy body dementia 10–20%

Rare causes include:

1. Genetic disorders (Huntington's disease, Pick's disease)
2. Infections (Creutzfeld–Jacob disease, see p.559, AIDS)

ALZHEIMER'S DISEASE

This disease accounts for around 70% of cases of dementia. While typically a disease of the elderly, especially females, it is also seen in patients under 60 years, in whom there is often a family history. Almost all patients with Down's syndrome who survive to 50 years develop Alzheimer's (suggesting that chromosome 21 is important).

Pathology

The changes of Alzheimer's resemble those of normal ageing, but are greatly exaggerated in the temporal and parietal lobes and in the hippocampus.

Parietal lobe - - - →

The lateral ventricles show compensatory dilatation.

Temporal lobe - - →

Hippocampus - - - -

The histological hallmarks are:

1. Extracellular senile plaques.

(Silver stain)

Tangled aggregates of distended neurites presenting as black dots and rods with a centre core of amyloid

2. Intracellular neuro-fibrillary tangles.

Paired helical filaments composed of tau protein form around the nuclei of neurones.

3. Amyloid angiopathy.

Deposited in meninges and blood vessel walls

Aetiology

This remains unclear, but there are both genetic and acquired factors.

Genetic factors – several genes are involved
1. Amyloid precursor protein (chromosome 21) – early onset Alzheimer's.
2. Presenilin 1 and 2 (chromosome 14 and 1) – proteins involved in binding amyloid precursor proteins.
3. Apolipoprotein E – the e4 allele is associated with late onset disease – it may determine the age of onset.
4. α-2 macroglobulin – may be involved in clearance of amyloid proteins.

Acquired factors
1. Toxic substances e.g. aluminium.
2. Reduced nerve growth factors and diminished repair.
3. Impairment of calcium dependent K^+ channels in neurones.
4. Repeated head injury.
5. Free radical injury.
6. Coexistent vascular disease.

Genetic factors → Deposition of amyloid

Environmental factors → Neuronal damage

Reduced neuronal function (especially cholinergic nerves)

DEMENTIA

549

DEMENTIA

MULTI-INFARCT DEMENTIA

This form of dementia is associated with vascular disease – with infarcts often in the middle cerebral arterial distribution. The volume of brain loss appears to be important.

Loss of >100 ml of brain correlates with dementia.

Hypertension is an important underlying factor.

LEWY BODY DEMENTIA

This disorder accounts for 10–20% of dementias. Clinically there are overlapping features with Parkinson's disease. There is widespread neuronal loss in the cerebral cortex. Characteristic Lewy bodies are identified in surviving neurones. Known components of Lewy bodies include alpha-synuclein and ubiquitin.

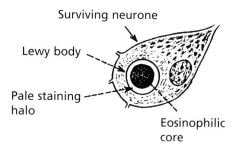

PICK'S DISEASE

This uncommon form of dementia has a strong familial (autosomal dominant) component. There is typically severe atrophy of the temporal and frontal lobes. The histological marker in the surviving neurones is the Pick body.

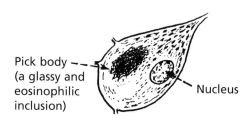

HUNTINGTON'S DISEASE

This is an uncommon autosomal dominant condition beginning in the 3rd or 4th decade and characterised by psychiatric disorders, progressive dementia and in some patients bizarre writhing movements (chorea).

Pathology

The caudate nucleus is severely atrophic. The genetic locus is on chromosome 4 and consists of a trinucleotide repeat with up to 34 copies in normal patients. In Huntington's disease the number of repeats increases with each successive generation resulting in earlier onset of symptoms (genetic anticipation). Genetic screening is available.

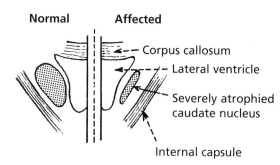

PUNCH DRUNK SYNDROME

Professional boxers may develop dementia due to neuronal damage caused by repeated blows to the head.

INFECTIONS

Compared with the high incidence of infection generally, infection of the central nervous system is uncommon. The pathological effects may be slight and wholly recoverable as in some virus infections, or severe, leading to permanent damage or death.

Anatomically, infections fall into two main groups which tend to remain separated due to the intervention of the **pial** barrier (see p.531).

Infections will be considered in three broad aetiological groups:
(1) Bacterial, (2) Viral and (3) Miscellaneous types.

BACTERIAL INFECTIONS

1. Most commonly by the blood stream

Bacteria settling in subarachnoid space

Meningitis

Common organisms include:
Infants – *Escherichia coli*
Children – *Haemophilus influenzae*
Adults – *Neisseria meningitidis*
Elderly – *Streptococcus pneumoniae*

Bacteria settling in brain substance

Brain abscess

Common organisms include:
Streptococcus species
Staphylococcus aureus
Others

2. From an adjacent local infected site – these are pyogenic infections.

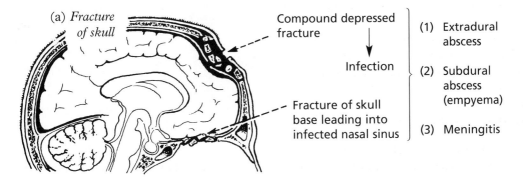

(a) *Fracture of skull*

Compound depressed fracture
↓
Infection

Fracture of skull base leading into infected nasal sinus

(1) Extradural abscess

(2) Subdural abscess (empyema)

(3) Meningitis

BACTERIAL INFECTION

Bacterial infections from an adjacent local infected site (*continued*)

(b) *Middle ear and mastoid disease*

In untreated purulent otitis media, three serious complications may arise from spread of the inflammation.

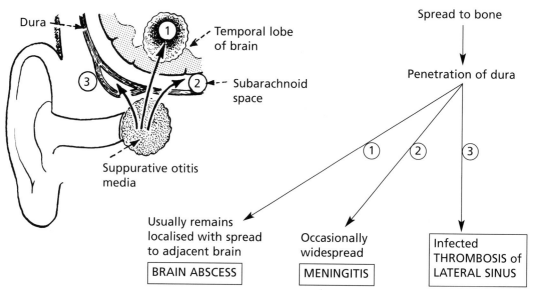

PYOGENIC MENINGITIS

The whole subarachnoid space contains purulent exudate which is maximal in sulci and around the brain base cisternae.

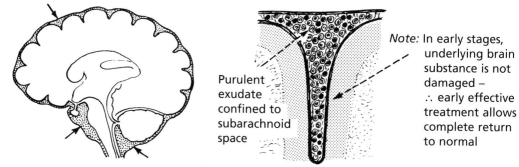

In untreated or ineffectively treated patients who survive, complications include cranial nerve damage, hydrocephalus and variable brain damage.

The CSF in the acute stage contains neutrophils and the infecting organism can usually be demonstrated.

BACTERIAL INFECTION

PYOGENIC BRAIN ABSCESS

The abscesses resulting from direct spread of adjacent infection or by blood borne infection – as seen particularly in bronchiectasis – are often well circumscribed by a pyogenic membrane.

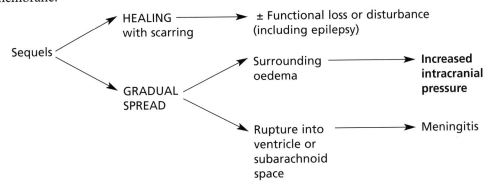

Sequels
- HEALING with scarring ⟶ ± Functional loss or disturbance (including epilepsy)
- GRADUAL SPREAD
  - Surrounding oedema ⟶ **Increased intracranial pressure**
  - Rupture into ventricle or subarachnoid space ⟶ Meningitis

Clinical note: An abscess is often silent early in its evolution, and the infection at the site of entry may have healed before the onset of serious complications causes clinical signs.

Multiple small abscesses occur in staphylococcal pyaemia and microabscesses may complicate bacterial endocarditis. The cerebral pathology in these circumstances is only one facet of serious systemic infection.

TUBERCULOSIS

Infection of the nervous system is always secondary to disease elsewhere and may be a component of miliary tuberculosis. It may complicate AIDS and remains prevalent in many parts of the world. Without treatment tuberculous meningitis is invariably fatal.

Tubercles appearing round vessels

Exudate of lymphocytes and fibrin

Creamy exudate obscuring anatomy of vessels and nerves at base of brain

TUBERCULOMA These localised tuberculous cerebral abscesses are now very rare.

SYPHILIS Neurological syphilis is rare nowadays. The main pathological lesions are described on p.76, 77.

VIRUS INFECTIONS

Compared with the incidence of virus infections in general, infection of the central nervous system is rare, even with viruses having an affinity for the CNS – **NEUROTROPIC VIRUSES.**

There are 3 broad groups:

1. **Acute**
   Cell lysis occurs towards the end of the viraemic phase of infection. This is the common type of disease. Herpes simplex, mumps, poliovirus and togaviruses are examples.

2. **Persistent**
   Viruses which usually cause damage outside the CNS behave uncharacteristically and cause continuing and active disease of the CNS over a long period (months – years). Measles, rubella and JC papovavirus are examples.

3. **Latent** virus infection is seen in herpes zoster and possibly plays a role in the demyelinating diseases.

Virus infection also has a possible role in oncogenesis within the CNS.

Routes of infection

Most viruses arrive at the CNS via the blood, but the factors which potentiate the establishment of disease within the CNS are poorly understood.

Primary portal of entry

In rabies, the virus travels from the wound up the peripheral nerves to the CNS; a similar mechanism may be involved in herpes simplex encephalitis.

VIRUS INFECTIONS

BASIC PATHOLOGICAL EFFECTS

(a) **VIRAL MENINGITIS** is the commonest form of meningitis; the disease is usually mild and only the meninges are affected. Recovery is usually complete.

(b) In more severe cases, the brain substance is also damaged in varying degree – ENCEPHALITIS (meningoencephalitis).

The meninges (CSF) contain increased protein, normal sugar and a mononuclear cellular infiltrate (particularly **lymphocytes**, plasma cells and large mononuclear cells).

In the brain the characteristic changes are:

1. PERIVASCULAR CUFFING (same infiltrate as meninges)
2. ACUTE NEURONAL DAMAGE up to complete lysis with accompaning neuronophagia and inflammatory changes. In some conditions, surviving neurones contain cytoplasmic and/or nuclear inclusions. Specific viral inclusions, e.g. HSV and CMV, may be detected by immunohistochemistry.

To these basic changes, damage to myelin and glial tissue may be added, and small focal haemorrhages may be seen. The damage is effected in two ways:

1. By the direct effects of virus on cells.
2. By a host cell-mediated and humoral response to the infected cell.

Diagnosis

Examination of the CSF is helpful in establishing a diagnosis of aseptic meningitis or meningoencephalitis.

Note: The findings in tuberculous meningitis are very similar except that in tuberculous meningitis the CSF **sugar is low.**

The specific virus aetiology is more difficult to establish and in severe cases brain biopsy may be required.

Clinical associations and progress

In viral meningitis, the illness is mild with fever, headache and neck stiffness the main signs. Recovery is almost always complete.

In meningoencephalitis, signs of cerebral 'irritation' and neuronal damage are seen, e.g. mental confusion, delusion, stupor, convulsions and coma, and there may be localising signs. In mild cases, recovery is complete, but in more severe cases residual paralysis and other signs indicative of permanent brain damage may follow. Death in coma with respiratory failure occurs in very severe cases.

VIRUS INFECTIONS

HERPES SIMPLEX VIRUS (HSV) ENCEPHALITIS

This is the commonest form of severe acute viral encephalitis and is almost always due to Herpes Simplex Virus Type 1. It occurs in 2 forms:

1. In infancy, as part of a generalised HSV infection.
2. In adults, due to reactivation of the virus in the trigeminal ganglion.

Most cases are sporadic but immunosuppression increases the risk.

The temporal lobes are most affected. Early treatment with antiviral drugs has now greatly reduced the previous high mortality.

HERPES ZOSTER (See also p.80)

This is a disease of adults, presenting as a painful vesicular rash, usually unilateral and affecting one or a few adjacent dermatomes only. It is due to recurrence of a latent varicella (chickenpox) infection.

Mechanism

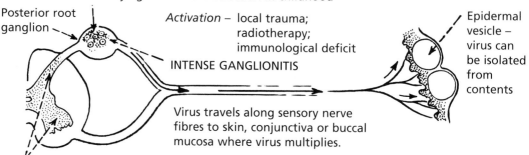

Virus lying latent from infection in childhood

Posterior root ganglion

Activation – local trauma; radiotherapy; immunological deficit

INTENSE GANGLIONITIS

Epidermal vesicle – virus can be isolated from contents

Virus travels along sensory nerve fibres to skin, conjunctiva or buccal mucosa where virus multiplies.

Minor secondary degenerative changes in cord

Sequels
1. An occasional sequel is intense pain with varying paraesthesiae and anaesthesia long after the acute phase has healed.
2. In cases of Vth nerve herpes, serious damage to the eye may result.

RABIES

The rabies virus shows marked neurotropism and can infect most mammals. Various wild carnivores (fox, jackal, skunk, vampire bats) are the natural reservoir. Many human cases are contracted from dogs.

Mechanism

Incubation period – usually 1–2 months may be up to 12 months

Entry of virus by bite or salivary contamination or abrasion → Local replication → Travels up sensory nerves to root ganglia → Spreads and replicates in CNS

Clinical signs appear

An unremitting encephalitis particularly affecting the grey matter is established. Diagnostic Negri bodies (virus inclusions) are found at autopsy in the pyramidal cells of the hippocampus and the Purkinje cells of the cerebellum.

Clinically, the encephalitis presents with extreme excitation of the sensory system. The classical hydrophobia (fear of water) is due to serious disturbance of the swallowing mechanism with muscular spasm. Without supportive therapy death occurs and is due to respiratory muscle spasm or paralysis.

VIRUS INFECTIONS

ENTEROVIRUSES

These are small RNA viruses (picornavirus group) and include POLIOVIRUSES, COXSACKIE VIRUSES and ECHOVIRUSES.

Infection is acquired by ingestion of faecally contaminated material followed by proliferation in the intestine. In only a small minority of infected cases does the virus pass the blood-brain barrier and cause disease of the CNS.

In addition to aseptic meningitis, the POLIOVIRUSES (and very occasionally Coxsackie and Echo viruses) cause the classic paralytic disease, **ANTERIOR POLIOMYELITIS**.

Pathological changes

The pathological changes are reflected in three clinical stages: (1) acute, (2) recovery and (3) permanent residual disability.

(1) **Acute** (up to 2 weeks)

Febrile illness — Viraemia

The virus shows tropism for motor nerve cells, particularly in the spinal cord

Perivascular cuffing

Aseptic meningitis

Partially damaged neurone

Dead neurone (neuronophagia)

Normal neurone

Damage to anterior horn is often localised and unilateral

Sometimes RESPIRATORY paralysis — — — — — — — — — — — — — — — — — — Damage to bulbar motor nuclei

(2) **Recovery**
(Several weeks/months)
Paralyses improve
– in mild cases functional recovery may be complete

Damaged neurone recovers — —

Dead neurone does not recover – gliosis

Inflammation has subsided

(3) **Permanent residual disability**
Wasting of muscles (neurogenic atrophy), varying deformities due to unopposed action of non-paralysed muscle

Shrunken anterior horn

Thin anterior nerve roots

VIRUS INFECTIONS

Persistent virus infections

Subacute sclerosing panencephalitis is a very rare disorder due to reactivation of latent measles virus. It affects children and young adults, often several years after uncomplicated measles, and is usually fatal within 6 months. The sequence is probably as follows:

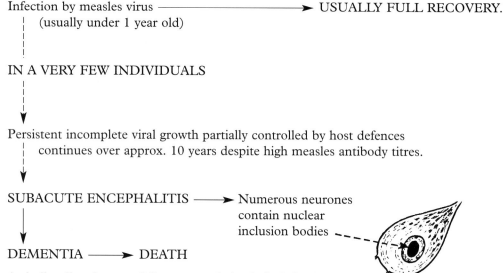

Infection by measles virus ⟶ USUALLY FULL RECOVERY.
    (usually under 1 year old)

IN A VERY FEW INDIVIDUALS

Persistent incomplete viral growth partially controlled by host defences
    continues over approx. 10 years despite high measles antibody titres.

SUBACUTE ENCEPHALITIS ⟶ Numerous neurones
                          contain nuclear
                          inclusion bodies

DEMENTIA ⟶ DEATH

A similar disorder may follow congenital rubella infection.

Progressive Multi-focal Leukoencephalopathy

JC papovavirus, a member of the polyoma virus group, may infect the oligodendrocytes of adults who are immunosuppressed. A rapidly progressive demyelinating disease follows – with degenerative changes in the deep white matter.

HIV and the Brain

Despite the introduction of highly active antiretroviral therapy (HAART), brain involvement is still a major cause of death in AIDS patients.

(a) HIV infection of the brain. This may lead to a subacute encephalitis often with dementia. The incidence has not decreased with HAART.
(b) Opportunistic infections including toxoplasma, fungi (cryptococcus), viruses (cytomegalovirus).
(c) Tumours – especially cerebral lymphoma.

The incidence of (b) and (c) has decreased dramatically with HAART.

PRION DISEASES

Also known as the transmissible spongiform encephalopathies, this group of diseases is caused by abnormal, distorted PRIONS. A prion is a small protein molecule found in the brain cell membrane. Normal cellular prion protein is termed PrP^c whereas the distorted protein is termed PrP^{sc} (originally referring to scrapie but now a generic term).

The PRION HYPOTHESIS

When a distorted prion molecule reaches the prions in the brain cell membrane of an individual, that molecule is able to act as a three-dimensional template to cause a normal prion molecule to adopt a similar distorted shape. This in turn can distort further proteins and so on.

TYPES OF PRION DISEASE

1. **Creutzfeld–Jacob Disease (CJD)** – this may be (i) **sporadic** (ii) **acquired** through contact with infected material e.g. pituitary derived hormones, corneal grafts or (iii) **familial** due a point mutation of the PrP gene.
2. **New-variant CJD** – This occurs in younger patients with early psychiatric symptoms and a longer clinical course. The strain of PrP responsible for nvCJD is identical to that of bovine spongiform encephalopathy (BSE) and is probably caused by ingestion of products from infected cattle.
3. **Other** – include KURU (historical) due to ingestion of human brain by cannibalism in New Guinea; GERSTMANN–STRAUSSLER–SCHEINKER disease; a familial dementia.

PATHOLOGY

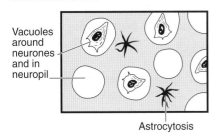

Vacuoles around neurones and in neuropil

Astrocytosis

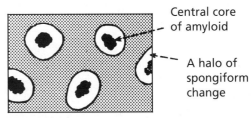

Central core of amyloid

A halo of spongiform change

Fibrillary plaques of PrP are numerous, particularly in the occipital cortex. These PrP plaques are most numerous in the cerebellum and can be detected by immunohistochemistry with antibodies to PrP^{sc}.

MISCELLANEOUS INFECTIONS AND INFESTATIONS

1. FUNGAL INFECTIONS

(a) **Primary infections.** In healthy adults, fungal infections are rare. Occasionally in the presence of heavy exposure to fungus, localised infection, often clinically insignificant, may occur, and in very rare cases CNS infection is a complication. In CRYPTOCOCCOSIS (C. *neoformans*), the fungus exhibits neurotropism and occasionally causes meningitis in otherwise healthy subjects.

(b) **Opportunistic infections** are becoming more common nowadays due to the use of immunosuppressive therapy and the increasing prevalence of AIDS. Various fungi including *Candida, Aspergillus, Nocardia* may cause serious cerebral damage. The incidence is decreasing in AIDS patients due to HAART.

2. PROTOZOAL INFECTIONS

(a) CEREBRAL MALARIA

Cerebral complications may occur in the severe acute malaria (falciparum type) which affects non-immune adults. Clinically, coma rapidly proceeds to death.

Mechanism

At autopsy the brain is swollen (oedema) and there may be petechial haemorrhages. Histologically, the capillaries are congested and malarial parasites and pigment are easily seen.

MISCELLANEOUS INFECTIONS AND INFESTATIONS

Protozoal infections (*continued*)

(b) TOXOPLASMOSIS

Although infection by *T. gondii* is common, serious nervous tissue damage is rare and is seen in two main circumstances. In both, it occurs as part of a systemic infection.

(i) In **congenital toxoplasmosis**, the infection is acquired by the fetus during a primary maternal infection.

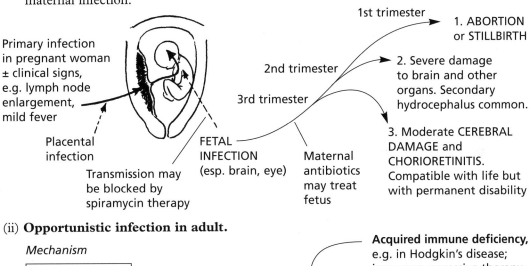

Primary infection in pregnant woman ± clinical signs, e.g. lymph node enlargement, mild fever

Placental infection

Transmission may be blocked by spiramycin therapy

FETAL INFECTION (esp. brain, eye)

Maternal antibiotics may treat fetus

1st trimester

2nd trimester

3rd trimester

1. ABORTION or STILLBIRTH

2. Severe damage to brain and other organs. Secondary hydrocephalus common.

3. Moderate CEREBRAL DAMAGE and CHORIORETINITIS. Compatible with life but with permanent disability

(ii) **Opportunistic infection in adult.**

Mechanism

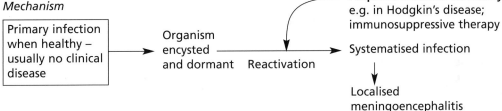

| Primary infection when healthy – usually no clinical disease |

Organism encysted and dormant → Reactivation

Acquired immune deficiency, e.g. in Hodgkin's disease; immunosuppressive therapy

Systematised infection

Localised meningoencephalitis

(c) TRYPANOSOMIASIS (AFRICAN SLEEPING SICKNESS)

T. brucei infection is transmitted to humans from animal reservoirs by the Tsetse fly. The organism is neurotropic and a meningoencephalitis results. The infection is associated with excessive IgM production. The 'cuffing' infiltrate has a high component of plasma cells and also 'Mott' cells – plasma cells distended by eosinophilic globules (denatured Ig).

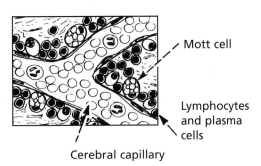

Mott cell

Lymphocytes and plasma cells

Cerebral capillary

3. METAZOAL INFESTATION

Cysticercosis.
The larvae of *Taenia solium* may encyst in the brain and can be the cause of epilepsy.
Hydatid cyst – also occurs in the brain (see p.361).

DEMYELINATING DISEASES

MULTIPLE SCLEROSIS (MS)

This is the commonest demyelinating disease – where the myelin sheath breaks down, leaving the axons healthy but with serious effects on their function.
Multiple sclerosis is a chronic disease of young adults.

The basic pathological change is a scattering of 'plaques' of demyelination most commonly adjacent to the lateral ventricles, optic nerve and chiasm, brainstem, cerebellum and spinal cord.

(Normal myelin stained black with Loyez stain or Weigert–Pal. No staining in areas of demyelination.)

In the early stages, there may be lymphocytic infiltration, but in the usually seen late lesions inflammation is absent

Clinical associations

The neurological signs reflect *white matter damage* – upper motor neurone weakness and paralysis; incoordination; visual disturbances; paraesthesia. ('Grey matter' signs, e.g. aphasia, fits and muscle atrophy are rare.)

Pons

Medulla

Spinal cord

Black staining normal myelin

Plaque – no myelin; axons remain; glial fibres increased; few oligodendrocytes

Course of disease

	Onset	Progress over many years
	Often acute; may be unnoticed.	Remission . . . Relapse . . . Remission → Incremental deterioration → Death

Variants are:
1. acute severe disease – rapid progress to death
2. chronic progression without remission
3. minimal signs with very long remissions.

Aetiology – This is unknown.
Geographically, the disease is common throughout temperate Europe and North America and is rare in the tropics.
A possible mechanism is:

LATENT VIRAL INFECTION
(? measles, ? EBV, ? Herpes)

GENETIC DISPOSITION
(High concordance in identical twins) increase in HLA A3, B7, DW2, DR2

Activation of CD4+ T cells

Autoimmune attack on myelin

DEMYELINATION

DEMYELINATING DISEASES

ACUTE DISSEMINATED ENCEPHALOMYELITIS

An acute encephalitis in which demyelination is a prominent and characteristic feature is a very rare sequel to many natural viral diseases such as mumps, measles, chickenpox and rubella and to vaccination, historically against smallpox and rabies.

Clinically, there is fever, headache, vomiting and drowsiness followed by coma. There may be clinical evidence of focal neurological damage. Pathological changes are widespread in the brain and cord and rapidly progressive.

Distribution throughout brain
or
cord, especially **deep white matter** and pons

Minimal cellular infiltration of meninges

(Normal myelin of white matter stained black)

Perivenular cellular infiltrate (lymphocytes: plasma cells and macrophages)

Perivenular **demyelination** (unstained)

In **ACUTE HAEMORRHAGIC LEUKOENCEPHALITIS,** to these are added actual petechial haemorrhages from damaged vessels, particularly in the white matter; not all cases follow virus infection.

Mechanism. It is thought that in these disorders the damage to the myelin is not the result of direct virus attack but is an *autoimmune* reaction in which the antigen is a component of myelin and the virus in some unknown way acts as a trigger.

DISEASES due to ABNORMAL MYELIN

In this group of rare 'leukodystrophies', the molecular structure of myelin is abnormal due usually to abnormal or deficient enzyme action. Most cases are genetically determined, present in early life and progress fairly rapidly.

Abnormal metabolites which can be specifically identified accumulate in macrophages, glial cells and sometimes neurones.

e.g. 1. In **metachromatic leukodystrophy,** the accumulation of a *sulphatide* gives a metachromatic staining reaction and characteristic EM appearance.

2. In **Krabbe's disease** there are typical multinucleated histiocytes (called globoid cells) containing *cerebroside*.

PARKINSON'S DISEASE

This is a disease of the extrapyramidal system which links the higher motor centres and effector motor cells of the spinal cord. Important neurotransmitters are DOPAMINE and γ-aminobutyric acid (GABA).

Aetiology – The disease occurs in 2 main circumstances:

(a) *Idiopathic:* The majority of cases occurring in the elderly population (1% of over 60s) are idiopathic and the cause remains unclear. Genetic and environmental factors may be involved.

Genetic: There is a 2–3 times increased risk of the development of Parkinson's disease in the first-degree relatives of patients.

Environmental: Some pesticides can cross the blood–brain barrier and may be associated with Parkinson's disease.

(b) *Secondary:* 1. **Postencephalitic** (historically) i.e. as a sequel to encephalitis lethargica which occurred in epidemic form in the 1920s. Very few patients now survive.
2. **Drug induced.** The use of neuroleptic drugs may induce the syndrome temporarily (occasionally permanently), by disturbing the balance of the chemical transmitters.
3. **Arteriopathy.**
4. **Heavy metal poisoning.**

Clinically, **Parkinsonism** illustrates the classical features of extrapyramidal damage.

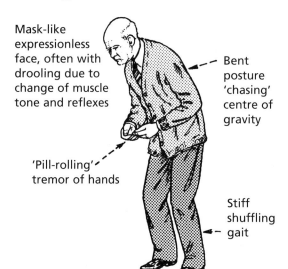

Mask-like expressionless face, often with drooling due to change of muscle tone and reflexes

Bent posture 'chasing' centre of gravity

'Pill-rolling' tremor of hands

Stiff shuffling gait

Pathological mechanism
In all cases of long-standing Parkinsonism of any type, degenerative changes are seen in the extrapyramidal nuclei. In particular, there is depigmentation of the substantia nigra.

Normal

Also there is a deficiency of DOPAMINE in affected nuclei.

Histologically, there is loss of neurones, and the surviving nerve cells contain inclusions known as Lewy bodies (p.550).

Other extrapyramidal disorders include the choreas, of which there are 2 main types. Sydenham's chorea occurs in children with rheumatic fever, while chorea is a manifestation in some patients with Huntington's disease.

MISCELLANEOUS DISORDERS

NUTRITIONAL AND METABOLIC DISORDERS (ENCEPHALOPATHIES)

In the last analysis, all disorders in this group are mediated by disturbed neuronal metabolism, so that exact classification may present some difficulty. However, it is convenient to consider them in 2 broad groups.

1. NUTRITIONAL DEFICIENCY

The vitamins of the B group are important coenzymes in several intracellular oxidative pathways. Deficiency, which may arise from primary malnutrition but more commonly in association with alcohol abuse, is the cause of degenerations of the brain, spinal cord and peripheral nerves.

Wernicke's encephalopathy

Clinically, this condition presents with disturbances of consciousness, ataxia and visual disturbances, and without prompt treatment progresses to death in coma.

In Western countries, chronic alcoholism is usually present; often a particularly heavy bout of drinking precipitates the condition.

Chronic alcoholism ⟶ Poor diet ⟶ NUTRITIONAL DEFICIENCY of vit B complex, esp. THIAMIN.

Bout of heavy drinking ⟶ Vomiting *Accentuates*

The blood PYRUVATE level is raised.

The lesions, which are focal, consist of glial proliferations with varying neurone loss. Petechial haemorrhages may be seen.

The lesions have a characteristic anatomical distribution:

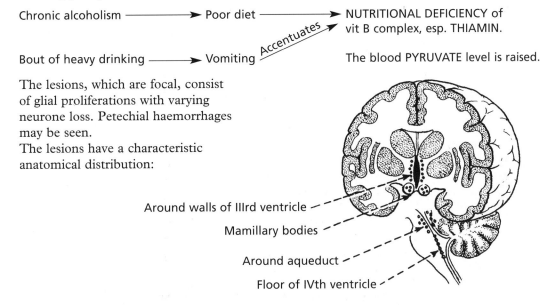

Around walls of IIIrd ventricle

Mamillary bodies

Around aqueduct

Floor of IVth ventricle

Prompt treatment with thiamin minimises the damage, but if treatment is omitted or delayed, permanent damage results. The patient may have a persistent Korsakoff's psychosis. At autopsy, there is visible shrinkage of the mamillary bodies.

MISCELLANEOUS DISORDERS

2. METABOLIC DISORDERS

In the following examples, the metabolic defect causes neurological disorder, but in addition, other organs are seriously disturbed.

(a) *Aminoacidopathies*

A wide variety of hepatic enzyme defects in the complex metabolism of amino acids has now been described. When neurological damage occurs, it is essentially non-specific and developing in the immediate postnatal period, a critical time in the development of the brain which leads to *mental retardation.*

Phenylketonuria is an example.

The importance of this disease is that the effects can be prevented by dietary restriction of phenylalanine-containing substances, provided the treatment is begun within 60 days of birth.

Mechanism

(b) In the *neuronal storage diseases*, which usually present during the first decade, deficiency of lysozomal enzymes leads to accumulation of intermediate metabolites in the neurones. The diagnosis of the condition often depends on the identification of the abnormal metabolite by histochemistry or EM.

Tay–Sach's disease (amaurotic familial idiocy) is an illustrative example.

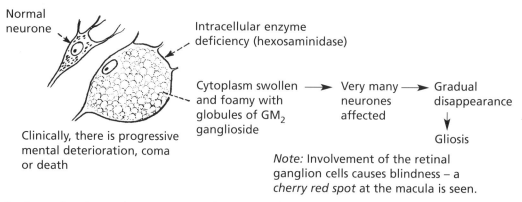

In these disorders, other organs may be mildly affected by the enzyme defect but the neurological effects are predominant.

DISEASES OF THE SPINAL CORD

In purely spinal lesions, basic disease processes have important anatomical and functional implications. Lack of space for expansion produces important compression effects. Examples are:

Fracture/
dislocation
of vertebra

Tumour (usually
secondary) in vertebrae
growing into canal

Prolapse of
intervertebral
disc

Tumour of
meninges or
nerve sheath

Effects

Normal

Cord, nerve roots and
blood vessels loosely
suspended in CSF 'water
bath'

Compression

(3) *Damage to nerve roots*
(radiculitis); a common
complication of spondylosis

(1) *Damage to neurones and
nerve tracts*
May be focal but is often
transverse and complete

(2) *Vascular compression*
Impairment of circulation
may cause infarction; this is
important particularly in
traumatic cases

At the level of the lesion, there is loss of the sensory and motor connections which constitute the spinal reflex.

In addition, severance of the longitudinal tracts cuts off the cerebral connections to all parts below the lesion.

Sensory
impulses
stop here

Motor impulses from
higher centres stop here

∴ LOSS OF SENSORY
APPRECIATION below
lesion

∴ PARALYSIS below lesion

Note: The spinal reflexes
remain intact below the lesion.

DISEASES OF THE SPINAL CORD

ASCENDING AND DESCENDING DEGENERATIONS

The long tract fibres which are cut off from their neurones progressively degenerate.

Ascending degeneration
in gracile and cuneate tracts
above the lesion extends as far
as their nuclei in the medulla

Cortical motor neurone

Level of lesion

Sensory neurone
in root ganglion

Descending degeneration
in lateral corticospinal tracts
(pyramidal) below the lesion

Note: In transverse lesions of the
cord, all the long tracts degenerate
either upwards (sensory) or
downwards (motor). These particular
tracts are shown for illustrative
convenience.

The commonest example of **descending degeneration** is seen following cerebral infarction
involving the internal capsule; the degeneration extends from the lesion along the
corticospinal axons to their terminations in the anterior horn.

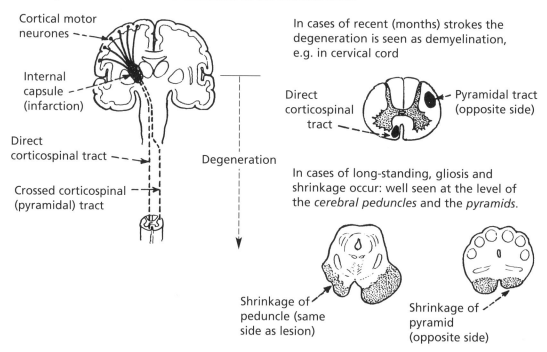

Cortical motor
neurones

Internal
capsule
(infarction)

Direct
corticospinal tract

Crossed corticospinal
(pyramidal) tract

Degeneration

In cases of recent (months) strokes the
degeneration is seen as demyelination,
e.g. in cervical cord

Direct
corticospinal
tract

Pyramidal tract
(opposite side)

In cases of long-standing, gliosis and
shrinkage occur: well seen at the level of
the *cerebral peduncles* and the *pyramids*.

Shrinkage of
peduncle (same
side as lesion)

Shrinkage of
pyramid
(opposite side)

DISORDERS OF MOTOR PATHWAYS

The concept of upper and lower motor neuronal activity, based on anatomical and physiological evidence, has great clinical value in diagnosis.

The **upper motor neurones** (UMN) synapse with the **lower motor neurones** (LMN)

Cortical motor neurones (pre-central gyrus)

Motor tracts in cerebrum (internal capsule)

Motor tracts in brain stem – fibres crossing to cranial nerves in opposite side

Decussation of pyramids

Small direct corticospinal tract (anterior)

Large crossed pyramidal tract (anterolateral)

Cranial nerve nuclei (motor) and their axons in the cranial nerves

Anterior horn cells and their axons in the spinal nerves

It will be appreciated that in its long course from the cerebral cortex to the anterior horn, the upper motor neurone is susceptible to damage from a variety of disease processes acting at various sites. The lower motor neurone may be damaged in the cord or in the peripheral nerve. Important illustrative examples are:

Upper motor neurone damage

Stroke

damaging internal capsule

Multiple sclerosis

– random demyelination damaging motor tracts at several sites.

Note: Clinically, tendon jerks are increased and the plantar reflex is extensor.

Lower motor neurone damage

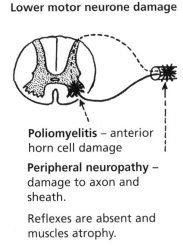

Poliomyelitis – anterior horn cell damage

Peripheral neuropathy – damage to axon and sheath.

Reflexes are absent and muscles atrophy.

MOTOR NEURONE DISEASE

This is a disease of unknown aetiology occurring predominantly in adult males. In a few cases motor neurone disease is familial and is caused by a mutation in the gene encoding a free radical scavenger, superoxide dismutase 1. Other susceptiblity genes have been identified.

Three variants of MND are recognised according to the distribution of the disease process.

1. In **progressive muscular atrophy,** as the name implies, the main signs are of neurogenic atrophy due to degeneration of the anterior horn cells (LMN).

Predilection for cervical cord

Gradual (several years) degeneration of anterior horn cells

↓

Gliosis

↓

Shrinkage

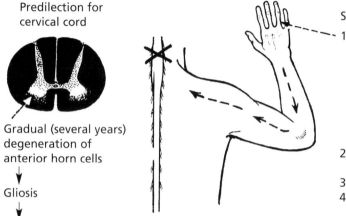

Sites particularly affected are:

1. Small muscles of hand – wasting ('simian hand')
   Note: While degeneration of neurones is proceeding spontaneous irregular discharges cause muscle twitching –
   FASCICULATION
2. Muscles of arm and shoulder girdle.
3. Spread towards medulla.
4. Later leg weakness and paralysis reflect both LMN and UMN damage.

2. In **amyotrophic lateral sclerosis** there is both UMN and LMN damage: 'lateral sclerosis' indicates the degeneration of the pyramidal tracts.

The degeneration affects the cortical motor cells – particularly those supplying the lower limbs but spreading over a few years to involve the neck and head centres. Voluntary movements of the face, jaw and tongue muscles are defective.
Corticospinal tracts showing degeneration and, later, gliosis.

The lesions are very rarely pure UMN type even initially, and with progression, the LMN lesions increase.

3. **Progressive bulbar palsy**
   In a few cases, the disease begins with signs of cranial nerve dysfunction – swallowing and facial movements are impaired.

Progress

In motor neurone disease after a long progressive illness the stage is reached when the bulbar degeneration is severe enough to prevent elimination of secretions from the respiratory tract. Death is usually due to aspiration bronchopneumonia or respiratory failure.

MIXED MOTOR AND SENSORY DISORDERS

SUBACUTE COMBINED DEGENERATION OF CORD

Due specifically to vit B_{12} deficiency. If replacement therapy is begun early enough, there is restoration to normal.

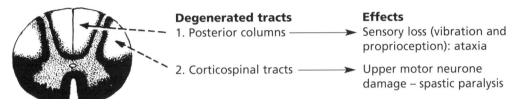

Degenerated tracts

1. Posterior columns ⟶ **Effects** Sensory loss (vibration and proprioception): ataxia

2. Corticospinal tracts ⟶ Upper motor neurone damage – spastic paralysis

SYRINGOMYELIA

In this condition, a glial-lined cystic space gradually expands within the cord, usually in the cervical region. The pathogenesis is not certain, but it is suggested that the lesion is essentially an expansion of the central canal associated with a mild developmental abnormality of the distal end of the IVth ventricle. Some cases follow spinal trauma.

Effects
Damage to sensory fibres decussating in the cord. Loss of temperature and touch in local segments (**dissociated anaesthesia**).

Early

Late

Destruction of grey matter and gradual affection of long tracts. Loss of local reflexes. Severe sensory loss. Spastic paralysis.

SPINOCEREBELLAR DEGENERATIONS

This is a large group of related disorders, usually familial, in which there is motor and sensory degeneration particularly affecting gait, posture, equilibrium and movement. There is sometimes optic nerve and retinal damage and intellectual disturbance.

Friedreich's ataxia is the most common hereditary ataxia and is caused by expansion of a trinucleotide triplet repeat in the FRATAXIN gene on chromosome 9. Deficiency of frataxin leads to mitochondrial respiratory chain dysfunction. In addition to the effects of spinocerebellar degeneration there may be cardiomyopathy with arrhythmia.

SENSORY DISORDERS

In **TABES DORSALIS**, a tertiary manifestation of syphilis in which the lumbar cord is commonly affected, there is degeneration of the posterior nerve roots and columns.

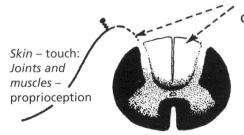

Skin – touch:
Joints and
muscles –
proprioception

Clinically
Loss of vibration sense and reflexes
Ataxia
Trophic skin ulcers
Severe joint derangement
(Charcot, p.617)

Additional features
Cranial and sympathetic nerve involvement – disturbance of pupillary reflex

Painful visceral crises

THE PERIPHERAL NERVES/THE NEUROPATHIES

There are 3 main reactions that occur in peripheral nerves.

1. Traumatic damage followed by regeneration or formation of a traumatic neuroma.
2. Damage to axons and myelin sheath.
   (a) Axonal degeneration

Damage to axon results in distal axonal degeneration

Secondary myelin breakdown

   (b) Demyelination

Segmental myelin degeneration between nodes of Ranvier indicating individual Schwann cell damage

3. Damage to supporting structures, e.g blood vessels or epi-, peri- or endoneurium.

CLINICAL MANIFESTATIONS OF PERIPHERAL NERVE DISORDERS

1. *Mononeuropathy:* single nerve damage by compression, e.g. compression of median nerve in carpal tunnel syndrome, compression of nerve root by prolapsed intervertebral disc

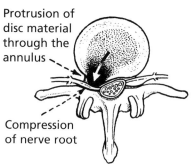

Protrusion of disc material through the annulus

Compression of nerve root

2. *Mononeuritis multiplex:* where several nerves are involved e.g. arteritis with inflammation of vasa nervorum leading to ischaemia

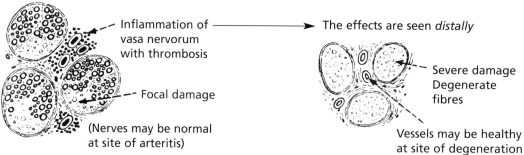

Inflammation of vasa nervorum with thrombosis

Focal damage

(Nerves may be normal at site of arteritis)

The effects are seen *distally*

Severe damage Degenerate fibres

Vessels may be healthy at site of degeneration

THE NEUROPATHIES

3. ***Polyneuropathy***: where there is extensive and symmetrical disturbance of function, often peripheral in distribution and especially affecting the legs. There are many causes:

    Toxic – diphtheria; lead; arsenic; drugs used in medicine

    Deficiency states – particularly vit B complex deficiency causing Beri-Beri

    Metabolic disorders – diabetes mellitus; porphyria, metachromatic leukodystrophy, associated with malignant tumours, in uraemia treated by dialysis.

    Inflammatory/Immunological – Guillain–Barré syndrome where ascending paralysis occurs usually after a mild febrile illness. Respiratory failure requires supportive treatment but recovery is usually complete.

Other Neuropathies

Bell's Palsy

This is a unilateral facial weakness of sudden onset. The cause is unclear but it may occur with draughts and chilling and is not uncommon in pregnancy. The mechanism is thought to be inflammation with swelling and compression of the facial nerve in its course in the bone adjacent to the internal auditory meatus. Progress: 75% of cases recover in about 4–8 weeks.

Note drooping and loss
of facial expression on
paralysed side.
Facial muscles pull
across the mid line
– mouth is distorted.

Leprosy

In the lepromatous form, there is a diffuse neuropathy involving the peripheries (which are at the lower temperature required for proliferation of *M. leprae*).

There is a low grade chronic inflammation of the nerve sheaths associated with fibrosis and nerve fibre degeneration.

HYDROCEPHALUS

In hydrocephalus, the volume of the CSF is increased and the ventricles are dilated. In the majority of cases, there is an increase in intracranial pressure. Three possible **mechanisms** are considered.

1. **Overproduction of CSF**
   The choroid plexus will secrete more CSF to compensate for any external leak, but overproduction is not a cause of hydrocephalus.
2. **Obstruction to the flow of CSF is the common mechanism.**

INTRACEREBRAL FLOW

Production (choroid plexuses)

Lateral vent.

Via foramen of Munro

III vent.

Via aqueduct of Sylvius

IV vent.

Via foramina of Magendie and Luschka

Sites of narrowing particularly vulnerable to obstruction
(1) Aqueduct of Sylvius
(2) Foramina of Magendie and Luschka
(3) The subarachnoid space between the midbrain and forebrain (interposition of tentorium cerebelli)

EXTRACEREBRAL FLOW

SUBARACHNOID SPACE

In cases of obstruction up to the IV ventricular foramina, the CSF cannot reach the subarachnoid space; e.g. sites 1 and 2. The hydrocephalus is **NON-COMMUNICATING.**

When the obstruction is beyond the foramina, e.g. site 3, the hydrocephalus is **COMMUNICATING.**

3. **Defective absorption of CSF** is a rare mechanism.

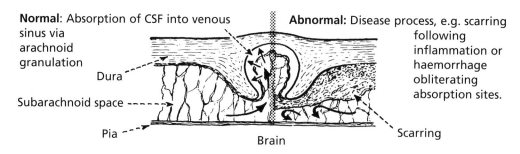

Normal: Absorption of CSF into venous sinus via arachnoid granulation

Dura

Subarachnoid space

Pia

Brain

Abnormal: Disease process, e.g. scarring following inflammation or haemorrhage obliterating absorption sites.

Scarring

HYDROCEPHALUS

CAUSES

The diseases causing hydrocephalus fall into two groups:

1. Congenital (developmental) abnormalities

The common conditions are:

(a) *The Arnold–Chiari malformation*

Prolongation
of cerebellum
and medulla
bulging
through
the foramen
magnum

Obstruction to
flow of CSF in
posterior fossa

Associated with
spina bifida, usually
meningomyelocele

Dura
deficient

Arachnoid and
nervous tissue
lying under
bulging skin

(b) *Congenital stenosis or atresia
of aqueduct of Sylvius*

Leads to
dilatation
of IIIrd
and lateral
ventricles

Stenosis

(c) *Atresia of foramina of
Magendie and Luschka*

Leads to
dilatation
of IVth,
IIIrd and
lateral
ventricles

Atresia

2. Acquired hydrocephalus

Of the many possible conditions causing hydrocephalus, the following are most common: (a) cerebral tumour (primary or secondary) and (b) scarring of the meninges following meningitis or subarachnoid haemorrhage.

As already explained, whether any particular disease produces hydrocephalus depends largely on the site affected.

HYDROCEPHALUS

EFFECTS

In the infant and young child, the pliable skull expands to accommodate the enlarging brain – but these extreme changes do not occur if an effective shunt is inserted.

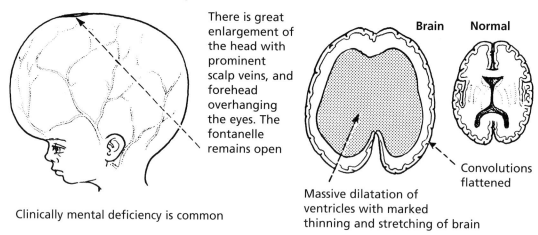

There is great enlargement of the head with prominent scalp veins, and forehead overhanging the eyes. The fontanelle remains open

Brain   **Normal**

Convolutions flattened

Massive dilatation of ventricles with marked thinning and stretching of brain

Clinically mental deficiency is common

In the **older child and adult**, enlargement of the brain is prevented by the inability of the skull to expand. The main change is dilatation of the ventricles associated with the effects on the brain of increased intracranial pressure.

SPECIAL TYPES OF HYDROCEPHALUS

1. In cases of generalised cerebral atrophy, the ventricular system enlarges to compensate for the loss of cerebral tissue. This also happens locally when cerebral tissue is lost, e.g. following infarction.

Primary atrophy of brain (deepened sulci, thinned convolutions)

Secondary dilatation

Local dilatation of ventricle

Old infarct

No increase in pressure is involved and the pathological and clinical effects wholly reflect the primary loss of cerebral tissue. The condition is sometimes called **secondary hydrocephalus.**

2. Normal pressure hydrocephalus

In this rare condition, progressive mental deterioration (dementia) and disturbances of gait and micturition are associated with ventricular dilatation. Random sampling often shows normal CSF pressures but continuous monitoring shows significant intermittent increases. (Some prefer the title Intermittent Hydrocephalus.) The diagnosis has assumed importance because in some cases CSF shunt procedures have arrested the progress. The aetiology is obscure.

DEVELOPMENTAL ABNORMALITIES

Developmental abnormalities of the brain and cranium are relatively common. They range from anencephaly (absence of brain) to minor malformations e.g. meningocele and encephalocele. There may be associated congenital defects elsewhere in the body.

Neural Tube Defects

Local defects in the development and closure of the neural tube are common and largely preventable by folic acid supplementation in pregnancy. They may be diagnosed in utero by increased α-fetoprotein in maternal blood. They include:

(a) **Spina bifida occulta**
Normal skin covering

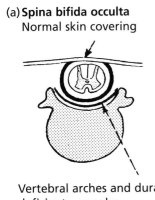

Vertebral arches and dura deficient – may be associated with minor nerve defects – particularly affecting bladder function

(b) **Meningocele**
Skin may be thin at apex

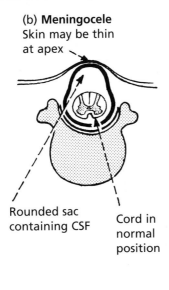

Rounded sac containing CSF

Cord in normal position

(c) **Meningomyelocele**
Skin usually defective

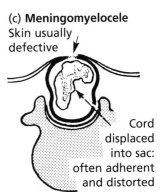

Cord displaced into sac: often adherent and distorted

May be associated with serious nerve deficit – especially in legs, bladder.

Infection through the deficient skin is a serious complication.

There is strong evidence that folic acid deficiency is the cause of these defects.

Diagnosis in utero

α-fetoprotein leaks through the defective skin covering and increased amounts are found in the amniotic fluid. Ultrasonography may also reveal the defect.

Complications

In addition to severe neurological deficits which are aggravated by infection, an important complication even in minor defects is **HYDROCEPHALUS**.

TUMOURS OF THE NERVOUS SYSTEM

The following scheme illustrates the various non-specific clinicopathological effects of a tumour within the skull.

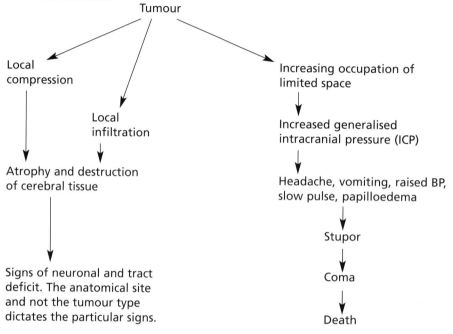

An important factor which materially influences the relative importance of each of these effects is the rate of tumour growth.

Tumours will be considered in a simplified form under the following broad headings:
1. Secondary neoplasms.
2. Neoplasms of neuroectodermal origin.
3. Neoplasms arising in supporting tissue (mesodermal).
4. Neoplasms and swellings of developmental origin.
5. Neoplasms of nerve sheaths.

SECONDARY BRAIN TUMOURS

In the general population the incidence of metastatic cerebral tumour is much higher than that of primary cerebral neoplasm. The two most common primary sites are lung and breast, but any malignant tumour can metastasise to the brain.

The common presentation is in the form of multiple, well-delineated spherical nodules, randomly distributed

Only occasionally is there a single nodule.

A less common distribution is by permeation of the subarachnoid space – **meningeal carcinomatosis.**

Brain surface covered by a layer of tumour tissue – – – – →

Carcinoma, leukaemia and lymphoreticular neoplasms may spread in this way (malignant cells may be seen in the CSF).

Secondary tumours may cause serious spinal damage by destroying the integrity of the vertebrae. The prostate and cervix, in addition to lung, breast and kidney, are usual primary sites.

In contrast to tumours causing neurological damage by their physical presence and growth, less commonly *non-metastatic effects of cancer* are seen.

There is a wide range of disorders which are conveniently divided into two groups:

1. Neurological disorders in which the mechanism and association with cancer are known:

Examples	Mechanism caused by cancer
Opportunistic infections	Immune depression
Metabolic and hormonal imbalance	Destruction of organs, e.g. liver, kidney Inappropriate secretion
Vascular accidents	Coagulation disorders

2. A group of conditions in which the mechanism is not known. This includes dementia, encephalopathy, cerebellar degeneration, neuropathies and a syndrome mimicking myasthenia gravis (Lambert–Eaton syndrome).

PRIMARY BRAIN TUMOURS

GLIOMAS

Astrocytoma

This is a low grade tumour derived from astrocytes and occurring most frequently in the cerebrum of young adults.

The tumour which has ill-defined margins grows irregularly into the surrounding brain tissue and only latterly causes increased ICP

Note enlargement of hemisphere by ill defined growth.

Because they have ill-defined margins, astrocytomas are difficult to eradicate and slowly but inexorably grow and eventually cause death. Many eventually transform to a high grade tumour (anaplastic astrocytoma or glioblastoma). The rare pilocytic astrocytoma occurs in the cerebellum or optic nerve of children and carries a good prognosis.

Glioblastoma

This is the commonest glial tumour and may occur de novo or following a history of low-grade astrocytoma. This is a highly malignant tumour and the cells are pleomorphic, with mitoses, necrosis and a striking proliferation of blood vessels.

The prognosis of these patients is very poor.

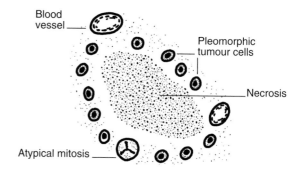

Oligodendroglioma

These tumours, derived from oligodendroglia, tend to occur in the cerebrum of adults and may present clinically with epilepsy. They are usually slow growing and often show calcification.

Ependymoma

These are also rare and arise from the lining of the ventricles and central spinal cord. They may block the flow of CSF and cause hydrocephalus.

Note: The above gliomas very rarely metastasise outside the nervous system.

TUMOURS OF THE NERVOUS SYSTEM

TUMOURS of NEURONAL TYPE CELLS

Fully differentiated neurones can neither multiply nor give rise to neoplasms. Tumours of this type, derived from primitive nerve precursors (blast cells), are seen in infancy and childhood before completion of differentiation.
They display a basic histological pattern.

Closely aggregated small cells with hyperchromatic round or oval nuclei and scanty cytoplasm

Rosettes, the centres of which are formed by rudimentary nerve fibres, are often seen and represent a step towards differentiation

Depending on the site of origin, specific names are given:

Cerebellum:
MEDULLOBLASTOMA

Retina:
RETINOBLASTOMA

Sympathetic ganglia (including adrenal medulla):
NEUROBLASTOMA and GANGLIONEUROMA

Medulloblastoma
This highly malignant tumour arises in and spreads over the surface of the cerebellum, often invading the IVth ventricle. Diffuse tumour nodules may develop on surfaces bathed by CSF.

Retinoblastoma
These tumours arise from the retina in children under 3 years. Around 40% of cases are inherited and the tumour may be bilateral. The remaining cases arise sporadically and are usually unilateral. The genetic mechanism involves inactivation of the retinoblastoma gene (RB gene), a tumour suppressor gene situated on the short arm of chromosome 13 (13q14). Untreated the tumour may fill the eye and spread locally into the brain via the optic nerve or systemically after invasion of the choroid. Modern therapy is curative in around 90% of cases.

Neuroblastoma
These tumours arise from the precursor cells of the autonomic system; the majority occur in the adrenal medulla. They grow rapidly to become large, soft, haemorrhagic and necrotic retroperitoneal masses soon metastasising to lymph nodes, liver and bones.

Ganglioneuroma
In some cases, neuronal differentiation proceeds, and mature ganglion cells appear and nerve fibres are formed. In some instances, differentiation is complete; such tumours are found in adult life particularly in the mediastinum where they may grow slowly, eventually causing signs due to their size, but never metastasising. With intermediate degrees of differentiation the name ganglioneuroblastoma is used.

TUMOURS OF THE NERVOUS SYSTEM

Meningiomas

These are thought to arise from arachnoid granulations and so are found most commonly adjacent to venous sinuses. They account for 15–20% of intracranial tumours. They are slow growing and essentially 'benign'. A few more aggressive tumours may metastasise.

A smooth firm lobulated tumour arising from a broad base adjacent to the sagittal sinus

The effects are due to local compression of nervous tissues.

The skull may be eroded.

Growth to large size is usually slow so that the compensating mechanisms prevent increased intracranial pressure. Occasional meningiomas arise in the spine.

The histological appearances are variable depending on the relative amounts of cells and collagen, and they mimic in varying degree the arachnoid granulations. Concentric calcified structures (psammoma bodies) are often seen.

Venous sinus

Normal arachnoid granulation projecting into lumen

Whorls of fibrous tissue and spindle cells

Sinus wall

Arachnoid membrane

Calcified psammoma bodies

Other mesodermal tumours

True vascular neoplasms are rare, but vascular HAMARTOMAS are fairly common and are a cause of intracranial haemorrhage and epilepsy. These lesions show great variation in site, size and complexity.

Primary microglial and lymphoid tumours are rare; the latter may be intrinsic to the CNS or be metastatic from a primary tumour outside the CNS. Primary cerebral lymphomas are an important complication of AIDS.

The incidence of CNS lymphomas is apparently increasing. This may be due to better diagnosis and/or to the more common use of therapeutic immunosuppression.

TUMOURS OF THE NERVOUS SYSTEM

Craniopharyngioma

This is a benign epithelial tumour arising in suprasellar areas. Similar benign cysts also occur.

Germ cell tumours

These occasionally arise in midline structures: they are derived from embryologically misplaced germ cells.

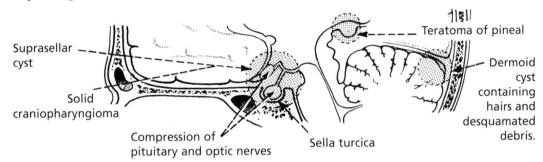

Suprasellar cyst

Solid craniopharyngioma

Compression of pituitary and optic nerves

Sella turcica

Teratoma of pineal

Dermoid cyst containing hairs and desquamated debris.

TUMOURS OF PERIPHERAL NERVES

These tumours arise in nerve roots within the skull and spine, or in the peripheral nerves. Nomenclature is based on the tissue of origin.

Neurofibroma
Derived from endoneurium

Schwannoma
Derived from Schwann cells intimately surrounding axons.

Spindle cells with wavy nuclei: fine collagen fibres: occasional nerve fibres

Note nuclear palisading in addition to whorls and fascicles of collagen

Note: Since neurones do not give rise to these neoplasms, the term neuroma is not used. Traumatic neuroma indicates proliferating nerve endings following injury and is not a true neoplasm (see p.57).

Nerve sheath tumours may be single or multiple; their effects are due to compression of adjacent neural tissue and are seen best within the skull or spinal cord.

583

TUMOURS OF PERIPHERAL NERVES

SCHWANNOMA

Acoustic Neuroma is a good example. This tumour arises from the VIIIth nerve in the cerebellopontine angle. Although this tumour is benign, it grows around adjacent structures and has an irregular surface so that it may be difficult to remove.

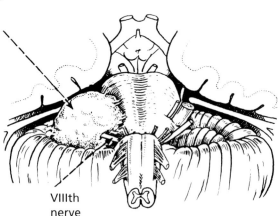

> The tumour exerts its effects by compression – distortion of the VIIIth nerve (tinnitus → deafness) and adjacent nerves. Pressure on IVth ventricle → hydrocephalus → increased intracranial pressure.

VIIIth nerve

These tumours are rarely multiple as part of neurofibromatosis Type 2 (associated with NF2 gene on chromosome 22).

Neurofibromas
These may be solitary or, in neurofibromatosis, multiple and affect peripheral nerves over a wide area or occupy a single group of nerves. They form either rounded nodules or fusiform swellings and may be cosmetically disfiguring.

Multiple neurofibromas occur in neurofibromatosis Type 1. This is an autosomal dominant condition caused by a mutation in the NF-1 gene on chromosome 17. Plexiform neurofibroma, which involves a group of nerves forming complex thickening, is considered pathognomonic of neurofibromatosis Type 1.

Unlike schwannomas, a small but significant proportion of neurofibromas undergo transformation to malignant peripheral nerve sheath tumours. The risk is highest when associated with NF-1.

CEREBROSPINAL FLUID

Although the CSF and extracellular fluid of the central nervous system are essentially similar in composition, changes in the CSF are not reliable indicators of disease within the brain parenchyma.

However, since the CSF reflects conditions in the subarachnoid space, in clinical practice detailed examination and analysis are important and are mandatory in suspected meningitis. The important observations using CSF obtained by lumbar puncture are grouped under headings as follows.

NORMAL	IN DISEASE			
	Meningitis		Virus infection	Miscellaneous
	Pyogenic	*Tuberculous*	*Meningo-encephalitis*	
Pressure 60–180 mmH$_2$O	↑ Over 200	↑ Over 200	↑High	↓ Below spinal block
Appearance Crystal clear *(for blood staining see below)	Turbid	Opalescent: may be fine fibrin web	Opalescent	–
Cell content 0–4 mononuclears/μl	+++ >1000 Neutrophils	+++ Lymphocytes	± + Lymphocytes	–
Biochemistry Protein 0.2–0.4 g/l	↑ 1–10 g/l	↑ 1–3 g/l	↑ 0.5–2 g/l	Very high in spinal block
Glucose 50–80 mg/100 ml (2.8-4.4 mmol/l)	greatly↓ or absent	Low 20–30 mg	Normal	Normal

* When the CSF is blood-stained, it is important to distinguish between contamination due to trauma caused by the tap and true intracranial haemorrhage.

	Contamination	True haemorrhage
Supernatant after centrifugation	Clear	Yellow due to bilirubin (red cell degeneration)
Cell count – leucocyte:RBC ratio	Normal	Increased

Microbiology. Identification of organisms is very important.

(1) Deposit and/or fibrin web – stained ⟨ Gram – pyogenic bacteria and fungi
⟨ ZN – tubercle bacilli

(2) Culture: virus isolation

(3) Tests for microbial antigens ⟨ Wassermann reaction for syphilis
⟨ Immunoelectrophoresis for other antigens

THE EYE

CATARACT

The normal lens consists of soluble crystalline proteins encased within elongated lens fibre cells surrounded by an elastic lens capsule. There is also a layer of lens epithelium beneath the anterior capsule. The metabolism of the lens depends on diffusion of nutrients from the aqueous. In cataract the lens is opaque and this is one of the most common and treatable causes of blindness worldwide.

Aetiology of Cataracts

Developmental: due to congenital malformation or toxic damage to lens fibres e.g. Rubella, Trauma, Inflammation, Metabolic disease e.g. hypocalcaemia, diabetes

Senile: due to degradation of lens proteins in the oldest central part of the lens

GLAUCOMA

This is a common cause of blindness in the Western World. Glaucoma occurs when intraocular pressure (IOP) rises to an extent which causes damage to tissues within the eye.

Normal

IOP is maintained by a balance between aqueous inflow from the ciliary body and outflow via the trabecular meshwork (TM) and canal of Schlemm.

Types

Open angle
(a) **Primary** – acquired disease due to increased resistance in the TM.
(b) **Secondary** – due to blockage of the TM by tumour cells, leaked lens protein etc.

Closed angle
(a) **Primary** – the iris root becomes opposed to the TM. The mechanism is unknown.
(b) **Secondary** – due to intraocular neovascularisation e.g. diabetes, ocular ischaemia

Congenital – due to malformation of the TM.

THE EYE

GLAUCOMA *(continued)*

Effects of increased IOP
Corneal oedema
Iris ischaemia
Ciliary body atrophy
Cataract
Retinal atrophy
Cupping of optic disc
Enlargement of the eye in children
(buphthalmos = ox eye)

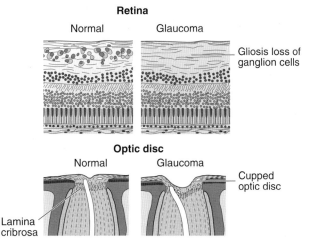

TUMOURS
Retinoblastoma is the most common primary intraocular tumour of childhood. This is
discussed on page 581.

Melanoma
This is the most common primary intraocular tumour in adults. It can occur anywhere in the
uveal tract. Iris melanomas usually present early, as they are visible. Ciliary body melanomas
present late with visual disturbances or glaucoma due to invasion of the trabecular
meshwork. Choroid melanomas may be asymptomatic and picked up at routine eye checks
or later present with symptoms secondary to associated retinal detachment.

Pathology
Mushroom shaped tumour due to spread beneath retina
Spindle cells (better prognosis)
Epithelioid cells – poorer prognosis)
(The majority of tumours are mixed)

Secondary Tumours
Metastasis is the commonest type of intraocular malignancy. The most common primary
sites are breast and lung.

MUSCULO-SKELETAL SYSTEM

SKELETAL MUSCLE

It is useful to consider the anatomy at various levels of magnification.

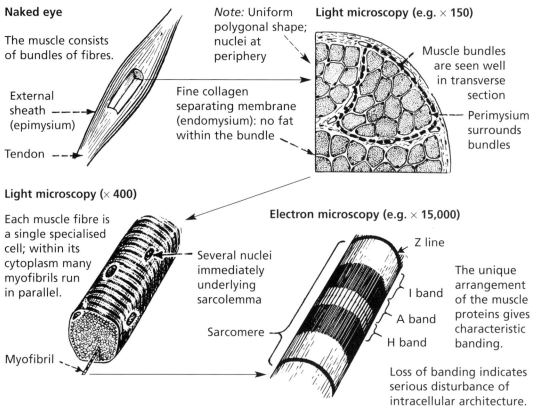

Naked eye

The muscle consists of bundles of fibres.

External sheath (epimysium)

Tendon

Note: Uniform polygonal shape; nuclei at periphery

Fine collagen separating membrane (endomysium): no fat within the bundle

Light microscopy (e.g. × 150)

Muscle bundles are seen well in transverse section

Perimysium surrounds bundles

Light microscopy (× 400)

Each muscle fibre is a single specialised cell; within its cytoplasm many myofibrils run in parallel.

Myofibril

Several nuclei immediately underlying sarcolemma

Sarcomere

Electron microscopy (e.g. × 15,000)

Z line

I band

A band

H band

The unique arrangement of the muscle proteins gives characteristic banding.

Loss of banding indicates serious disturbance of intracellular architecture.

MUSCLE CONTRACTION

Within each muscle cell the basic mechanism by which energy is mobilised and released is as follows:

In mitochondrion

Glucose
Amino acids + O_2
Fat

→ ATP →

ADP + P + ENERGY

At myofibril

Contraction

Complex enzyme systems including particularly creatine kinase (CK) and aldolase (ALS)

SKELETAL MUSCLE

There are 3 types of muscle fibre, related to differences in functional activity.

	Type of contraction	Location	Myoglobin	Mitochondria	Metabolism
Type I (red muscle)	SLOW twitch, FATIGUE RESISTANT	POSTURAL MUSCLES	+++	+++	AEROBIC
Type IIa (red muscle)	FAST twitch, FATIGUE RESISTANT	e.g. in LEGS of SPRINTERS	+++	+++	AEROBIC
Type IIb (white muscle)	FAST twitch, FATIGUABLE	ARM MUSCLES	+	+	ANAEROBIC

Note: Most muscles are a mixture of the 3 fibre types, but the proportion varies according to the function of the muscle.

In section, the three fibre types are identified by their ATPase activity.

Normal muscle stained H & E

Normal muscle stained for ATPase activity

Type I = black
Type IIa = white
Type IIb = stipple
Note random mosaic pattern.

It is of interest that the muscle fibre function is not intrinsic but is conditioned by its type of nerve supply: any single anterior horn cell innervates fibres of only one type.

MUSCLE INNERVATION
The motor unit consists of:
 a single lower
 motor neurone (**LMN**) — and the
  muscle fibres
  it supplies.

Muscle spindles

← Muscle fibres – a few to hundreds

Anterior horn cell   Nerve root   Peripheral nerve

Muscle spindles are bundles of specialised fibres which control and refine muscle contraction and are important for proprioception. They are separately innervated from the surrounding fibres.

591

ATROPHY AND HYPERTROPHY

Generalised disuse atrophy occurs as a result of prolonged immobilisation in bed. Local atrophy follows immobilisation due to joint disease or after bone fractures.

Hypertrophy of muscle tissue in response to increased work load is well seen in heavy event athletes. Localised hypertrophy can compensate for damage to adjacent muscular tissues.

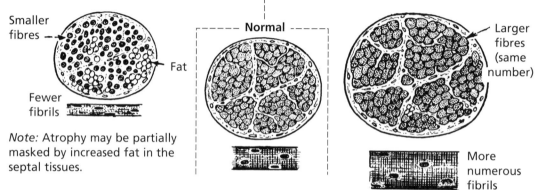

Smaller fibres

Fat

Fewer fibrils

Normal

Larger fibres (same number)

More numerous fibrils

Note: Atrophy may be partially masked by increased fat in the septal tissues.

NEUROGENIC ATROPHY

This is a special form of atrophy seen when the nerve supply is damaged. The distribution of nerve fibres within the muscle is important and is represented diagrammatically in respect of two motor units: A and B.

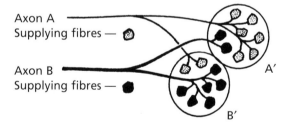

Axon A
Supplying fibres —

Axon B
Supplying fibres —

A'

B'

Note that while A and B respectively innervate the majority of fibres in bundles A' and B', there is overlap between bundles. Since many axons supply a muscle the overlap is considerable.

Apart from complete traumatic section of a peripheral nerve, it is unusual for all motor fibres to a muscle to be destroyed. Both the basic pattern of innervation and the variations in nerve fibre damage are reflected in the histological appearances in the denervated muscle.

1. **Pattern of atrophy**

Groups of atrophic denervated fibres with adjacent groups of normal fibres.

Note the overlap – atrophic fibres among normal, and vice versa.

This is the striking basic pattern seen in most diseases of the LMN.

NEUROGENIC ATROPHY

2. Re-innervation

In an area of denervation, the terminal axonal branches of intact neurones sprout and can re-innervate the atrophic fibres. The effects of denervation and re-innervation are shown in a muscle bundle supplied by 2 axons A and B.

Denervation of A

A

B

Fibres supplied by A atrophy

Fibres supplied by B remain normal

This explains

Re-innervation and **restoration** of fibre size

B

The terminal fibres of B now sprout and innervate the atrophic fibres which are restored to normal size.

3. Change in muscle type which may occur.

Since the type (fast or slow) of each muscle fibre is conditioned by its nerve supply, the pattern of distribution of fast and slow fibres within a muscle may be changed by reinnervation.

Thus, although a muscle may be restored to normal in terms of routine histological assessment, slight changes in functional activity may be present.

MYASTHENIA GRAVIS

The **MOTOR END-PLATE** is the specialised neuromuscular junction situated at the middle of each muscle fibre. The nervous impulse causes release of **ACETYLCHOLINE** at the specialised nerve endings – depolarisation at this site is the stimulus to contraction. The sarcolemma at this site contains abundant **CHOLINESTERASE**. In MYASTHENIA GRAVIS, the essential disorder is at the motor end-plate where there is a defect in the action of acetylcholine. This rare disease occurs mainly in young females, the important clinical features being muscle weakness and early fatigue of the ocular and head and neck muscles particularly.

Aetiology and mechanism

This is essentially an auto-immune disease (see p.109).
1. Antibodies to ACETYLCHOLINE RECEPTORS are present in 90% of cases.
2. There is a strong association with THYMIC abnormalities. In young women this is usually *thymic germinal centre hyperplasia*: in middle aged males a *thymoma* may be present.
3. There is an association with hyperthyroidism (this has an autoimmune basis).

In the affected muscles, aggregates of lymphocytes with occasional single necrotic fibres may be seen.

MUSCLE DAMAGE

(a) Trauma and ischaemia

In severe cases where trauma and ischaemia combine to cause necrosis of a considerable mass of muscle, the effects may be serious.

The latter situation is well exemplified in the CRUSH SYNDROME – classically seen in building collapse.

Repair of massive muscle damage

The basic inflammatory response is followed by organisation with removal of the dead muscle.

There are two possible results:

(i) If the gap is not too great, regeneration effects restoration to normal.

(ii) If the gap is too great, scar tissue prevents the regeneration.

(b) Inflammation

In most inflammatory processes, including the common pyogenic infections, the intermuscular fascial planes are involved and muscle damage is negligible and superficial, consisting of degeneration and necrosis of individual fibres.

Abscess formation may follow intramuscular injections.

Viral myositis

A true myositis with focal necrosis of fibres, lymphocyte and macrophage infiltration can be caused by the Coxsackie group of viruses. The muscles of the upper thorax are particularly affected.

Parasitic myositis

In trichinosis, the parasitic larvae encyst in the interstitial tissues within muscles. The adjacent muscle fibres become necrotic; focal calcification is often a late sequel.

MUSCULAR DYSTROPHY

Muscular dystrophies are inherited diseases, causing muscle damage and weakness.

Duchenne Muscular Dystrophy

This is the commonest and most serious form.

Clinical features: Muscle weakness in early childhood; typically wheelchair-bound by 12 years of age and death by late teens or early twenties.

Pathology: The main features are
    (1) muscle fibre necrosis and
    (2) regeneration.

In time, fibres are atrophic and there is fibrosis and fatty replacement.

Biopsy shows:

Moderately affected muscle

A group of normal fibres

Fat cells

Neuro-muscle spindle

Fibres showing various degrees of atrophy

Late stage muscle

Almost complete replacement of muscle by fat; only a few atrophic fibres remain.

Prominent winging of scapulae

Scoliosis (due to muscle weakness)

Pseudo-hypertrophy in calf muscles (due to fatty infiltration)

Aetiology: This is an X-linked recessive disease occurring almost exclusively in boys. The dystrophin gene lies on the short arm of chromosome X.

Chromosome X

Mutations especially deletions

Lack of DYSTROPHIN

Sarcolemma

Muscle cytoplasm

Muscle cell degeneration (? by apoptosis)

Biopsy in early stages shows a lack of dystrophin using immuno-staining (anti-dystrophin antibodies).

Normal

Dystrophin lies inside cell membrane

Dystrophic muscle

No staining

Genetic screening for mutations of the dystrophin gene is now available.

Becker type muscular dystrophy is a milder form caused by mutation in the dystrophin gene resulting in diminished levels of the protein.

Other muscular dystrophies include the facio-scapulohumoral, limb girdle and myotonic dystrophy forms.

595

INHERITED MYOPATHIES

Specific metabolic defects

An enlarging group of genetic myopathies with specific biochemical or morphological abnormalities is emerging due to the application of modern biochemical, histochemical and morphological (e.g. EM) techniques.

In some, the specific inborn error of metabolism is generalised and includes muscle; in others it is confined to the muscle fibre. Some examples will be given under broad headings:

(1) **Glycogen storage**	(2) **Lipid metabolism**	(3) **Periodic paralysis**
Type 2 (Pompe) – deficiency of acid maltase Type 5 (McArdle) – muscle phosphorylase Type 7 – phospho-fructokinase (PFK)	Defect in free fatty acid transport into and utilisation within fibre. (a) carnitine palmityl transferase (CPT) (b) muscle carnitine deficiency	Associated with hypo- and hyperkalaemia – the muscle defect is a vacuolar degeneration of the sarcolemma

(4) Morphological abnormalities

(a) *Mitochondrial*

(b) *Others*

(a) Mitochondrial	(b)(i) Central core myopathy	(b)(iii) Centronuclear myopathy
Large or increased numbers of mitochondria – abnormal oxidative processes	Central area is abnormal	Nucleus in middle of cell
	(ii) Rod body myopathy (nemaline) Rods of tropomysin under sarcolemma	(iv) Disproportion of fibre types I and II

These various myopathies exhibit a wide range in respect of age of onset, clinical presentation and prognosis.

A further rare but interesting autosomal dominant genetic abnormality of muscle is malignant hyperpyrexia. In this condition the administration of a general anaesthetic precipitates acute muscle damage. Clinically, there is very high fever, muscle stiffness, cyanosis and acidosis very often resulting in death.

ACQUIRED MYOPATHIES

Inflammatory myopathies – polymyositis and dermatomyositis – are two similar **inflammatory** disorders of muscle.

POLYMYOSITIS – occurs in both sexes and at any age, but especially in middle age. It is characterised by muscle pain and weakness – especially of proximal muscle groups. Progress is variable – deterioration may be rapid or slow.

DERMATOMYOSITIS – has similar muscle changes and also skin lesions often on the face and hands. In adults, dermatomyositis may herald malignancy – often bronchial carcinoma – and there is often evidence of other connective tissue diseases e.g. rheumatoid arthritis.

Pathology:

Muscle fibres show damage varying from atrophy to necrosis and some hypertrophied fibres are seen.

There is a lymphocytic infiltrate.

Aetiology

These are both autoimmune diseases although the precise details differ. Polymyositis is a T cell mediated attack on muscle fibres, while dermatomyositis is an immune complex disorder with vascular damage.

CACHECTIC MYOPATHY

In any wasting disease, loss of muscle with weakness is seen.

Endocrine, toxic and nutritional myopathies

(a) Myopathy is seen in acromegaly, hyperthyroidism, hypothyroidism, hyperaldosteronism (due to hypokalaemia), hyperparathyroidism and in corticosteroid excess.
(b) In alcoholics and a variety of drugs in addition to corticosteroids, e.g. chloroquine, vincristine; and in vitamin D deficiency.

MUSCLE DISEASES – DIAGNOSIS

In clinical practice, although in only a few conditions is curative therapy available, accurate diagnosis of cases of muscular weakness and atrophy is important since there is considerable variation in prognosis and management of these diverse disorders.

A diagnosis is usually reached from a synthesis of the information obtained from investigations under three main headings:

1. **General clinical considerations are fundamental.** Of particular importance are *family history, age of onset, distribution of muscle weakness and rate of progress.* To these are added clinical neurological assessment.

2. **Special investigation of neuromuscular electrical activity.** The rate of motor and sensory nerve conduction can be measured electrically.

The ELECTROMYOGRAM records the activity of groups of muscle fibres and even of individual fibres (usually fine needle electrodes). The broad basic pathological changes already described are reflected in variations of the electrical potential within the muscle during various types of activity.

These methods are particularly useful in distinguishing primary myopathies, including myotonias, from denervation atrophy.

3. **Laboratory tests**
   (a) *MUSCLE BIOPSY.* The motor unit area of a moderately weak muscle is chosen (end-stage muscle should not be taken). Special precautions must be taken to minimise artefacts. Routine histological examination will usually distinguish the broad groups of disorders and identify the occasional rare myopathy with specific morphological features.

   Histochemical and EM examination and biochemical analysis may identify specific disorders.

   (b) *SERUM ENZYMES.* In the myopathies where actual muscle fibre destruction is proceeding, increased levels of creatine kinase (CK) and aldolase (ALS) are found.

598

POST-VIRAL FATIGUE SYNDROME

This syndrome has recently come to prominence due to an increased prevalence, both in sporadic cases and in small epidemics. For many years, post-viral depression (e.g. after influenza) and fatigue (e.g. after glandular fever) have been recognised and these symptoms are self-limiting and usually last only a few weeks; the pathological mechanisms are obscure.

The syndrome now so prevalent may be associated with **enterovirus** e.g. coxsackie and other infections and leads to severe functional deficits which are often long-lasting (years). Alternative names for the syndrome are **myalgic encephalomyelitis (ME)** or **chronic fatigue syndrome.**

The clinical signs and symptoms are protean, but the major complaint is extreme fatigue made worse by exercise. For many years the condition was considered to be psychologically induced and was labelled a form of hysteria, but has now been accepted as an organic condition.

The mechanisms however are not yet established with certainty. The flow diagram illustrates the possible mechanisms:

BONE

Normal adult bone shows two gross anatomical forms in varying proportions, depending on the particular type of supportive function required of it. Both have a lamellar structure.

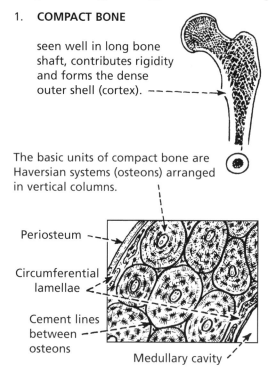

1. COMPACT BONE

seen well in long bone shaft, contributes rigidity and forms the dense outer shell (cortex). - - - - - - →

The basic units of compact bone are Haversian systems (osteons) arranged in vertical columns.

Periosteum - - -

Circumferential lamellae <

Cement lines between - - osteons

Medullary cavity

2. CANCELLOUS BONE

(along with marrow) occupies the medullary cavities. This arrangement as exemplified in a vertebral body contributes some compressibility and pliability.

Haemopoietic marrow

The basic unit of cancellous bone is the trabecula, arranged along lines of stress.

Note: Cancellous bone comprises 20% of bone mass but 80% of bone turnover due to its large surface area

WOVEN BONE (non-lamellar), a primitive form laid down in fetal development.

Osteoblasts on surface

Irregular trabeculae - - in primitive matrix

Osteocytes within trabeculae

Interwoven collagen -

In adult life, this type is seen in bone repair and tumours. Later, it may be replaced by lamellar bone.

Bone and calcium

Bone acts as a reservoir for calcium, which is maintained within a narrow range (2.1–2.6 mmol/l). Hypocalcaemia stimulates parathyroids to produce parathormone (PTH) which promotes bone resorption, calcium absorption from the gut and reabsorption from the kidney. As the serum calcium rises, PTH production is switched off.

BONE TURNOVER

There are two main types of bone cell:

OSTEOBLASTS

– derived from osteoprogenitor cells.
– produce Type I collagen and other proteins.
– secrete alkaline phosphatase – a marker of bone formation.
– stimulated by mechanical stress, androgens, cytokines, e.g. TGF-β

OSTEOCLASTS

– derived from marrow precursors.
– produce acid and enzymes to remove bone.
– produce collagen degradation products e.g. urinary HO proline – a marker of bone destruction.
– stimulated by cytokines e.g. IL-1, IL-6 (indirectly by PTH).
– inhibited by oestrogens.

The activities of the two cell types are closely 'coupled' in the normal process of bone turnover. In the adult 10% of the skeleton is replaced annually. The process has *activating* and *inhibitory* arms.

ACTIVATION

Osteoblasts bear RANKL (**R**eceptor **A**ctivator of **NF-κB L**igand)

Binds to RANK

Proliferation and differentiation into osteoclasts

INHIBITION

Under other circumstances osteoblasts and other cells produce osteoprotegerin (OPG) a soluble molecule which blocks activation through RANK.

Howship's lacunae are formed.

Release of cytokines (eg TGF- β) from bone matrix stimulates osteoblasts.

Osteoblasts lay down osteoid which is then mineralised and the bone cycle is complete.

OSTEOPOROSIS

OSTEOPOROSIS is the commonest disorder of bone.
It is defined as a systemic disease characterised by:

(1) low bone mass.
(2) microarchitectural deterioration of bone, with
(3) an increase in bone fragility and susceptibility to fracture.

A patient is said to have osteoporosis if BONE MINERAL DENSITY >2.5 standard deviations below the mean of normal young subjects.

Clinical effects: – osteoporosis is a disease predominantly of post-menopausal females, but men are also affected.

1. Compression (collapse) of vertebral bodies (usually preceded by gradual loss of height and kyphosis); often associated with sudden pain on weight lifting.
2. Fracture of neck of femur or other long bones (especially Colles' fracture of distal radius).

Note: In osteoporosis, the routine serum biochemical tests – particularly the calcium levels – are within the normal range.

Leverage applied at weakened neck

Pathology: The changes in the vertebral bodies are illustrative.

Normal

Naked eye and Microscopic appearances

Disc bulging into bone.

Porotic bone: wide honey-comb spaces.

Collapse of vertebral body

Sparse thin trabeculae appear disconnected in 2 dimensions 'Microarchitectural deterioration'.

Note: (i) The atrophied trabeculae have a normal calcium content.
(ii) Bone loss is most marked in cancellous bone with its high turnover, but cortical bone is also affected.

OSTEOPOROSIS

Aetiology

In *normal* bones the dynamic processes of formation and resorption are in balance.

In *osteoporosis* the balance is upset by
(1) diminished formation
(2) increased resorption
(3) both 1 and 2 together

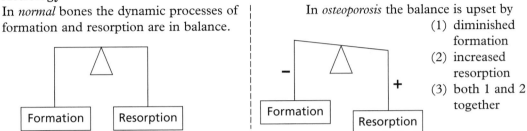

However, bone mass decreases with age in both sexes: in old age, osteoblastic activity falls.

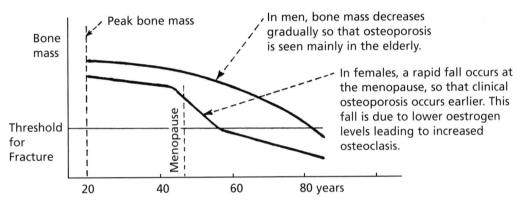

Bone mass
Threshold for Fracture

Peak bone mass

In men, bone mass decreases gradually so that osteoporosis is seen mainly in the elderly.

In females, a rapid fall occurs at the menopause, so that clinical osteoporosis occurs earlier. This fall is due to lower oestrogen levels leading to increased osteoclasis.

Menopause

20   40   60   80 years

PEAK BONE MASS is important – a high initial figure makes osteoporosis less likely. This depends on factors including:
(a) Genetic predisposition – polymorphisms of Type I collagen gene and other genes regulating bone cell activity.
(b) Nutrition – especially calcium intake.
(c) Exercise.

The **aetiology** can be summarised as follows:

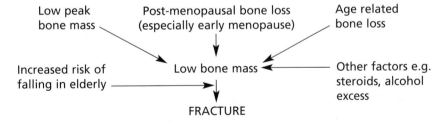

Low peak bone mass   Post-menopausal bone loss (especially early menopause)   Age related bone loss

Increased risk of falling in elderly   Low bone mass   Other factors e.g. steroids, alcohol excess

FRACTURE

Localised osteoporosis is commonly due to disuse and is seen as a complication of other disorders, e.g. local IMMOBILISATION following fracture; limb paralysis and adjacent to severe joint disease with limitation of movement.

This process can be acute with active osteoclasis, but when function is resumed, normal bone structure is often restored.

OSTEOMALACIA AND RICKETS

Osteomalacia and rickets are disorders of bone in which the essential defect is failure of calcification in newly formed osteoid, caused by vitamin D deficiency in almost all cases.

Osteomalacia occurs in adult life and affects the osteoid which is being continually laid down in the normal remodelling of bone.

Rickets affects the growing child, and serious additional disturbances are seen at the growing ends of long bones. Clinically there is pain, weakness of bones with a tendency to distortion and even fracture. Looser's zones, seen in X-ray, are linear partial fractures of long bones which have failed to calcify.

The following simplified diagrams indicate the causes of vitamin D deficiency and its effects on bone.

(a) **Causes of deficiency:**

(b) **Effects on bone**

Note: A compensatory increase in parathyroid activity tends to restore serum calcium towards normal.

METABOLIC BONE DISEASE

In **rickets** there are important changes at the growing ends of long bones.

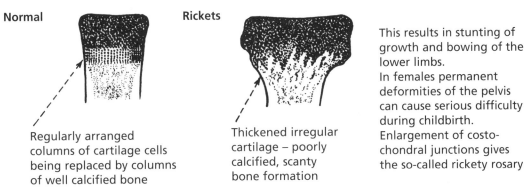

Normal

Regularly arranged columns of cartilage cells being replaced by columns of well calcified bone

Rickets

Thickened irregular cartilage – poorly calcified, scanty bone formation

This results in stunting of growth and bowing of the lower limbs.
In females permanent deformities of the pelvis can cause serious difficulty during childbirth.
Enlargement of costo-chondral junctions gives the so-called rickety rosary

HYPERPARATHYROIDISM

Bone changes may be seen in hyperparathyroidism, especially when severe or long-standing. The essential change is increased bone resorption due to greatly increased osteoclastic activity; usually osteoblastic activity is also increased but the net effect is bone loss.

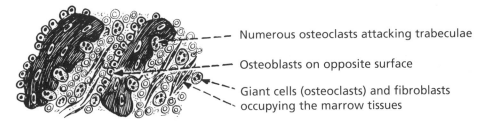

Numerous osteoclasts attacking trabeculae

Osteoblasts on opposite surface

Giant cells (osteoclasts) and fibroblasts occupying the marrow tissues

These changes, although generalised, may be locally severe causing cystic spaces – the fully developed disorder is called **osteitis fibrosa cystica**. In some cases giant cell tumour of bone may be mimicked (so-called BROWN TUMOUR of hyperparathyroidism).

RENAL OSTEODYSTROPHY

In chronic renal failure abnormalities of bone occur. The essential factors are failure of kidneys to produce 1,25 vitamin D, and the failure of the kidneys to eliminate phosphate. These lead to important secondary effects:

Reduced 1,25 D_3 ⟶ **OSTEOMALACIA**

Decreased plasma CALCIUM ⟶ **'SECONDARY' HYPERPARATHYROIDISM** ⟶ RENAL OSTEODYSTROPHY

Increased OSTEOCLASIS

Reduced bone formation ⟶ 'ADYNAMIC BONE DISEASE'

PAGET'S DISEASE OF BONE

This disease of unknown aetiology usually presents after the age of 50 years and affects males predominantly. It is fairly common (3% of autopsies), but only in its more severe forms are there clinical symptoms. The disorder is focal: the bones particularly affected are the pelvis, vertebrae, skull and lower limbs. It has been suggested that virus infection (e.g. measles, distemper) of osteoclasts is responsible. Genetic factors are important.

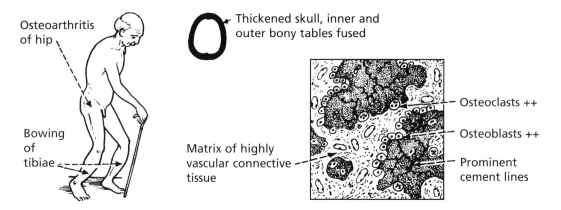

To begin with, there is a localised increase in **osteoclastic** activity causing bone resorption; soon there is a marked **osteoblastic** reaction with bone resorption and deposition proceeding chaotically, so that irregular bone trabeculae with mosaic cement lines are formed. The bone may be thickened, but its structure is defective and weak. Biochemical changes reflect the cellular activity at trabecular level: *Alkaline phosphatase* ↑(osteoblastic); *urinary hydroxyproline* ↑(collagen destruction).

The important **complications** are:

1. **Fracture** of weakened bones (including partial long bone fracture and vertebral compression).
2. **Osteoarthritis** of joints due to abnormal stresses caused by bony deformity.
3. An increased risk (×30) of the development of **bone sarcoma.**
4. The increased circulatory load through the vascular stroma may cause high output cardiac failure in patients with compromised cardiac function.
5. Nerve compression causing deafness.

The use of bisphosphonates offers effective therapy in many cases.

BONE – MISCELLANEOUS

AVASCULAR OSTEONECROSIS (BONE NECROSIS)

(a) The usual processes involved in fracture healing have been dealt with (p.58). Due to details of vascular anatomy at particular sites, fractures may be complicated by severance of the blood supply to one of the bone fragments. This results in a high incidence of avascular bone necrosis. Fractures of the femoral neck and scaphoid bone are good examples.

(b) Other causes include decompression in those working in increased atmospheric pressure (caisson disease), alcoholism, Gaucher's disease, sickle cell anaemia and prolonged corticosteroid therapy. Bone necrosis of this type has important effects when it occurs at an articular surface: serious degenerative arthritis may ensue.

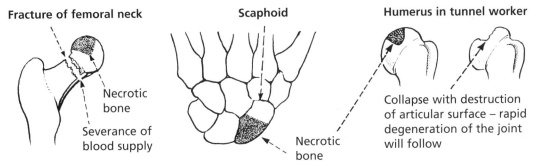

Fracture of femoral neck

Necrotic bone

Severance of blood supply

Scaphoid

Necrotic bone

Humerus in tunnel worker

Collapse with destruction of articular surface – rapid degeneration of the joint will follow

Note: These areas of necrotic bone may be relatively radiodense due to disuse osteoporosis of the adjacent living bone.

(c) In children and adolescents osteonecrosis occurs at several epiphyseal sites for no known cause (repeated minor trauma may be operative in some cases). The commonest is Perthes' disease in which necrosis of one or both femoral heads occurs in children aged 4–10 years: (male: female = 5:1).

FIBROUS DYSPLASIA OF BONE

This disorder may affect a single (monostotic) or several bones (polyostotic). The lesion is of well demarcated fibrous tissue containing small abnormal woven bone trabeculae. Somatic mutations of the GNAS1 gene which encodes the α subunit of a stimulatory G-protein are responsible. Whether the disease is polyostotic or monostotic depends on the stage of development of the embryo when the mutation occurs, a state known as mosaicism.

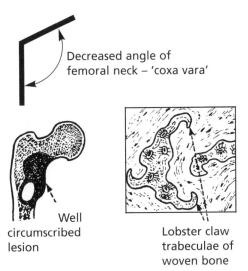

Decreased angle of femoral neck – 'coxa vara'

Well circumscribed lesion

Lobster claw trabeculae of woven bone

Complications

Fracture or deformity of the weakened bone.

INFECTIONS OF BONE

The following basic pathological processes occur in all bone infections.

1. Destruction of bone due to necrosis.

2. Reactive and reparative processes.

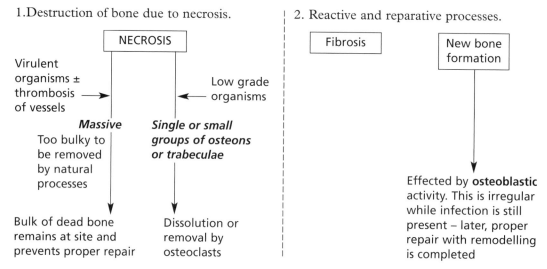

As the infection progresses, the balance between the various components changes. In chronic infections, fibrosis and reparative new bone growth may be very striking.

In addition to the usual accompaniments of inflammation, other important complications are: (1) weakening of bone resulting in deformity or fracture and (2) local complications of the inflammation, particularly abscess and sinus formation.

The following bone infections are illustrative:

ACUTE OSTEOMYELITIS

Classically caused by the *Staphylococcus aureus* and affects the growing ends of the metaphyses of long bones in children. Nowadays the incidence has been greatly reduced and the use of antibiotics aborts the development of the disease. The organisms are blood borne and settle in the cancellous bone of the metaphysis. The effects are dramatic and rapidly progressive.

INFECTIONS OF BONE

Acute Osteomyelitis (*continued*)

Unless treatment is started promptly, the expanding inflammatory process within the rigid bone is seriously complicated.

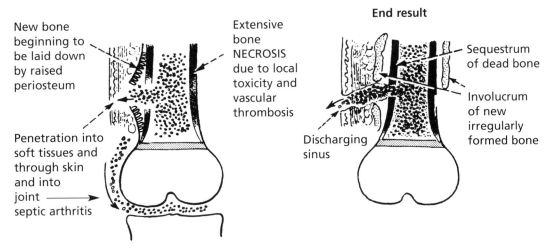

End result

New bone beginning to be laid down by raised periosteum

Extensive bone NECROSIS due to local toxicity and vascular thrombosis

Penetration into soft tissues and through skin and into joint → septic arthritis

Discharging sinus

Sequestrum of dead bone

Involucrum of new irregularly formed bone

The presence of necrotic bone ensures that the inflammation and sinus discharge continue. With large sequestra, the usual natural methods of removal of dead tissue are inadequate so that surgical treatment is necessary.

At a late chronic stage, in addition to the local disability and disturbance of bone growth, **AMYLOID** disease may supervene and occasionally squamous carcinoma arises in a sinus.

Other pyogenic bacteria can cause osteitis – the salmonella group (esp. *S. typhi*) and brucella, the latter often causing a low grade osteitis of the spine.

With inadequate antibiotic treatment, acute inflammatory processes may be converted into low grade osteitis. Staphylococcal infection of the spine may present in adults in this way.

TUBERCULOSIS

The incidence of bone and joint infection parallels the incidence of the more common pulmonary and intestinal infections. It is therefore low in developed countries but still significant elsewhere, and has risen in association with HIV infection.

The spine and growing ends of long bones including the epiphyses are commonly affected by blood borne spread and, because of the proximity of joints, tuberculous arthritis is a frequent concomitant.

The basic pathological process is destruction of bone and replacement with tuberculous granulation tissue. Caseous necrosis is common and tracking and spread into adjacent tissues, particularly in relation to spinal tuberculosis, leads to 'cold abscess' formation.

Although the progress is much less rapid than in acute osteomyelitis, without adequate treatment serious damage to bones and joints occurs.

DEVELOPMENTAL ABNORMALITIES

Local abnormalities are fairly common and include cleft palate, spina bifida and many structural variations of limb development. In the majority the aetiology is uncertain: the presence of teratogens (e.g. thalidomide) is suspected in many and, in a few, genetic inheritance has been established.

Generalised abnormalities are rare and usually inherited.

1. **ACHONDROPLASIA** causes a particularly striking dwarfism. Short, deformed limbs cause a waddling gait. The bones at the skull base are underdeveloped.
The basic abnormality is defective, irregular development of cartilage cells, particularly at the growing epiphyseal plate. This results in stunted long bones.
A mutation of the fibroblast growth factor receptor gene is responsible.

2. In **OSTEOGENESIS IMPERFECTA,** if there is survival beyond infancy, the thin brittle bones fracture easily and a history of multiple fractures with minimal cause is the usual presentation.
The basic defect is in the osteoblasts which fail to synthesise collagen properly. The defects are due to mutations affecting the Type I collagen genes on chromosomes 7 and 17. The severity of the disorder depends on the type of mutation.

A long bone showing three fractures.

| Old, with deformity | More recent, with exuberant callus | Recent, with displacement |

Associated conditions due to the same defect are:
(a) very thin sclerae which appear blue
(b) abnormal tooth development due to defective dentine formation.

3. **OSTEOPETROSIS** (Marble bone disease of Albers–Schönberg) is a disorder in which osteoclasts are absent or defective. This results in failure of bone remodelling and abnormal conversion of cartilage to bone. The whole skeleton becomes dense and the bones thickened.

Complications are: (a) anaemia due to marrow replacement
(b) fractures
(c) cranial nerve compression.

Replacement of osteoclasts by marrow transplant has been done with success.

CYSTIC LESIONS IN BONE

True simple (unicameral) cysts in bone are not uncommon. They have a thin fibrous lining and occur in the proximal humeral and femoral metaphyses in children. As they expand, the risk of fracture increases and this is the most usual presenting sign.

Other true cysts include aneurysmal bone cysts (expanding blood-filled cysts in adolescents) and cysts adjacent to osteoarthritic joints.

Many lesions of bone in which bone is replaced by non-calcified material appear 'lytic' or 'cystic' on X-ray. These include myeloma and metastatic carcinoma.

Contains clear watery fluid

Lining

Eosinophilic granuloma (at the benign end of the spectrum of Langerhans histiocytosis) usually presents as single osteolytic radiolucent lesions of bone in children. Vertebral collapse and pathological fractures are sometimes seen.

The prognosis is usually good.
The histological appearances are typical.

Eosinophils

Langerhans cells

Multinucleate giant cells

TUMOURS IN BONE

Benign tumours present as proliferations of a variety of tissues, varying from rounded excrescences of cartilage and hard bone (simple exostoses and osteomas) through multiple intraosseous irregular nodules of cartilage (enchondromas) to areas of replacement of bone by fibrous or myxomatous tissue. In the field of benign bone tumours, the borderland between true neoplasia and developmental defect is ill-defined.

The importance of benign bone tumours is that:

1. They may cause cosmetic and slight functional defects.
2. Pathological fracture may occur.
3. In some conditions (e.g. multiple enchondroma and exostoses), there is a tendency to malignant transformation.

TUMOURS IN BONE

OSTEOID OSTEOMA

This uncommon benign tumour has a striking clinical presentation and a distinctive pathology.

Clinical: Classically, an adolescent complains of well localised, increasingly severe pain in a lower limb long bone. Aspirin gives relief.

Pathological: The essential lesion is a small focus of newly formed irregular trabeculae of osteoid or poorly calcified woven bone in a highly vascular stroma.

Radiologically a very small radiolucent nidus (<1.5 cm diameter) is surrounded by densely calcified bone

Note: Reaction in surrounding bone; sclerosis of adjacent cortex and periosteal bone thickening.

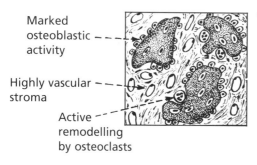

Marked osteoblastic activity

Highly vascular stroma

Active remodelling by osteoclasts

GIANT CELL TUMOUR (osteoclastoma)

This is not a common tumour but presents characteristic histological appearances. The tumour arises in adult life (age 20–40 years), usually at the end of a long bone – especially adjacent to the knee. The basic pathological process is destructive of bone so that the cortex, gradually expanded by the tumour, becomes egg-shell thin. Pathological fracture is common.

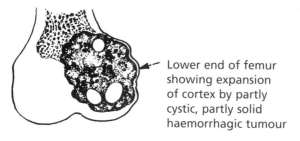

Lower end of femur showing expansion of cortex by partly cystic, partly solid haemorrhagic tumour

Numerous osteoclast-like giant cells and ovoid tumour cells in a vascular stroma

Behaviour: Almost all giant cell tumours are benign. Most are cured by thorough removal: approximately 20% recur: well under 5% are malignant or become malignant after radiotherapy and metastasise to the lungs.

TUMOURS IN BONE

MALIGNANT TUMOURS

Primary malignant tumours of bone are not common, but they assume importance because some arise in young people and are highly malignant and in a few, specific pre-existing bone disorders are known precursors, e.g. Paget's disease, previous irradiation.

Osteosarcoma

This highly malignant tumour is the commonest primary malignant tumour of bone (excluding myeloma). It affects two distinct age groups and there is a preponderance of males over females.

Young age group – majority of cases (10–25 years)
The tumour usually arises near the end of a limb long bone (particularly around the knee).

Elderly subjects (over 60 yrs.)
In 50% of this group, Paget's disease is associated. Long bones, vertebrae and pelvis are often affected, and tumours may be multicentric in origin.

The 'classic' tumour in an adolescent will be described: tumour growth begins in the metaphysis of the medullary cavity. When the cortex has been destroyed and penetrated there is swelling. Most patients complain of bone pain.

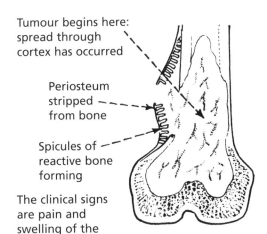

Tumour begins here: spread through cortex has occurred

Periosteum stripped from bone

Spicules of reactive bone forming

The clinical signs are pain and swelling of the lower thigh

The radiological counterpart is a patchily radiolucent tumour

Sun-ray appearance due to new bone spicules

Codman's triangle (new bone forming where periosteum is being stripped)

Note: At this stage lung metastases may be present.

The tumour arises from primitive cells which retain to a varying extent the ability to form bone. Histologically, varying amounts of osteoid, irregularly woven bone and sometimes islands of primitive cartilage are seen. The tumour cells are pleomorphic and mitotically active. With modern chemotherapy 50–60% of patients survive for 5 years.

TUMOURS IN BONE

Chondrosarcoma

This shows a much slower growth pattern and affects the age group 40–70 years. Multiple enchondromatosis pre-exists in a small number of cases. The tumours arise particularly in the limb girdles and proximal long bones and consist of primitive cartilage. Progressive local destruction is usual. Metastases to the lung are rare.

Ewing's tumour

This rare malignant tumour affects young subjects (age 5–20 years): it arises in long bones, pelvis, ribs and scapulae. The tumour is very aggressive, metastasising early to lungs and other bones.

The tumour cells are small and uniform with pale, open nuclei: the cytoplasm contains glycogen. The histological appearances may mimic lymphoma.

Histogenesis

It is known to be a primitive neuro-ectodermal tumour and is associated with translocation and fusion of genes, typically the *EWS* and *Fli-1* genes, on chromosomes 11 and 22. With chemotherapy, survival is similar to that of osteosarcoma.

Lymphoid tumours

Lymphoma and myeloma (see p.438) arise in bone, causing osteolysis. In myeloma IL-6 (interleukin 6) in the main mediator of bone destruction.

SECONDARY TUMOURS IN BONE

THIS IS THE MOST COMMON TYPE OF TUMOUR IN BONE.

Metastases are usually multiple: occasionally latent renal and thyroid cancers present as a single bony metastasis with pathological fracture. Tumours which show a predilection for spread to bone are carcinoma of the PROSTATE, BREAST, LUNG, KIDNEY and THYROID particularly. The incidence of bone secondaries ESPECIALLY IN THE SPINE is very high when these tumours become widespread.

Metastases are usually osteolytic with extensive destruction of bone. In a minority of cases, osteoblastic activity is stimulated by the presence of the tumour so that dense reactive bone is formed. Osteosclerotic secondaries of this type are seen particularly in cancers of the PROSTATE and BREAST.

JOINTS

The diagram illustrates the important components of a **diarthrodial joint.**

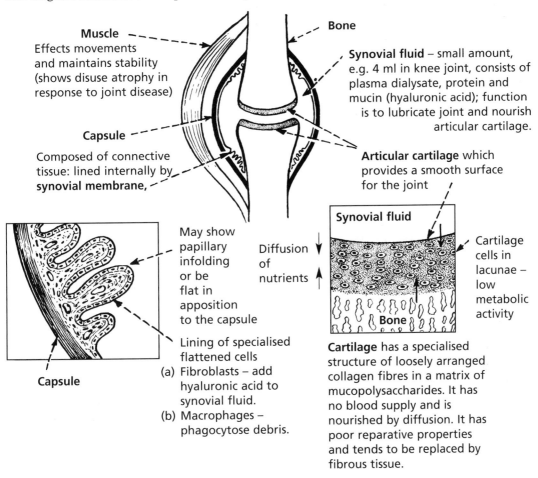

Muscle
Effects movements and maintains stability (shows disuse atrophy in response to joint disease)

Bone

Synovial fluid – small amount, e.g. 4 ml in knee joint, consists of plasma dialysate, protein and mucin (hyaluronic acid); function is to lubricate joint and nourish articular cartilage.

Capsule
Composed of connective tissue: lined internally by **synovial membrane,**

Articular cartilage which provides a smooth surface for the joint

Synovial fluid

Cartilage cells in lacunae – low metabolic activity

Bone

May show papillary infolding or be flat in apposition to the capsule

Diffusion of nutrients

Capsule

Lining of specialised flattened cells
(a) Fibroblasts – add hyaluronic acid to synovial fluid.
(b) Macrophages – phagocytose debris.

Cartilage has a specialised structure of loosely arranged collagen fibres in a matrix of mucopolysaccharides. It has no blood supply and is nourished by diffusion. It has poor reparative properties and tends to be replaced by fibrous tissue.

The two most common joint diseases illustrate how individual components of a joint may be initially affected:

Rheumatoid Arthritis essentially an inflammation of **synovial membrane**	**Osteoarthritis** essentially a degeneration of **articular cartilage**

As the diseases progress, other secondary effects are added and may obscure the basic pathology.

615

JOINT TRAUMA

Trauma is very variable in its severity and effects.

At one end of the scale a single incident of 'sprain' or 'strain' involves only minor soft tissue damage with minimal associated haemorrhage – in these circumstances the healing capacity of joints is rapid and complete.

In contrast, many modern road traffic accidents involve serious damage to joints.

These include:

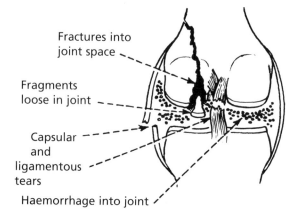

Fractures into joint space

Fragments loose in joint

Capsular and ligamentous tears

Haemorrhage into joint

Possible sequels are:
1. The articular surface is permanently deformed (ineffective repair of cartilage).
2. Loose body continues to cause traumatic damage to synovium of cartilage.
3. Ligaments may not heal or are united by poor scar tissue.
4. Haemorrhagic exudate may not be resorbed – adhesions form within the joint.

With lesser degrees of trauma, particularly if repeated, the synovial membrane shows non-specific reactive changes which include hyperaemia and a mild chronic inflammatory cellular infiltrate. There is often a joint **effusion**.

The knee joint is susceptible to a particular type of injury in which one (particularly the medial) of the fibrocartilagenous menisci is torn.

Medial meniscus

Movement of sudden flexion and rotation – cartilage caught between femur and tibia.

Linear tear

Locking of the joint and effusion are common.

Apart from damage directly attributable to trauma, the most important sequel is that the scene is set within the joint for the more rapid development of **DEGENERATIVE JOINT DISEASE**.

OSTEOARTHRITIS (OA)

OSTEOARTHRITIS (OA)

This is the commonest disorder of joints and, by causing pain and stiffness, is the commonest cause of chronic disability after middle age. The basic pathological progress is degenerative and is similar to that seen in lesser degree in simple ageing. The suffix 'itis' is really inappropriate since any inflammatory changes are secondary.

The disorder is divided into two main groups:

1. In **secondary OA** there is a clear association with some predisposing condition which may be virtually any abnormality of a joint. Of particular importance are:
   (a) alterations to the joint mechanics (e.g. abnormal alignments and angulations); a particularly severe form (Charcot's joint) is seen when the nerve supply to a joint is defective – neuropathic arthropathy.
   (b) abnormality of the articular surfaces (e.g. following injury).
   (c) abnormal stresses on the joint (e.g. the increased weight-bearing demanded by obesity; association with particular occupations and sports).
   (d) previous inflammation e.g. sepsis, rheumatoid arthritis.

2. In **primary OA**, no obvious predisposing cause is evident; there is a presumptive abnormality of chondrocyte metabolism but its essential nature remains obscure. A familial pattern is apparent is some cases – in some, mutation of Type II collagen gene is found. In both types of osteoarthritis the basic pathological processes are the same.

Normal

The integrity of the articular cartilagenous surface represents a fine balance between 'wear and tear' losses and replacement by chondrocytes of the specialised matrix.

The earliest change in ageing and OA is in the chemical composition of the matrix which becomes softer. This is followed by progressive characteristic morphological changes.

At site of pressure

Early OA

Flaking and fibrillation of surface

Later OA

Areas of cystic degeneration

Loss of cartilage; exposure of bone which becomes hard and polished (eburnated)

OSTEOARTHRITIS (OA)

OSTEOARTHRITIS (*continued*)

At edge of joint

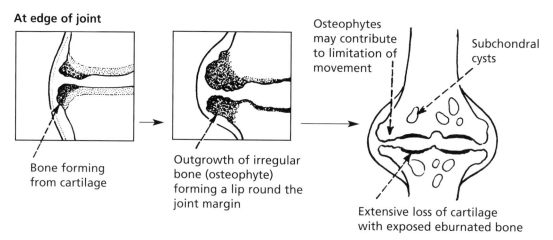

Bone forming from cartilage

Outgrowth of irregular bone (osteophyte) forming a lip round the joint margin

Osteophytes may contribute to limitation of movement

Subchondral cysts

Extensive loss of cartilage with exposed eburnated bone

The synovial membrane may show mild, non-specific inflammation and effusion may occur but these changes are secondary.

Distribution: secondary OA often affects a single predisposed joint.

In primary OA, the larger weight bearing joints and the spine in particular are susceptible, but interphalangeal joints bear osteophytic outgrowths (Heberden's and Bouchard's nodes). Osteoarthritis is the main indication for hip and knee replacement surgery.

Cervical spondylosis. When osteophytes form around the various intervertebral joints, particularly in the cervical spine, neurological complications ranging from compression of individual nerves to actual spinal cord damage are seen.

Note: OA is a local degenerative disease; there is no associated systemic illness.

GOUT. The arthritis of gout begins as an acute inflammatory process often affecting a great toe; with repeated attacks, degenerative arthritis supervenes.

Aetiology: the disease is a disorder of purine metabolism. There is hyperuricaemia (serum uric acid >7 mg/dl). Periodically, urate crystals are deposited within the affected joint, at first in the articular cartilage, but later both in the adjacent bone and soft tissues. Joint aspiration shows characteristic appearances.

Needle shaped crystal

Neutrophil polymorph

PSEUDO-GOUT. In this condition of the elderly, rhomboid crystals of calcium pyrophosphate are deposited in the joint, evoking a similar inflammatory reaction. Larger joints such as the knee tend to be affected; chronic degenerative arthritis often supervenes or co-exists.

RHEUMATOID ARTHRITIS (RA)

Rheumatoid arthritis (RA) is a fairly common systemic disease (1–3% of population in Europe). The main target tissue is the synovial membrane of joints (polyarthritis). The typical clinical course is insidious in its onset and progression. In a minority of cases, the onset is acute and the progress rapid. Frequently there are remissions and exacerbations.

Incidence: female > male
2–3:1

Age of onset: usually 35–55 years, but also in childhood – usually severe.

Typically, the joints of the hands and feet and the knee joints are affected; less commonly there is involvement of the cervical spine and temporomandibular joints.

Pathology: The essential condition is chronic inflammation of the synovial membrane.

Early

Swollen inflamed synovium

Fibrinous exudate

Intense infiltration with lymphocytes and plasma cells

Fluid contains fibrin and neutrophils

Signs of inflammation with swelling over joints

A raised ESR and normochromic anaemia are evidence of the systemic illness.

Intermediate

Laxity of capsule and soft tissue – inflammation in periarticular tissues

Joints swollen + marked muscle wasting (interosseous and thenar muscles)

Destruction of cartilage by enzymatic action and granulation tissue spreading over the articular surface (pannus)

Late

Severely distorted joint

Inflammation usually less marked – fibrous adhesions across joint – may be irregular bony union

Permanent deformity due to contracture and often subluxation

Severe muscle wasting

RHEUMATOID ARTHRITIS (RA)

Rheumatoid arthritis is an autoimmune disease, with no single provoking factor. A possible hypothesis is:

Joint destruction is due to a complex cascade of cytokines, inflammatory cell interaction, and alteration of activity of chondrocytes, osteoblasts and osteoclasts.

Rheumatoid factors

These are antibodies, mainly of IgM and IgG class, which are directed against the patient's IgG, and may form immune complexes which may contribute to the joint inflammation. Patients in whom these autoantibodies can be found in the serum are described as seropositive. Around 85% of RA patients are seropositive.

The systemic nature of the disease is illustrated by inflammatory processes affecting the connective tissues at other sites.

1. **Rheumatoid nodules** occur under the skin at pressure points, particularly in the forearms and elbow joints in 1/5 of cases. They range in size up to a few centimetres in diameter. The histological appearance is striking.

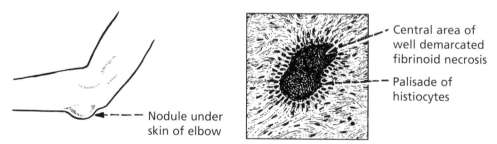

2. The lung may be diffusely affected or, in some cases, lesions similar to rheumatoid nodules are seen. In coal miners, the mixture of coal dust and collagen gives characteristic radiological and pathological appearances – Caplan's nodules.
3. Necrotising arteritis is a serious complication in a few cases.
4. A mild interstitial myocarditis, polymyositis or neuritis may be seen in some cases.
5. Lymphoid and splenic reactive enlargements are seen (particularly in juvenile rheumatoid arthritis). Splenomegaly may cause hypersplenism – so-called Felty's syndrome.
6. Amyloid disease – may complicate long standing RA.

SERO-NEGATIVE ARTHRITIS

Ankylosing spondylitis (AS) is an arthritis affecting particularly the sacroiliac, costovertebral and vertebral joints, but peripheral arthritis is also seen.

Incidence: 0.05% of population
male:female; 3:1

Age of onset: Young adults progressing into middle age.
Rheumatoid factor negative

The disorder is, like RA, an active chronic arthritis, but differs in that it may proceed to osseous ankylosis, so that no movement of the affected joints is possible.

 Bony union on the periphery of the intervertebral discs gives the characteristic radiological appearance – bamboo spine.

Aortitis leading to aortic incompetence and uveitis may be seen.

Psoriatic arthritis affects the axial and peripheral joints. Typically the distal interphalangeal joints are involved and the adjacent nails are affected.

Reiter's syndrome: This is a syndrome of polyarthritis, urethritis and conjunctivitis following infections e.g. chlamydia, yersinia and salmonella. The detailed mechanisms are unclear.

HLA association. It is of great interest in that ankylosing spondylitis, psoriatic patients with arthritis and Reiter's syndrome all have a close association with HLA-B27 (>95% in AS). This suggests that a genetic susceptibility is an important factor predisposing to the arthritis.

No such association with HLA-B27 is evident with RA, which however shows an association with HLA-DR4, twice that of the general population.

Arthritis in acute rheumatic fever

During this stage, arthritis of the knee, ankle and wrist joints is common. The synovial tissues are inflamed and there is an inflammatory cellular infiltrate: the joint fluid contains neutrophils but is sterile. The arthritis is usually self-limiting and without sequelae, in contrast to the cardiac valvular lesions.

OSTEO- AND RHEUMATOID ARTHRITIS – COMPARISON

	OSTEOARTHRITIS	RHEUMATOID ARTHRITIS
Type of disorder	Degenerative	Inflammatory
Site of initial damage	Articular cartilage	Synovial membrane
Age	Late middle age +	3rd decade (any age)
Joints affected	Large weight bearing often single, pre-existing local factors in some cases	Small joints of hands and feet, multiple
Systemic disease	None ESR – normal Rheumatoid factor – absent	++ ESR ↑ Rheumatoid factor positive Secondary anaemia

INFECTIONS OF JOINTS

1. **Acute infective arthritis**

(a) Primary pyogenic haematogenous infection is now rare. It remains, however, a serious complication in joints already damaged. *S. aureus* is the common infecting organism. The essential changes are:

(b) Arthritis complicating **gonorrhoea** and **brucellosis**.
In both of these conditions, a polyarthritis may occur in the acute phase and, in a small number, continues as a low grade arthritis. The spine particularly is affected in brucellosis.

2. **Tuberculous arthritis**
In Western countries the incidence is low: a few cases arise complicating reactivated pulmonary tuberculosis in the elderly. If untreated, there is a low grade chronic inflammation with effusion and progressive destruction of tissues.
The diagnosis requires culture of joint fluid and/or biopsy when the typical histology of tuberculosis is seen.

3. **Lyme disease** is a polyarthritis due to *Borrelia burgdorferi* transmitted by bites from deer ticks.

JOINT AND SOFT TISSUES – MISCELLANEOUS

Pigmented villonodular synovitis (PVNS) (tenosynovial giant cell tumour)

This may affect any synovial tissue, but the knee and hip joints are most commonly involved. There is a strong male predominance (age 20–50). The synovial membrane shows a striking proliferation either in the form of brown pigmented large villi or rounded nodules.

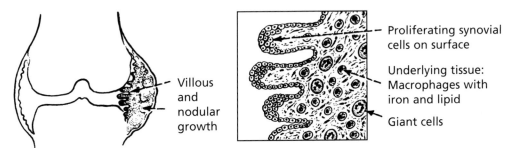

Villous and nodular growth

Proliferating synovial cells on surface

Underlying tissue: Macrophages with iron and lipid

Giant cells

The exact nature of the lesion is not certain. It is now thought to be neoplastic **but to all intents it never metastasises.**
The so-called benign giant cell tumour of tendon sheath is now considered to be a solitary variant of PVNS.

SOFT TISSUE TUMOURS
These are dealt with on pages 123 and 124: 128–130.

Note: The term synovial sarcoma is a misnomer: the tumour does not arise from synovium but from adjacent soft tissues. It is often a biphasic tumour (see p.131).

LOOSE BODIES IN JOINTS
Loose bodies are usually found in diseased or damaged joints and their presence tends to aggravate any existing disease. Clinically, there is often recurrent 'locking' of the joint.

Traumatic:
Fragments derived from fractures: tearing of cartilage and synovium

Degenerative:
Melon seed bodies } Products
Fragments of osteophytes } of arthritis

Synovial chondromatosis – numerous polypoidal projections of cartilage formed by metaplasia within the synovium.

PARA-ARTICULAR TISSUES – MISCELLANEOUS

Bursae

These are synovial-lined spaces usually overlying bony prominences and often connected with adjacent joint spaces. They are subject to traumatic and inflammatory disorders as have been described in joints.

Ganglion

This is a swelling which forms in relation to joint synovium or more usually, tendon sheath. The essential lesion is a myxomatous degeneration of the sheath substance; it is not lined by synovium. Ganglia are classically seen around the wrist.

This type of myxomatous cystic degeneration may occur at other less prominent sites, e.g. within the cartilagenous menisci of the knee.

Dupuytren's Contracture. See page 124.

CONNECTIVE TISSUE DISEASES

This term describes a group of multisystem diseases, many autoimmune in origin.

The group includes rheumatoid arthritis (RA); systemic lupus erythematosus (SLE); scleroderma; polyarteritis nodosa (PAN) and dermatomyositis.

Some of these disorders have already been described (RA p.619; PAN p.227; dermatomyositis p.597).

Systemic lupus erythematosus (SLE)

This is a rare disease predominantly affecting young women. The clinical progress varies from acute and rapid to insidious and slow. Most frequently the skin, kidneys, joints, serous membranes and endocardium are damaged and, in 20% of cases, the central nervous system. The essential lesion is a vasculitis affecting arterioles, capillaries and venules with fibrinoid necrosis and a variable inflammatory cellular infiltrate. In the kidney the lesion is a glomerulitis (see p.463).

SLE is an autoimmune disorder. Antibodies against many cellular constituents may be found e.g. anti-nuclear, anti-DNA.

Immune complexes activate complement so that low serum levels e.g. of C3, C4 are found.

Progressive systemic sclerosis

This is a rare, slowly progressive disease in which there is gradual fibrosis of various organs including the skin (face and hands), gastrointestinal tract, heart and lungs. Raynaud's disease is a common concomitant. The basic abnormality is in the small blood vessels, which show sclerosis with intimal thickening. The change is associated with fibrosis of the surrounding tissues. Auto-antibodies, typically against nuclear components, are often found.

From the description of these various disorders it will be seen that the basic mechanisms are essentially inflammatory and are mediated by autoimmune processes. The inflammatory damage is very variable in its severity, its site of predilection and even its local effects. Multiple factors, of which inherited susceptibility and resistance are important, are involved. The following diagram illustrates the basic mechanisms.

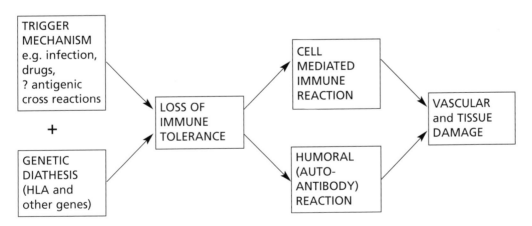

ENDOCRINE SYSTEM

ENDOCRINE DISEASES

Most endocrine glands are controlled by hormones produced in the anterior pituitary, themselves under control of substances produced in the hypothalamus. A variety of stimuli control pituitary and hypothalamic hormone release, especially feedback control from hormone levels from the target glands. Levels of pituitary hormones show a circadian rhythm.

Endocrine diseases can be broadly classified as:

Hormone excess
– primary overproduction by gland
– secondary to excessive trophic hormone

Hormone deficiency
– primary underproduction by gland, e.g. due to inflammation, post surgery
– secondary to insufficient trophic hormones

Hormone resistance
– target organ resistance
– failure to activate hormone

Effects of non-functioning tumours
– local pressure and invasion
– metastatic disease

PITUITARY GLAND

The pituitary has two divisions, the anterior (adenohypophysis) and the posterior (neurohypophysis).

Anterior pituitary (adenohypophysis)

Adeno-hypophysis

Neuro-hypophysis

The blood supply is via a portal system from the hypothalamus bringing peptides which stimulate or inhibit pituitary hormone production. The cells producing each hormone can be identified by immunohistochemistry (for stored hormone) or in situ hybridisation (for mRNA).

Posterior pituitary

This is composed of neural tissue and secretes two hormones made in the hypothalamus (oxytocin and antidiuretic hormone).

Thyrotrophs produce thyroid stimulating hormone (TSH) which stimulates thyroid follicle cells
Lactotrophs produce prolactin which initiates and maintains lactation

Oxytocin
– causes expulsion of milk during lactation
– aids contraction of uterine smooth muscle during labour

Corticotrophs produce adrenocorticotrophic hormone (ACTH) which stimulates glucocorticoid secretion
Antidiuretic hormone (ADH) helps control water balance by altering the permeability of the renal collecting tubules. Deficiency leads to diabetes insipidus

Gonadotrophs produce follicle stimulating hormone (FSH) which stimulates spermatogenesis, ovarian follicle development and luteinising hormone (LH) which controls Leydig cell function and promotes ovulation

Note

1. ACTH (39 amino acids long) is synthesised as part of a large molecule proopiomelanocortin (POMC) from which other molecules including melanocyte stimulating hormone (MSH) are derived.

2. Hypothalamic releasing hormones have been found for TSH (TRH), LH/FSH (GnRH), ACTH (CRH) and GH (GHRH); somatostatin inhibits release of GH.

Somatotrophs produce growth hormone which stimulates liver and muscle protein synthesis and, indirectly through insulin-like growth factors (IGF-1), skeletal growth

629

PITUITARY HYPERFUNCTION

In most cases, this is associated with PITUITARY ADENOMA.

Pituitary adenomas are divided on the basis of size into MACROADENOMAS (>10 mm) and MICROADENOMAS (<10 mm).

Small tumours present only if they produce excess hormones, while larger tumours may cause pressure effects (e.g. on optic chiasma, page 141) or with hypopituitarism due to destruction of normal pituitary. Occasionally haemorrhage into a pituitary adenoma causes raised intracranial pressure (PITUITARY APOPLEXY).

Gigantism and acromegaly

These are both the result of excess production of growth hormone by a somatotroph (acidophil) adenoma. Gigantism arises in children before the epiphyses have fused; acromegaly occurs in adult life.

Gigantism

The excess growth hormone induces skeletal growth, the bones retaining their normal shape and relative proportions. Fusion of epiphyses is delayed, but eventually occurs and the features of acromegaly appear.

Acromegaly

There is overgrowth of bone and soft tissue.

Clinical signs
Features coarsened: nose enlarged.
Prognathic (projecting jaw).
Irregular bone formation – interferes with
    joint function – leads to osteoarthritis.
Limbs enlarged.

Pain due to nerve compression is common. Glucose tolerance is diminished and diabetes occurs in 10%. High blood pressure with cardiac hypertrophy and extensive atheroma is common, and the patient may die in cardiac failure. There is a 2–3 fold increased risk of colonic cancer.

HYPERPROLACTINAEMIA

Prolactin secreting adenomas are often small. They cause amenorrhoea, infertility and occasionally galactorrhoea in younger women, but are usually asymptomatic in older women and men.

CUSHING'S SYNDROME is frequently due to an ACTH secreting adenoma when it is known as Cushing's disease. The effects are described on p.640.

HYPOPITUITARISM

Failure of pituitary secretion may affect one or several hormones. Causes include:
(a) Pituitary tumour.
(b) Pituitary surgery/cranial irradiation.
(c) Head injury.
(d) Hypothalamic dysfunction, including craniopharyngioma.
(e) Sheehan's syndrome: is used as an example. It is still an important cause where obstetric services are poor.

This syndrome occurs in women and is due to ischaemic necrosis of the pituitary following post-partum haemorrhage. The normally low pressure in the pituitary portal vascular supply increases the susceptibility of the gland. The results vary with the extent of necrosis and may include the following:

Lack of TSH – low BMR, features of hypothyroidism, sensitivity to cold, coarsening and loss of hair

Lack of prolactin
– failure of lactation, and later breast atrophy

Lack of ACTH – deficiency of glucocorticoids – weakness, low BP, hypoglycaemia

Lack of gonadotrophins – amenorrhoea, sterility, loss of libido (usually earliest symptoms).

Loss of pubic hair

In time, the peripheral endocrine organs – thyroid, adrenals, ovaries – show atrophy.

In childhood, growth hormone deficiency is a cause of dwarfism. Skeletal growth is diminished with retarded sexual development but normal intelligence. Hypothalamic GHRH deficiency may be responsible.

Note: Some individuals treated with human growth hormone have developed Creutzfeld–Jacob disease (p.559).

In adults, GH deficiency leads to lethargy, diminished muscle mass, obesity and premature atheroma.

Inflammation of the pituitary gland
Apart from involvement in acute meningitis, inflammation, acute or chronic, is uncommon. Tuberculosis, syphilis and sarcoidosis all rarely occur.

THYROID GLAND

Normal bilobed gland weighs approximately 25 g

Colloid storing thyroid hormones

Follicles lined by cuboidal epithelium

Parafollicular cells (source of calcitonin)

Rich capillary network

The thyroid gland is under the control of the pituitary thyroid-stimulating hormone (TSH p.629).

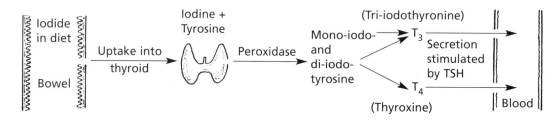

Iodide in diet

Bowel

Uptake into thyroid

Iodine + Tyrosine

Peroxidase

Mono-iodo- and di-iodo-tyrosine

(Tri-iodothyronine)

T_3

Secretion stimulated by TSH

T_4

(Thyroxine)

Blood

T_4 can be regarded as a prohormone, which is converted to active T_3 by deiodination in liver, muscle and kidney.

THYROID HYPOFUNCTION

Insufficient thyroid hormone is produced, resulting in myxoedema in adults and cretinism in children.

Adults – MYXOEDEMA

Clinical signs

Basal metabolic rate reduced, weight gain.

Body temperature falls, cold intolerance.

Lethargy and apathy.

Appetite reduced.

Constipation.

Respiratory and heart rates reduced.

Diminished libido.

Lack of ovulation.

Skin thickened, non-pitting oedema due to increase in mucopolysaccharide ground substance.

Hair brittle, dry and falls out.

Blood cholesterol is raised.

TSH secretion is increased.

T_3 and T_4 blood levels low.

THYROID GLAND

Myxoedema (*continued*)

Causes

1. Autoimmune thyroiditis
   (a) Atrophic form – so-called
       primary myxoedema – the
       commonest cause of hypothyroidism
   (b) Goitrous form –
       Hashimoto's disease.
2. Severe iodine deficiency.

3. Dyshormonogenesis – inborn errors
   in the formation of thyroid hormones.
4. Anti-thyroid drugs, e.g. lithium
5. Excessive surgical resection
   of thyroid gland.
6. Treatment with radioiodine.
7. Hypopituitarism → reduced TSH.

Pathological changes in primary myxoedema

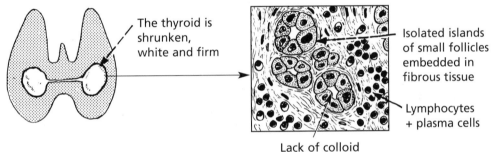

The thyroid is shrunken, white and firm

Isolated islands of small follicles embedded in fibrous tissue

Lymphocytes + plasma cells

Lack of colloid

Children – CRETINISM

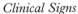

Infants normal at birth, but abnormality appears within weeks.

Clinical Signs

Protruding tongue

Dwarf with short limbs
Coarse dry skin
Lack of hair and teeth
Mental deficiency

Pot belly – often umbilical hernia

Changes are irreversible unless treatment is given early.
Two forms are recognised:

(1) endemic and (2) sporadic cretinism.

THYROID GLAND

Endemic cretinism

This occurs in districts where goitre is common due to iodine deficiency. It rarely appears until the 3rd generation of a goitrous family and the mother almost always has a goitre. The infantile thyroid is usually enlarged and nodular. Histologically, there are hyperplastic foci containing colloid which compress the intervening tissue. The incidence of this disorder has reduced following addition of iodine to salt.

Sporadic cretinism

This is usually due to congenital hypoplasia or absence of the thyroid. Deaf mutism is often present.

Dyshormonogenesis

In this condition, cretinism is due to a congenital familial recessive enzyme defect leading to inability to complete the formation of thyroid hormone. The thyroid gland is enlarged and shows epithelial hyperplasia. TSH is increased.

THYROID HYPERFUNCTION

Excessive quantities of circulating thyroid hormone (T_3 and T_4) cause thyrotoxicosis. Three types of thyroid lesion can give rise to thyrotoxicosis.

1. Graves' disease (exophthalmic goitre) >80%.
2. Toxic nodular goitre 10%
3. Toxic adenoma <5%.

Graves' Disease (Exophthalmic goitre)

Clinical signs
Exophthalmos
Prominent thyroid.
BMR increased.
Skin warm and sweaty: heat intolerance.
Weakness, hyperkinesia and emotional instability.
Loss of weight.
Glucose tolerance diminished, glycosuria.
Rapid pulse.
Cardiac arrhythmia, especially atrial fibrillation, and heart failure in older patients.
TSH low.

THYROID GLAND

Graves' disease

Gland is diffusely enlarged; pale pink in colour

Gland is hyperplastic; numerous closely packed acini of various sizes

Sometimes intra-acinar papilliform growths

Colloid absent

Cells columnar

In some cases there are foci of thyroiditis with lymphocytes and plasma cells.

Other changes: 1. Patches of myxoedema – usually on pre-tibial aspect of legs.
               2. Exophthalmos, due to autoimmune damage to the eye muscles.

Aetiology: 1. Usually in females, peak 20–40 years.
           2. More common in families showing high incidence of autoimmune disease, e.g. thyroiditis, pernicious anaemia.
           3. The stimulation of the thyroid is due to an autoantibody (thyroid stimulating immunoglobulin/TSH antibody also known as TRAb) which reacts with and activates the surface receptor for TSH on thyroid epithelium. Cyclic AMP is formed and this stimulates hyperplasia of the epithelium and increased formation of thyroid hormone. With the increase in hormone, the blood TSH falls.

Toxic adenoma

Most adenomas are non-active; only a small proportion (1%) give rise to toxic symptoms. Most patients are women over 40 years.

There is usually only one large adenoma present. The histological features are of follicles which may be small or of normal size. Increased production of thyroid hormone by the adenoma, which is autonomous, causes a fall in TSH, and the remainder of the thyroid is inactive.

Toxic nodular goitre

This develops in some cases of non-toxic nodular goitre. Nodules of hyperplasia are interspersed with inactive tissue. The condition is more common over the age of 50 especially in women. Exophthalmos is absent. Cardiac arrhythmias and heart failure is common.

THYROID GLAND

Non-toxic goitre

This is a simple enlargement of the thyroid gland, not associated with increased secretion of thyroid hormone.

Two morphological forms are found: (1) parenchymatous and (2) colloid: they are components of a disease spectrum and are separated only on morphological appearances.

1. *Parenchymatous goitre.* The gland is enlarged and pale pink. Two phases can be recognised:

    (a) **Diffuse hyperplasia:** The gland consists mainly of small closely packed acini lined by columnar epithelium and containing a small amount of poorly stained colloid. Occasional intra-acinar papilliform epithelial projections may be seen.

    (b) **Nodular hyperplasia:** This is a later stage. Areas of marked hyperplasia cause atrophy of intervening parenchyma. It appears to be related to continuing severity of iodine deficiency.

2. *Colloid goitre.* The enlarged gland is translucent and brown due to the large amount of stored colloid.

    This is common in women and appears at puberty or during pregnancy. There are usually no symptoms, but pressure symptoms develop if the thyroid is retrosternal, e.g. pressure on trachea causing stridor, pressure on recurrent laryngeal nerve → hoarseness.

Vesicles large and full of dense colloid

Small cysts common

Epithelium flattened

Aetiology. In most regions the aetiology is unknown. Goitre is endemic in central areas of the world, mountainous regions remote from the sea – Switzerland, Himalayas, Andes, etc. There is a lack of iodine in the soil, hence in the food. Addition of iodine to salt has lowered the prevalence.

(1) Lack of iodine in food   (2) Inhibited by drugs

Iodine + I
Tyrosine
Mono-iodo- Di-iodo-
tyrosine
Thyroid gland T_3 T_4

(3) Inhibited by inherited congenital lack of enzymes

Mechanism of goitre production

Lack of iodine ⟶ Deficient production of thyroid hormone ⟶ ↑TSH secretion ⟶ Enlargement of thyroid to extract maximum amount of iodine from blood

Where the lack of iodine is severe, proliferation is marked (parenchymatous goitre). In colloid goitre, the process is milder.

THYROID GLAND

AUTOIMMUNE THYROIDITIS

This type of disease is associated with the appearance of thyroid antibodies in the blood and inflammatory changes with lymphocytes and plasma cell reaction in the thyroid gland. The degree of pathological change and the clinical effects form a spectrum, but three conditions can be defined. There is an associated risk of development of non-Hodgkin's lymphoma in each.

1. **Hashimoto's thyroiditis (lymphadenoid goitre)**

    This is the most distinctive type of autoimmune thyroid disease, and the changes are widespread.

Lymphocytic infiltrate

Germinal centre

Many small acini

Acini lined by pink cells (Askanazy or Hürthle cells)

Lymphocytes and plasma cells

Nuclei often large and irregular

Clinical effects: While the patient may be euthyroid, it is obvious that the balance is precarious. In 80%, the patient, usually a middle-aged female, develops hypothyroidism. Any attempt to reduce the size of the goitre by surgery inevitably causes hypothyroidism.

In a small proportion of cases the patient has thyrotoxicosis in the early stages of the disease.

2. **Primary Myxoedema**

    Antibodies to thyroid hormones and epithelium are found in this disease (p.632).

3. **Focal thyroiditis**

    This extremely common form of autoimmune disease is usually asymptomatic, but again the balance is disturbed and surgical interference may precipitate hypothyroidism. The concentration of antibodies in the plasma is always low. The thyroid in Graves' disease often shows a form of focal thyroiditis and this may account for the occasional occurrence of hypothyroidism as a late complication in that disease.

    Patients with autoimmune thyroiditis are apt to have other organ-specific antibodies, e.g. gastric, adrenal etc., and pernicious anaemia and adrenal insufficiency may occur.

4. **Graves' disease** (p.634).

TUMOURS OF THYROID

Follicular Adenoma

This fairly common benign tumour is usually single and is encapsulated with compression of the surrounding gland. Very occasionally there is hypersecretion with thyrotoxicosis. Degenerative changes including haemorrhage into the tumour are common.

MALIGNANT TUMOURS are common. Five forms are recognised:

1. ***Papillary carcinoma*** 60–70%. This affects particularly young women: the tumours are usually small and may be multiple within the thyroid. They metastasise readily to local lymph nodes and the first clinical sign may be an enlarged cervical lymph node containing metastatic papillary tumour. Remote spread is unusual.

The histological appearances are typical:

(1) Small papillary structures - - - - - - - →
(2) Uniform, optically clear
    (Orphan Annie) or grooved nuclei - - - ▸
(3) Psammoma bodies - - - - - - - - -
    – concentric calcification

2. ***Follicular carcinoma*** 15–20%. These tumours have their highest incidence in women over middle age. They present in 2 forms:

   (a) Minimally invasive, well encapsulated and can only be differentiated from adenoma by invasion of the capsule and/or veins.

   (b) As a tumour of varying degrees of follicular differentiation, which spreads widely in the thyroid and invades venules.

Invasion - - - of vessel

Breach of - - - - capsule

Follicular tumour - - - spreading within thyroid

Blood spread particularly to BONES and LUNGS is usual in follicular carcinoma.

3. ***Medullary carcinoma*** 5–10%. This is a rare tumour arising from the calcitonin-producing cells of the thyroid. Blood calcitonin is high. In addition, there may be production of other hormones resulting in a carcinoid or Cushing's syndrome. There is a familial form in which there are multiple tumours of a number of endocrine organs (MEN 2, p.649).

4. ***Anaplastic carcinoma*** This occurs in the elderly and may cause stridor. Distant metastases are common.

5. ***Lymphoma*** B cell lymphoma occasionally arises in long-standing autoimmune thyroiditis (particularly Hashimoto's disease).

ADRENAL GLAND

The adrenal glands consist of several glands within one structure.

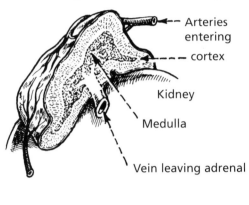

- Arteries entering
- cortex
- Kidney
- Medulla
- Vein leaving adrenal

Mineralocorticoids

The main one is aldosterone. It is involved with the renin-angiotensin system and ADH in the maintenance of blood volume. The mechanism is as follows:

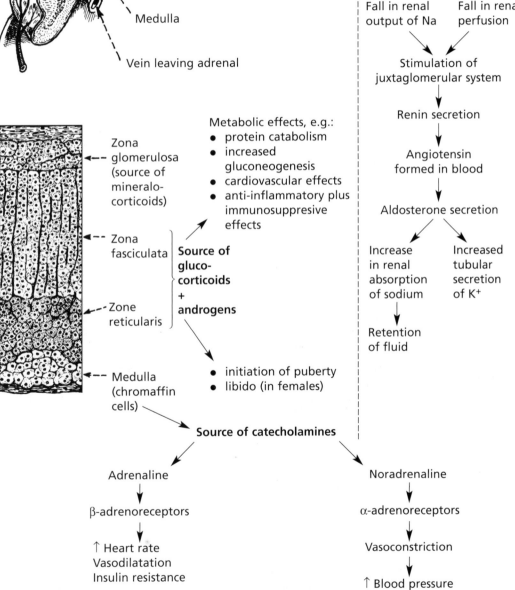

Fall in renal output of Na   Fall in renal perfusion

↓

Stimulation of juxtaglomerular system

↓

Renin secretion

↓

Angiotensin formed in blood

↓

Aldosterone secretion

Increase in renal absorption of sodium   Increased tubular secretion of K$^+$

↓

Retention of fluid

Zona glomerulosa (source of mineralo-corticoids)

Zona fasciculata

Zone reticularis

Source of gluco-corticoids + androgens

Metabolic effects, e.g.:
- protein catabolism
- increased gluconeogenesis
- cardiovascular effects
- anti-inflammatory plus immunosuppresive effects

- initiation of puberty
- libido (in females)

Medulla (chromaffin cells)

Source of catecholamines

Adrenaline

↓

β-adrenoreceptors

↓

↑ Heart rate
Vasodilatation
Insulin resistance

Noradrenaline

↓

α-adrenoreceptors

↓

Vasoconstriction

↓

↑ Blood pressure

ADRENAL CORTEX

HYPERACTIVITY

This manifests itself in three ways:

1. **Cushing's syndrome** (hypersecretion of cortisol)

This condition is commonest in women, but occurs also in men and rarely in children.

Clinical effects

In addition: 1. Osteoporosis → kyphosis
2. Hypertension
3. Degree of virilism common in women.

Causes
1. Excessive secretion of ACTH by pituitary adenoma, 70%.
2. Adenoma or carcinoma of adrenal cortex, 20%.
3. Inappropriate secretion of ACTH e.g. by bronchial carcinoma, carcinoids, pancreatic tumours.
4. Prolonged administration of glucocorticoids or ACTH as therapy.

2. **Primary hyperaldosteronism** (Conn's syndrome).

This is due to an adenoma (>80%) or hyperplasia of the zona glomerulosa.

Effects

Note: Secondary hyperaldosteronism is a consequence of any high renin state e.g. renal ischaemia.

3. **Excessive sex hormone secretion**

This can occur occasionally with an adrenal cortical adenoma; usually excessive androgens are secreted. (a) In children it causes precocious puberty; (b) In adult females – virilism, oligomenorrhoea.

ADRENAL CORTEX – HYPOFUNCTION

Adrenal cortical insufficiency may be due to panhypopituitarism or destruction of about 90% of the adrenal cortex. *Acute adrenal failure* is usually due to septicaemia, especially meningococcal (Waterhouse–Friderichsen syndrome).

Septicaemia ⟶ Endotoxaemia ⟶ Adrenal haemorrhage and necrosis

Shock

Chronic Hypofunction

Causes

1. Addison's disease. This is an autoimmune adrenalitis with humoral or cell mediated damage to the adrenal gland. It is responsible for at least 75% of cases.
2. Tuberculous destruction of adrenals – remains an important cause, especially in developing countries.
3. Pituitary failure.

Other autoimmune diseases affecting other endocrine glands are commonly associated with Addison's disease, e.g. thyroid, parathyroid disease, diabetes.

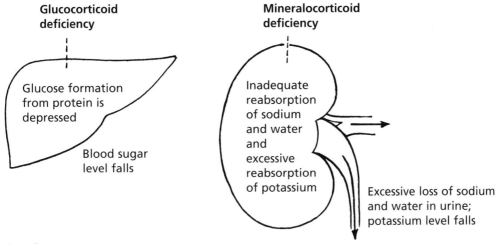

Glucocorticoid deficiency

Glucose formation from protein is depressed

Blood sugar level falls

Mineralocorticoid deficiency

Inadequate reabsorption of sodium and water and excessive reabsorption of potassium

Excessive loss of sodium and water in urine; potassium level falls

Other features

Muscular weakness and wasting.
Loss of weight.
Gastrointestinal upsets (vomiting, diarrhoea).
Anaemia.
Pigmentation of exposed and pressure areas of skin (↑ MSH).
Dehydration.
Crises occur especially if acute infection complicates the condition.

Administration of adrenal hormones restores individual to normal.

Note: In adrenal gland failure, a high level of ACTH results. Melanocyte stimulating hormone is derived from the same precursor pro-opiomelanocortin.

ADRENAL CORTEX AND MEDULLA

Congenital Adrenocortical Enzyme Defects

These are rare, inherited conditions due to autosomal recessive traits.
Each transformation step in the pathways of steroid formation in the adrenal cortex requires the activity of one or more enzymes. Deficiency of any enzyme will interfere with production of the end product.

21 hydroxylase deficiency

This is the commonest type, and the lack of this enzyme prevents the production of cortisol and aldosterone. The low blood cortisol activates ACTH secretion. Adrenal hyperplasia follows and, although cortisol is not formed, other steroids are produced in excess. The resulting clinical syndrome varies with the severity of the defect, e.g:

1. Symptoms of Addison's disease.
2. Lesser degrees of adrenal failure plus symptoms due to excess of sex steroids.
    (a) Pseudohermaphroditism in females; precocious puberty in males.
    (b) Virilism in female.
3. No signs of adrenal failure but sex disturbance, e.g. amenorrhoea, hirsutism.

ADRENAL MEDULLA

Excess production of catecholamines may occur with some tumours of the medulla. Three are described:

1. Phaeochromocytoma. This tumour is composed of chromaffin cells. Symptoms are due to paroxysmal overproduction of the amines with hypertension, raised metabolic rate and blood sugar. Cerebral haemorrhage may occur. About 10% of phaeochromocytomas are familial, 10% are bilateral and 10% are malignant. It is very difficult to predict behaviour on histological grounds.

Familial cases may be associated with: (a) MEN syndromes.
                                            (b) Neurofibromatosis.
                                            (c) Von Hippel–Lindau syndrome.

2. Ganglioneuroma: a benign tumour, composed of well-differentiated ganglion cells (p.581).

3. Neuroblastoma: a very malignant tumour of primitive nerve cells, occurring in children.

ENDOCRINE PANCREAS

The islets of Langerhans form 1–2% of the pancreatic tissue. Four types of cell make up the islets. The majority are β cells.

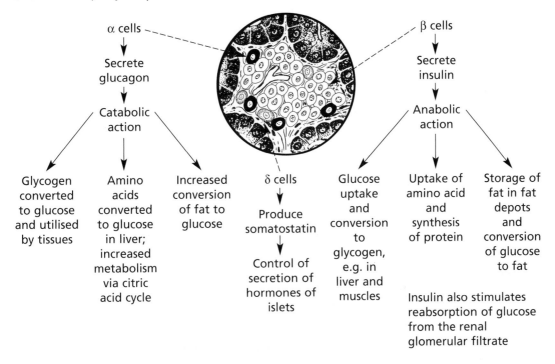

Insulin and glucagon have virtually opposite actions. The action of insulin is also opposed by growth hormone and glucocorticoids.

The fourth type of cell is the pancreatic polypeptide (PP) cell, found in highest concentration in the head of the pancreas.

DIABETES MELLITUS

This condition is due to an absolute or relative lack of insulin activity. The American Diabetic Association suggest that the classification of diabetes should be:

Type 1 – immune mediated β cell dysfunction ➝ absolute insulin deficiency.

Type 2 – adult onset due to insulin resistance, relative insulin deficiency or from a secretory defect.

Type 3 – a range of causes including genetic defects of β cell function and diseases of the exocrine pancreas.

Type 4 – gestational diabetes.

ENDOCRINE PANCREAS

BIOCHEMICAL CHANGES AND CLINICAL EFFECTS
The main results of insulin lack are:

1. **Inability to control carbohydrate metabolism, causing:**

Hyperglycaemia ⟶ Glycosuria

Hyperglycaemia ↓ Increased plasma osmolarity ⟵ Osmotic diuresis

Glycosuria ↓ Osmotic diuresis

Osmotic diuresis ⟶ Hypovolaemia Loss of Na$^+$ and K$^+$

2. **Increased fat catabolism**

Leads to:
Excess production of acetyl CoA

Increased plasma osmolarity and Hypovolaemia ⟶ Thirst ⟶ Polydipsia

↳ Conversion to ketone bodies (acetone + hydroxybutyric acid)

  ↳ Ketosis ⟶ Acidosis ⟶ Acid excreted in combination with Na$^+$ and K$^+$

  ↓ Further electrolyte depletion

3. **Increased catabolism of amino acids** prevents proper protein synthesis and this, together with (1) and (2) above, leads to loss of weight despite polyphagia.

TYPES OF DIABETES
Primary forms
TYPE 1 Insulin-Dependent Diabetes (juvenile 'immune-mediated' diabetes)

This form is due to destruction of β cells in the islets of Langerhans.

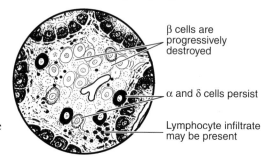

β cells are progressively destroyed

α and δ cells persist

Lymphocyte infiltrate may be present

The onset is acute and the peak of incidence is around 13 years. Three factors appear to be of importance in the aetiology:

1. There is a familial incidence and in 80% of cases there is an association with Class II HLA antigens (particularly HLA DR3, DR4).
2. The onset of the condition is commonest in autumn and winter.
3. Cell-mediated immunity against islet antigens and humoral antibodies are present in most cases.
   This has given rise to a theory of pathogenesis:

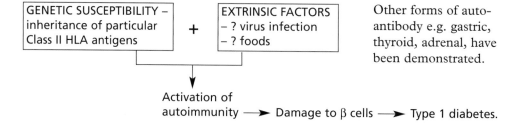

| GENETIC SUSCEPTIBILITY –
inheritance of particular
Class II HLA antigens | + | EXTRINSIC FACTORS
– ? virus infection
– ? foods |

Other forms of auto-antibody e.g. gastric, thyroid, adrenal, have been demonstrated.

Activation of autoimmunity ⟶ Damage to β cells ⟶ Type 1 diabetes.

ENDOCRINE PANCREAS

Types of diabetes (*continued*)

Primary forms

TYPE 2 Non-Insulin-Dependent Diabetes Mellitus (NIDDM)

This is the commonest form of diabetes affecting 10% of adults over 65 in Western society. It is commoner in Asians and Afro-Caribbeans within Western societies. It is more frequent in females and the incidence increases with age. In contrast to Type 1, the onset is slow and the changes in glucose metabolism mild. (Diet restriction to reduce OBESITY and oral hypoglycaemic drugs usually control the blood sugar.) Clinical presentation is often due to complications, particularly vascular, or the disorder is detected at community screening.

Aetiology

This is a multifactorial disorder involving environmental and strong genetic factors. The basic mechanism is prolonged INSULIN RESISTANCE in the tissues leading eventually to inadequate secretion of insulin by β cells. The term 'syndrome X' has been applied to the combination of obesity, NIDDM and hyperlipidaemia leading to an increased risk of cardiovascular disease.

The following theory accommodates the known facts:

Note 1: The concordance rate for identical twins is over 85% in some studies.
Note 2: β cells secrete islet amyloid protein along with insulin. **Amyloid** is deposited in islets in Type 2 diabetes probably reflecting the prolonged β cell activity.

ENDOCRINE PANCREAS

Types of diabetes (*continued*)

Secondary forms **(Type 3)**

Diabetes may complicate:

1. A number of endocrine diseases (acromegaly, Cushing's syndrome, phaeochromocytoma)
2. Metabolic diseases (haemochromatosis)
3. Drug therapy (steroids, thiazide diuretics)
4. Pancreatic inflammation, etc. (chronic pancreatitis, mumps, cystic fibrosis).

Gestational Diabetes (Type 4)

This is associated with glycosuria during pregnancy and the birth of overweight babies. Control of the maternal blood sugar reduces birth weight to normal. Permanent diabetes is apt to develop at a later date.

COMPLICATIONS OF DIABETES

1. **Diabetic Coma.** 2 forms occur:

    (a) **Keto-acidotic coma.** This is common in Type 1 diabetes. Hyperosmolarity, hypovolaemia, acidosis and loss of electrolytes if unchecked lead to coma.

    (b) **Hyperosmolar non-ketotic coma.** This develops slowly in Type 2 diabetes. Hyperglycaemia builds up and produces profound dehydration.

2. **Hypoglycaemic coma.** This complication of treatment occurs when insulin intake is excessive for the amount of food consumed.

3. **Cardiovascular lesions**

    (a) Atheroma develops at an earlier age and with increased severity. Coronary thrombosis is common.

    (b) Microangiopathy causing occlusion of arterioles and capillaries. These vascular lesions are responsible for many of the clinical lesions e.g. cardiac failure, retinopathy, neuropathy, gangrene of limbs, Kimmelstiel–Wilson lesions in the kidney.

    The frequency of cardiovascular lesions can be minimised by tight control of blood glucose levels (usually by monitoring glycated haemoglobin) and blood pressure.

4. **Renal failure** is common. It may be due to glomerulosclerosis, but pyelonephritis and renal papillary necrosis are other causes.

5. **Infections.** There is an increased susceptibility to sepsis, fungal infections and tuberculosis.

6. **Neuropathy.** (a) Peripheral ⎫ Possibly due to direct metabolic
                                    damage
                   (b) Autonomic ⎭ ± microvascular occlusion

ENDOCRINE PANCREAS

ISLET CELL TUMOURS

These are uncommon. Most are benign and are asymptomatic unless they secrete excess hormones. 10% are malignant. The clinical effects vary with the hormone produced.

1. Insulin-secreting tumours arising from β cells produce attacks of hypoglycaemia.
2. Gastrin-secreting tumours cause multiple peptice ulcers (Zollinger–Ellison syndrome).
3. Glucagonoma and somatostatinoma induce diabetes.
4. Inappropriate hormone secretion, e.g. carcinoid syndrome, Cushing's syndrome, etc.

These tumours may form part of multiple endocrine neoplasia syndromes (p.649).

PARATHYROID GLANDS

The parathyroids are four small glands lying posterior to the thyroid gland.

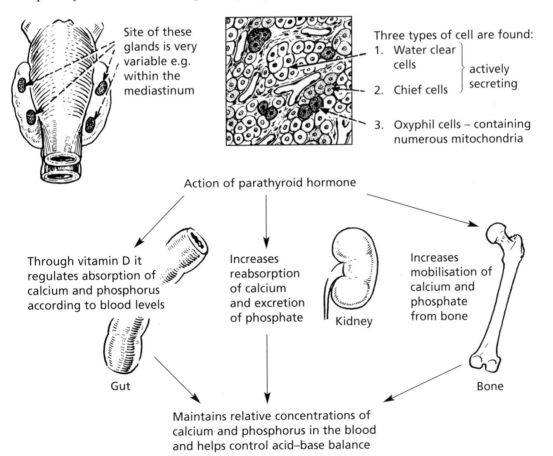

Site of these glands is very variable e.g. within the mediastinum

Three types of cell are found:
1. Water clear cells ⎫ actively secreting
2. Chief cells ⎭
3. Oxyphil cells – containing numerous mitochondria

Action of parathyroid hormone

Through vitamin D it regulates absorption of calcium and phosphorus according to blood levels

Gut

Increases reabsorption of calcium and excretion of phosphate

Kidney

Increases mobilisation of calcium and phosphate from bone

Bone

Maintains relative concentrations of calcium and phosphorus in the blood and helps control acid–base balance

647

PARATHYROID GLANDS

HYPERFUNCTION (see p.605)

There are 3 forms:

1. **Primary**

   This is due to **adenoma** (> 80%), **hyperplasia** (approx. 15%) and **carcinoma** (approx. 2%).

   The **blood calcium** is **raised.**

   The effects are:

   (a) Formation of renal calculi sometimes leading to renal failure.

   (b) Parathyroid bone disease (osteitis fibrosa cystica), now uncommon

   (c) General muscle weakness.

   (d) Metastatic calcification.

2. **Secondary**

   Parathyroid hyperplasia is a response to the low blood calcium from various causes as follows:

   CHRONIC RENAL FAILURE ⎱
   Malabsorption syndromes ⎰ HYPOCALCAEMIA ⟶ PARATHYROID
   Vitamin D deficiency   HYPERPLASIA

3. **Tertiary**

   In a few cases of secondary hyperparathyroidism an autonomous nodule develops in the hyperplastic gland and HYPERCALCAEMIA results.

Note: **Humoral Hypercalcaemia of Malignancy.**

   Carcinomas, particularly of the lung and kidney may produce **Parathyroid hormone related peptide** (PTHrP) which causes **hypercalcaemia.** This is not related to parathyroid disease.

HYPOPARATHYROIDISM

This occurs in 3 circumstances:

1. Surgical removal, sometimes accidentally during thyroidectomy
2. Auto-immune disease (very rare).
3. Congenital deficiency (e.g. DiGeorge syndrome).

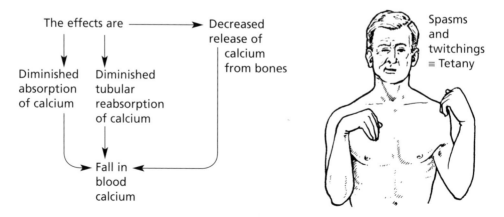

The effects are ⟶ Decreased release of calcium from bones

Diminished absorption of calcium

Diminished tubular reabsorption of calcium

Fall in blood calcium

Spasms and twitchings ≡ Tetany

MULTIPLE ENDOCRINE NEOPLASIA SYNDROMES (MENS)

This is a group of familial conditions (autosomal dominant inheritance) characterised by multiple endocrine tumours.

The main syndromes are:

MEN 1 – Parathyroid adenoma,
Pancreatic islet cell tumours,
Pituitary adenomas.

This is due to mutation of the MEN 1 gene on chromosome 11, which encodes menin, a nuclear protein.

MEN 2A – Medullary carcinoma of thyroid,
Phaeochromocytoma,
Parathyroid adenoma or hyperplasia.

MEN 2B – Medullary carcinoma of thyroid (poor prognosis),
Phaeochromocytoma,
Mucosal 'neuromas',
Ganglioneuromas of gut.

These are due to mutations activating the *ret* oncogene on chromosome 10 which encodes a cell surface receptor with tyrosine kinase activity.

Their importance is that family screening may pick up tumours at an early stage, indeed at the stage of hyperplasia which often precedes the development of tumours.

Illustrative family history:

†55 cerebral haemorrhage (FAMILY HISTORY)

INDEX CASE –
PHAEOCHROMOCYTOMA

Also → needing to be screened

Bilateral phaeochromocytoma

Medullary Ca of thyroid

Screening – 'C' cell hyperplasia of thyroid → prophylactic thyroidectomy and adrenal surveillance.